AF597495

1998
YEAR BOOK OF
RHEUMATOLOGY®

Statement of Purpose

The YEAR BOOK Service

The YEAR BOOK series was devised in 1901 by practicing health professionals who observed that the literature of medicine and related disciplines had become so voluminous that no one individual could read and place in perspective every potential advance in a major specialty. In the final decade of the 20th century, this recognition is more acutely true than it was in 1901.

More than merely a series of books, YEAR BOOK volumes are the tangible results of a unique service designed to accomplish the following:

- to *survey* a wide range of journals of proven value
- to *select* from those journals papers representing significant advances and statements of important clinical principles
- to provide *abstracts* of those articles that are readable, convenient summaries of their key points
- to provide *commentary* about those articles to place them in perspective

These publications grow out of a unique process that calls on the talents of outstanding authorities in clinical and fundamental disciplines, trained literature specialists, and professional writers, all supported by the resources of Mosby, the world's preeminent publisher for the health professions.

The Literature Base

Mosby and its editors survey more than 1,000 journals published worldwide, covering the full range of the health professions. On an annual basis, the publisher examines usage patterns and polls its expert authorities to add new journals to the literature base and to delete journals that are no longer useful as potential YEAR BOOK sources.

The Literature Survey

The publisher's team of literature specialists, all of whom are trained and experienced health professionals, examines every original, peer-reviewed article in each journal issue. More than 250,000 articles per year are scanned systematically, including title, text, illustrations, tables, and references. Each scan is compared, article by article, to the search strategies that the publisher has developed in consultation with the 270 outside experts who form the pool of YEAR BOOK editors. A given article may be reviewed by any number of editors, from one to a dozen or more, regardless of the discipline for which the paper was originally published. In turn, each editor who receives the article reviews it to determine whether the article should be included in the YEAR BOOK. This decision is based on the article's inherent quality, its probable usefulness to readers of that YEAR BOOK, and the editor's goal to represent a balanced picture of a given field in each volume of the YEAR BOOK. In addition, the editor indicates when to include figures and tables from the article to help the YEAR BOOK reader better understand the information.

Of the quarter million articles scanned each year, only 5% are selected for detailed analysis within the YEAR BOOK series, thereby assuring readers of the high value of every selection.

The Abstract

The publisher's abstracting staff is headed by a seasoned medical professional and includes individuals with training in the life sciences, medicine, and other areas, plus extensive experience in writing for the health professions and related industries. Each selected article is assigned to a specific writer on this abstracting staff. The abstracter, guided in many cases by notations supplied by the expert editor, writes a structured, condensed summary designed so that the reader can rapidly acquire the essential information contained in the article.

The Commentary

The YEAR BOOK editorial boards, sometimes assisted by guest commentators, write comments that place each article in perspective for the reader. This provides the reader with the equivalent of a personal consultation with a leading international authority—an opportunity to better understand the value of the article and to benefit from the authority's thought processes in assessing the article.

Additional Editorial Features

The editorial boards of each YEAR BOOK organize the abstracts and comments to provide a logical and satisfying sequence of information. To enhance the organization, editors also provide introductions to sections or individual chapters, comments linking a number of abstracts, citations to additional literature, and other features.

The published YEAR BOOK contains enhanced bibliographic citations for each selected article, including extended listings of multiple authors and identification of author affiliations. Each YEAR BOOK contains a Table of Contents specific to that year's volume. From year to year, the Table of Contents for a given YEAR BOOK will vary depending on developments within the field.

Every YEAR BOOK contains a list of the journals from which papers have been selected. This list represents a subset of the more than 1,000 journals surveyed by the publisher and occasionally reflects a particularly pertinent article from a journal that is not surveyed on a routine basis.

Finally, each volume contains a comprehensive subject index and an index to authors of each selected paper.

The 1998 Year Book Series

Year Book of Allergy, Asthma, and Clinical Immunology: Drs. Rosenwasser, Borish, Gelfand, Leung, Nelson, and Szefler

Year Book of Anesthesiology and Pain Management®: Drs. Tinker, Abram, Chestnut, Roizen, Rothenberg, and Wood

Year Book of Cardiology®: Drs. Schlant, Collins, Gersh, Graham, Kaplan, and Waldo

Year Book of Chiropractic®: Dr. Lawrence

Year Book of Critical Care Medicine®: Drs. Parrillo, Balk, Calvin, Franklin, and Shapiro

Year Book of Dentistry®: Drs. Meskin, Berry, Jeffcoat, Leinfelder, Roser, Summitt, and Zakariasen

Year Book of Dermatologic Surgery®: Drs. Greenway, Papadopoulos, Whitaker, and Barrett

Year Book of Dermatology®: Drs. Sober and Fitzpatrick

Year Book of Diagnostic Radiology®: Drs. Osborn, Groskin, Dalinka, Maynard, Pentecost, Rebner, Ros, Smirniotopoulos, and Young

Year Book of Digestive Diseases®: Dr. Aliperti

Year Book of Drug Therapy®: Drs. Lasagna and Weintraub

Year Book of Emergency Medicine®: Drs. Wagner, Dronen, Davidson, King, Niemann, and Roberts

Year Book of Endocrinology®: Drs. Bagdade, Braverman, Horton, Kannan, Landsberg, Molitch, Morley, Nathan, Odell, Poehlman, Rogol, and Ryan

Year Book of Family Practice®: Drs. Berg, Bowman, Davidson, Dexter, and Scherger

Year Book of Geriatrics and Gerontology®: Drs. Beck, Burton, Ostwald, Rabins, Reuben, Roth, Shapiro, and Whitehouse

Year Book of Hand Surgery®: Drs. Amadio and Hentz

Year Book of Hematology®: Drs. Spivak, Bell, Ness, Quesenberry, Wiernik, and Horowitz

Year Book of Infectious Diseases: Drs. Keusch, Barza, Bennish, Poutsiaka, Skolnik, and Snydman

Year Book of Medicine®: Drs. Klahr, Cline, McCallum, Frishman, Utiger, Malawista, Mandell, and Jett

Year Book of Neonatal and Perinatal Medicine®: Drs. Fanaroff, Maisels, and Stevenson

Year Book of Nephrology, Hypertension, and Mineral Metabolism: Drs. Schwab, Bennett, Emmett, Hostetter, Kuman, and Toto

Year Book of Neurology and Neurosurgery®: Drs. Bradley and Gibbs

Year Book of Nuclear Medicine®: Drs. Gottschalk, Blaufox, Neumann, Strauss, and Zubal

Year Book of Obstetrics, Gynecology, and Women's Health: Drs. Mishell, Herbst, and Kirschbaum

Year Book of Occupational and Environmental Medicine®: Drs. Emmett, Frank, Gochfeld, and Hessl

Year Book of Oncology®: Drs. Ozols, Eisenberg, Glatstein, Loehrer, Tallman, and Wiersma

Year Book of Ophthalmology®: Drs. Wilson, Augsburger, Cohen, Eagle, Flanagan, Grossman, Laibson, Maguire, Nelson, Penne, Rapuano, Sergott, Spaeth, Tipperman, Ms. Gosfield, and Ms. Salmon

Year Book of Orthopedics®: Dr. Morrey

Year Book of Otolaryngology–Head and Neck Surgery®: Drs. Paparella and Holt

Year Book of Pathology and Laboratory Medicine: Drs. Raab, Cohen, Olson, Sirgi, and Stanley

Year Book of Pediatrics®: Dr. Stockman

Year Book of Plastic, Reconstructive, and Aesthetic Surgery®: Drs. Miller, Bartlett, Garner, McKinney, Ruberg, Salisbury, and Smith

Year Book of Podiatric Medicine and Surgery®: Dr. Kominsky

Year Book of Psychiatry and Applied Mental Health®: Drs. Talbott, Ballanger, Frances, Lydiard, Meltzer, Schowalter, and Tasman

Year Book of Pulmonary Disease®: Drs. Jett, Mauer, Ryu, Strollo, and Wenzel

Year Book of Rheumatology®: Drs. Panush, Hadler, LeRoy, Liang, Reichlin, Simon, and Weinblatt

Year Book of Sports Medicine®: Drs. Shephard, Drinkwater, Eichner, Torg, Alexander, and Mr. George

Year Book of Surgery®: Drs. Copeland, Bland, Deitch, Eberlein, Howard, Luce, Seeger, Souba, and Sugarbaker

Year Book of Thoracic and Cardiovascular Surgery®: Drs. Ginsberg, Wechsler, and Williams

Year Book of Urology®: Drs. Andriole and Coplen

Year Book of Vascular Surgery®: Dr. Porter

1998
The Year Book of RHEUMATOLOGY®

Editor-in-Chief
Richard S. Panush, M.D.

Associate Editors
Nortin M. Hadler, M.D.
E. Carwile LeRoy, M.D.
Matthew H. Liang, M.D., M.P.H.
Morris Reichlin, M.D.
Lee S. Simon, M.D.
Michael E. Weinblatt, M.D.

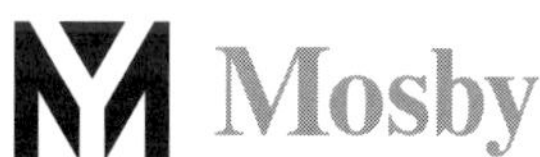

St. Louis Baltimore Boston Carlsbad Naples New York Philadelphia Portland London
Madrid Mexico City Singapore Sydney Tokyo Toronto Wiesbaden

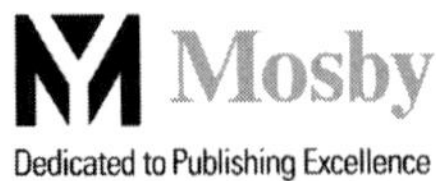

A Times Mirror
Company

Associate Publisher: Gretchen C. Murphy
Developmental Editor: JoEllen Tomlinson
Manuscript Editor: Stephanie M. Geels
Production Assistant: Laura Bayless
Illustrations and Permissions Specialist: Steve Ramay

1998 EDITION

Printed in the United States of America
Composition by Reed Technology and Information Services, Inc.
Printing/binding by Maple-Vail

Editorial Office:
Mosby, Inc.
11830 Westline Industrial Drive
St. Louis, MO 63146

International Standard Serial Number: 1070-5406
International Standard Book Number: 0-8151-7864-6

Editorial Board

Table of Contents

Journals Represented xiii
Publisher's Preface xv
Introduction xvii

1. Health Sciences, Epidemiology, and Economics 1
- Introduction 1
- Lead Article 2
- Economics 6
- Outcomes 8
- Healthcare 15

2. Rheumatoid Arthritis 19
- Introduction 19
- Immunogenetics and Pathophysiology 20
- Clinical Aspects 26
- Therapy 40
- Experimental Models 66
- Juvenile Rheumatoid Arthritis 70

3. Systemic Lupus Erythematosus and Related Disorders 81
- Introduction 81
- Lead Article 81
- Immunogenetics and Pathophysiology 82
- Antinuclear Antibodies and Other Autoantibodies 97
- Antiphospholipid Syndrome and Antibodies 105
- Clinical Aspects 116
- Therapy 120
- Sjögren's Syndrome 129

4. Systemic Sclerosis and Related Disorders 141
- Introduction 141
- Lead Article 142
- Immunogenetics and Pathophysiology 143
- Clinical Aspects 163
- Raynaud's Phenomenon 180

5. Vasculitis, Systemic Rheumatic Diseases, and Other Related Disorders 187
Introduction 187
Lead Article 188
Systemic Vasculitides 191
Eosinophilic Fasciitis 203
Behçet's Syndrome 204
Myopathies 207
Polychronditis 210

6. Osteoarthritis, Crystal-related Arthropathies, Osteoporosis, Infectious Arthritides 213
Introduction 213
Osteoarthritis 213
Epidemiology 213
Biology 217
Clinical Aspects 219
Crystal-related Arthropathies 220
Osteoporosis 225
Infectious Arthritis 232
Lyme Disease 235

7. Regional Pain Syndromes, Non-Articular Musculoskeletal Disorders, Fibromyalgia, and Miscellaneous Topics 245
Introduction 245
Regional Pain Syndromes and Non-Articular Musculoskeletal Disorders 246
Fibromyalgia 250
Miscellaneous Disorders 261
Lead Article 261

SUBJECT INDEX. 281

AUTHOR INDEX 343

Journals Represented

Mosby and its editors survey more than 1,000 journals for its abstract and commentary publications. From these journals, the editors select the articles to be abstracted. Journals represented in this YEAR BOOK are listed below.

Acta Dermato-Venereologica
Acta Radiologica
American Journal of Clinical Pathology
American Journal of Epidemiology
American Journal of Gastroenterology
American Journal of Medicine
American Journal of Pathology
Angiology: The Journal of Vascular Diseases
Annals of Internal Medicine
Annals of Rheumatic Diseases
Archives of Dermatology
Arthritis and Rheumatism
Bone
British Medical Journal
Canadian Medical Association Journal
Cancer
Chest
European Journal of Cancer
European Respiratory Journal
Gastroenterology
Human Pathology
Journal of Clinical Investigation
Journal of Clinical Oncology
Journal of Clinical Rheumatology
Journal of Experimental Medicine
Journal of Immunology
Journal of Medical Genetics
Journal of Pain and Symptom Management
Journal of Rheumatology
Journal of the American Academy of Dermatology
Journal of the American Medical Association
Lancet
Mayo Clinic Proceedings
Nephrology, Dialysis, Transplantation
Neurology
New England Journal of Medicine
Obstetrics and Gynecology
Occupational Medicine
Pain
Proceedings of the Association of American Physicians
Proceedings of the National Academy of Sciences
Radiology
Regional Anesthesia
Respiratory Medicine
Scandinavian Journal of Rheumatology
Science
Southern Medical Journal

Surgery
Thorax

Standard Abbreviations

The following terms are abbreviated in this edition: acquired immunodeficiency syndrome (AIDS), cardiopulmonary resuscitation (CPR), central nervous system (CNS), cerebrospinal fluid (CSF), computed tomography (CT), deoxyribonucleic acid (DNA), electrocardiography (ECG), health maintenance organization (HMO), human immunodeficiency virus (HIV), intensive care unit (ICU), intramuscular (IM), intravenous (IV), magnetic resonance (MR) imaging (MRI), rheumatoid arthritis (RA), and ribonucleic acid (RNA).

Note

The Year Book of Rheumatology is a literature survey service providing abstracts of articles published in the professional literature. Every effort is made to assure the accuracy of the information presented in these pages. Neither the editors nor the publisher of the Year Book of Rheumatology can be responsible for errors in the original materials. The editors' comments are their own opinions. Mention of specific products within this publication does not constitute endorsement.

To facilitate the use of the Year Book of Rheumatology as a reference tool, all illustrations and tables included in this publication are now identified as they appear in the original article. This change is meant to help the reader recognize that any illustration or table appearing in the Year Book of Rheumatology may be only one of many in the original article. For this reason, figure and table numbers will often appear to be out of sequence within the Year Book of Rheumatology.

Publisher's Preface

The 1998 YEAR BOOK OF RHEUMATOLOGY marks the first volume under the leadership of Richard S. Panush, M.D. He brings to this YEAR BOOK a great deal of enthusiam, vision, and experience. We at Mosby cordially welcome him to this position. Dr. Panush has been a member of the editorial board since the debut edition in 1994. We also welcome Dr. Nortin Hadler and Dr. Lee Simon, who have added insightful and thought-provoking commentary to this volume.

With this edition, we say goodbye to our esteemed colleagues Dr. Matthew H. Liang, Dr. Morris Reichlin, and Dr. Michael E. Weinblatt. We would like to thank them for their hard work and dedication. Dr. Liang and Dr. Weinblatt both served on the board for one year. Dr. Reichlin, a member of the board since the first volume, has provided thorough, insightful commentary for the YEAR BOOK, and he will be greatly missed.

This is the last edition of this book under the title "YEAR BOOK OF RHEUMATOLOGY." The new title for the 1999 edition will be the "YEAR BOOK OF RHEUMATOLOGY, ARTHRITIS, AND MUSCULOSKELETAL DISEASE." This title change reflects an expansion of subject matter that will make the YEAR BOOK of interest not only to rheumatologists, but to all who seek information on disorders affecting the musculoskeletal system. This reflects the commitment of the editorial board to provide pertinent information to all physicians caring for patients with rheumatic and musculoskeletal problems.

Introduction

This is my first year as editor-in-chief of the YEAR BOOK OF RHEUMATOLOGY. I am deeply honored to be offered this privilege. The responsibility of identifying important contributions to rheumatology, and presenting these to colleagues, is a duanting, and humbling, one.

I have tried to learn from watching John Sergent do this during the first 4 years of this YEAR BOOK. John has a unique ability to simultaneously take on a number of difficult tasks. He made editing the YEAR BOOK seem easy. It's not. But it is great fun and very satisfying to see all the editors' efforts come together to address topical issues in rheumatology. We all owe John a tremendous debt of gratitude for his skills and leadership as the first editor of this YEAR BOOK—he is a good friend and wonderful person with an unusual combination of vision, imagination, wisdom, discerning judgment, humor, and warmth. I will miss working with him on this. The success of the YEAR BOOK reflects not only John's superb efforts but also the invaluable contributions of his original editors, one of whom, Moe Reichlin, leaves the editorial board with this volume; Moe's insights and expositions have been illuminating in a difficult area (and we've enjoyed some places and nice runs together, which I hope will continue).

I am excited about this volume of the YEAR BOOK, and certainly about its future. I appreciate Carwile LeRoy again sharing his knowledgeable perspectives about scleroderma, as he has done so ably in the previous editions. And it is with great pleasure that I introduce several new associate editors. Nortin Hadler has reviewed vasculitis, certain aspects of regional pain syndromes, and anything controversial; they don't come any brighter, perceptive, or provocative than Nortin. Matt Liang has reviewed epidemiology and health services/sciences, and related areas; Matt deservedly has a reputation as one of the scions in this area and is a clear and lucid thinker. Lee Simon has reviewed osteoporosis and nonsteroidal anti-inflammatory drugs and other related topics; Lee has boundless energy and enthusiasm, and great expertise and perspective about emerging trends in these areas. Mike Weinblatt has reviewed RA and its therapy; Mike is clearly among our leaders in thinking about how to best confront the vexing problems of RA and is respected and articulate in his presentations.

I'm proud to work with this group of editors—they are critical thinkers, talented physicians, and eloquent, refreshing, and provocative writers. I hope readers enjoy their selections and commentaries as much as I have. Science isn't about knowing, it's about not knowing. We hope the 1998 YEAR BOOK OF RHEUMATOLOGY adds to our knowing so that we can better care for our patients.

Richard S. Panush, M.D.
Editor-in-Chief

1 Health Sciences, Epidemiology, and Economics

Introduction

Plus c'est la meme chose, plus ça change (the more we stay the same, the more things change). Times are still turbulent for rheumatology.[1] We still struggle to retain and redefine our identity and our roles in health care. Are we specialists? Primary care physicians? Principal physicians? Do we see only systemic rheumatic diseases? Or all musculoskeletal disorders? Do we do better than nonspecialists? Will guidelines help us and our patients? What is the American College of Rheumatology (ACR) doing for us? I don't have all the answers (my kids told me that years ago), nor do the other editors, nor does the literature. The selections (and comments) in this section offer some perspectives. My own thoughts this year, evolving from my comments in prior YEAR BOOKS (1995, pp xvii–xix; 1996, pp 1–2; 1997, pp 25–27), and elsewhere,[2] are that most of us will see patients broadly with musculoskeletal disorders, that many of us will want to be principal physicians for our patients, that we do provide measurably better care to our patients than nonrheumatologists,[3, 4] that guidelines will help some, and that changes may not be as sweeping as we originally thought.[5] And the ACR initiatives (guidelines, marketing the rheumatologist, and promoting rheumatologic care for musculoskeletal conditions) may prove more salutary than anticipated. I am optimistic about our future.

Richard S. Panush, M.D.

References

1. Panush RS: A rude awakening. *JAMA* 7:515–516, 1997.
2. Panush RS, Kaplan H: Who will care for our patients? *J Rheumatol* 12:2197–2199, 1995.
3. Solomon DH, Bates DW, Panush RS, et al: Costs, outcomes and patient satisfaction by provider type for patients with rheumatic and musculoskeletal conditions: A critical review of the literature and proposed methodologic standards. *Ann Intern Med* 1:52–60, 1997.

4. Remensone EL, Abraham VJ, Sigal LH, et al: Who knows how to care for fibromyalgia? Presented at the 61st Annual ACR Meeting, November 8–12, 1997. Washington, D.C., *Arthritis Rheum* (abstract) in press.
5. McDonald WJ: Specialists are back! *The Scribe*. Philadelphia, American College of Physicians, July 1997.

Lead Article *

Guidelines for Monitoring Drug Therapy in Rheumatoid Arthritis
Simms RW, and the American College of Rheumatology Ad Hoc Committee on Clinical Guidelines (Boston Univ)
Arthritis Rheum 39:723–731, 1996 1–1

Background.—Serious adverse effects, including death, can result from treatment with the drugs used to treat RA. This is particularly true if treatment continues in a patient with unrecognized toxic effects. Careful pretreatment assessment and patient and physician education can prevent many of these complications. Patient and physician alike must know the signs and symptoms of toxicity that necessitate discontinuation of treatment. Sometimes, laboratory monitoring tests can detect toxicity before it becomes clinically apparent. The Ad Hoc Committee on Clinical Guidelines of the American College of Rheumatology presented guidelines for monitoring drug treatment in patients with RA (Table 1).

Methods.—The guidelines were developed by a combination of expert opinion; a survey of rheumatologists; previously published guidelines; and, whenever possible, published toxicity data. The guidelines will be useful for all health care professionals involved in the care of patients with RA. Recommendations on the extent and frequency of monitoring are not entirely based on research evidence. Given the frequency of the toxic effects of drugs used to treat RA, no such studies are likely to be performed. Where conflicting recommendations existed and no supporting data were available, the option that reduced cost and inconvenience was selected.

Recommendations—Recommendations were developed for the 3 major categories of drugs used to treat RA: nonsteroidal anti-inflammatory drugs (NSAIDs); disease-modifying antirheumatic drugs (DMARDs) including hydroxychloroquine, sulfasalazine, methotrexate, gold compounds, D-penicillamine, and azathioprine; and glucocorticoids. All NSAIDs have gastrointestinal and renal toxic effects. These can be prevented through careful patient selection and treatment. Each of the DMARDs has specific toxic effects requiring specific monitoring protocols. Most of the potentially serious toxicity of glucocorticoid drugs is related to the dose and duration of treatment. The specific recommendations focus on the basic

*In 1996, we initiated the feature of "lead articles" (also called "picks of the year"). We ask each editor to pick an article that stands out as the best of the year among those reviewed and selected by each editor, one that will be important, one that will influence the way we think about and practice rheumatology. Our choices are indicated in the context of the presentation of our selections.

TABLE 1.—Recommended Monitoring Strategies for Drug Treatment of RA

Drugs	Toxicities requiring monitoring*	Monitoring: Baseline evaluation	Monitoring: System review/examination	Monitoring: Laboratory
Salicylates, nonsteroidal antiinflammatory drugs	Gastrointestinal ulceration and bleeding	CBC, creatinine, AST, ALT	Dark/black stool, dyspepsia, nausea/vomiting, abdominal pain, edema, shortness of breath	CBC yearly, LFTs, creatinine testing may be required†
Hydroxychloroquine	Macular damage	None unless patient is over age 40 or has previous eye disease	Visual changes, funduscopic and visual fields every 6–12 months	—
Sulfasalazine	Myelosuppression	CBC, and AST or ALT in patients at risk, G6PD	Symptoms of myelosuppression‡, photosensitivity, rash	CBC every 2–4 weeks for first 3 months, then every 3 months
Methotrexate	Myelosuppression, hepatic fibrosis, cirrhosis, pulmonary infiltrates or fibrosis	CBC, chest radiography within past year, hepatitis B and C serology in high-risk patients, AST or ALT, albumin, alkaline phosphatase, and creatinine	Symptoms of myelosuppression†, shortness of breath, nausea/vomiting, lymph node swelling	CBC, platelet count, AST, albumin, creatinine every 4–8 weeks
Gold, intramuscular	Myelosuppression, proteinuria	CBC, platelet count, creatinine, urine dipstick for protein	Symptoms of myelosuppression‡, edema, rash, oral ulcers, diarrhea	CBC, platelet count, urine dipstick every 1–2 weeks for first 20 weeks, then at the time of each (or every other) injection
Gold, oral	Myelosuppression, proteinuria	CBC, platelet count, urine dipstick for protein	Symptoms of myelosuppression‡, edema, rash, diarrhea	CBC, platelet count, urine dipstick for protein every 4–12 weeks
D-penicillamine	Myelosuppression, proteinuria	CBC, platelet count, creatinine, urine dipstick for protein	Symptoms of myelosuppression‡, edema, rash	CBC, urine dipstick for protein every 2 weeks until dosage stable, then every 1–3 months
Azathioprine	Myelosuppression, hepatotoxicity, lymphoproliferative disorders	CBC, platelet count, creatinine, AST or ALT	Symptoms of myelosuppression‡	CBC and platelet count every 1–2 weeks with changes in dosage, and every 1–3 months thereafter

(*Continued*)

TABLE 1 (cont.)

Drugs	Toxicities requiring monitoring*	Monitoring: Baseline evaluation	Monitoring: System review/examination	Monitoring: Laboratory
Corticosteroids (oral ≤10 mg of prednisone or equivalent)	Hypertension, hyperglycemia	BP, chemistry panel, bone densitometry in high-risk patients	BP at each visit, polyuria, polydipsia, edema, shortness of breath, visual changes, weight gain	Urinalysis for glucose yearly
Agents for refractory RA or severe extraarticular complications				
Cyclophosphamide	Myelosuppression, myeloproliferative disorders, malignancy, hemorrhagic cystitis	CBC, platelet count, urinalysis, creatinine, AST or ALT	Symptoms of myelosuppression‡, hematuria	CBC and platelet count every 1–2 weeks with changes in dosage, and every 1–3 months therafter, urinalysis and urine cytology every 6–12 months after cessation
Chlorambucil	Myelosuppression, myeloproliferative disorders, malignancy	CBC, urianalysis, creatinine, AST or ALT	Symptoms of myelosuppression‡	CBC and platelet count every 1–2 weeks with changes in dosage, and every 1–3 months thereafter
Cyclosporin A	Renal insufficiency, anemia, hypertension	CBC, creatinine, uric acid, LFTs, BP	Edema, BP every 2 weeks until dosage stable, then monthly	Creatinine every 2 weeks until dose is stable, then monthly; periodic CBC, potassium, and LFTs

*Potential serious toxicities that may be detected by monitoring before they have become clinically apparent or harmful to the patient. The list mentions toxicities that occur frequently enough to justify monitoring. Patients with comorbidity, concurrent medications, and other specific risk factors may need further studies to monitor for specific toxicity.

†Package insert for diclofenac (Voltaren) recommends that aspartate aminotransferase and alanine aminotransferase be monitored within the first 8 weeks of treatment and periodically thereafter. Monitoring of serum creatinine should be performed weekly for at least 3 weeks in patients receiving concomitant angiotensin-converting enzyme inhibitors or diuretics.

‡Symptoms of myelosuppression include fever, symptoms of infection, easy bruisability, and bleeding.

Abbreviations: CBC, complete blood cell count including differential cell and platelet counts; *ALT*, alanine aminotransferase; *AST*, aspartate aminotransferase; *LFTs*, liver function tests; *BP*, blood pressure.

(Courtesy of Simms RW, and the American College of Rheumatology Ad Hoc Committee on Clinical Guidelines: Guidelines for monitoring drug therapy in rheumatoid arthritis. *Arthritis Rheum* 39:723–731, 1996. Copyright American College of Rheumatology.)

monitoring requirements for patients with uncomplicated RA. Certain patients may need more intensive monitoring, such as those with comorbid conditions, other medications, or other risk factors.

▶ This is a reference article for monitoring drug therapy in patients with RA. An ad hoc committee developed these guidelines under the direction of the American College of Rheumatology (ACR). The guidelines are quite useful in the day-to-day management of our patients with rheumatoid arthritis and support our laboratory monitoring. This is not science but is extremely practical and valuable in the management of our patients and in dealing with the business of medicine. This will be helpful when dealing with health care agencies and managed care companies [and may help define and assert the prominent role of the rheumatologist in managing these patients...R.S. Panush, M.D.]

I have never been an advocate of most guidelines; however, these guidelines (and the guidelines for hepatic monitoring for methotrexate, for which I was a co-author) are important to physicians treating patients with RA. There may be variations in monitoring philosophies, but I view guidelines, in most cases, as the minimum recommendations for reducing the potential for drug toxicity. Managed care organizations and the insurance companies should not view these recommendations as the holy grail for monitoring because more frequent monitoring may be appropriate in individual patients.

M.E. Weinblatt, M.D.

▶ There has been a proliferation of guidelines for the approach to diagnosis and treatment of many diseases promulgated by subspecialty and specialty societies as well as other groups. The ACR has now developed and published at least 6 sets of guidelines with the prevention and treatment of glucocorticoid-induced osteoporosis as the newest. Guideline development requires a committee to achieve consensus about something, and in this case the ACR has reached an important consensus about the approach to the diagnosis, prevention and treatment of corticosteroid induced osteoporosis. This is an area uniquely applicable to rheumatologists. Not only are they well versed in metabolic bone disease, but they are often the treating physician who initiates therapy with glucocorticoids and thus induce unwanted changes in bone metabolism. This important area is also one that is changing constantly and rapidly—so much so, that although these thoughtful and reasonable guidelines were just produced and published they have very recently received some very important scientific validation.

It seems the development committee was clearly impressed with the effect of glucocorticoids on bone. They were also impressed with the necessity to use adequate doses of calcium supplementation along with vitamin D to decrease the biological effects of secondary hyperparathyroidism due to the decreased absorption of calcium induced by the use of the anti-inflammatory drug. Calcium supplementation clearly decreases this secondary hyperparathyroidism which serves to accelerate early increased bone resorption associated with glucocorticoid therapy. Furthermore, they also recommended the use of anti-resorptive therapy with bisphosphonates, although that had not yet been proven experimentally. Now Adachi et al. have demonstrated, in a series of patients with heterogeneous diseases requiring glucocorticoid therapy, that cyclical etidronate (14 days on and 76 days off repeated 3 times per year) reduced bone loss in the vertebrae and the trochanter but not in the femoral neck.[1] Presumably, other manufacturers of competing bisphosphonates will soon be releasing data describing the results of other clinical studies. It will be interesting to note whether the effects of other bisphosphonates will be similar or if there will be improved effects on non-vertebral sites using the other drugs.

Ultimately, these guidelines have proven their utility and are important for clinicians to consult as an excellent resource for information. Of course, they should be viewed by all interested parties as guidelines. Since each patient at times does not accurately fit into immutable "pigeonholes," it is hard to envision a diagnostic or treatment set of guidelines which fits every patient. Therefore each patient should be approached as though his or her problem is unique, and the guidelines should be used as a broad template not as "gospel." However, this set of guidelines is actually well written, well referenced, and is a useful tool for the practicing clinician. [These guidelines, too, may support an expanding role for rheumatologists in caring for patients with osteoporosis....R.S. Panush, M.D.]

L.S. Simon, M.D.

Reference

1. Adachi JD, Bensen WG, Brown J, et al.: Intermittent etidronate therapy to prevent corticosteroid-induced osteoporosis. *N Engl J Med* 337:382–387, 1997.

Economics

Indirect and Nonmedical Costs Among People With Rheumatoid Arthritis and Osteoarthritis Compared With Nonarthritic Controls

Gabriel SE, Crowson CS, Campion ME, et al (Mayo Clinic and Found, Rochester, Minn)

J Rheumatol 24:43–48, 1997 1–2

Introduction.—Osteoarthritis (OA) is more common than RA and is considered to be more benign and less costly than RA. Reported are results of a postal survey designed to estimate the indirect and nonmedical costs among 2 randomly selected, community-based samples of 200 each residents with RA and OA and 200 residents who were nonarthritic.

Methods.—The 3 major categories of estimated health expenditures were direct medical expenditures, nonmedical expenditures (transportation, home care, child care), and indirect expenditures (lost work days). These expenditures were compared for all 3 groups of residents.

Results.—There were 123, 116, and 94 respondents from the RA, OA, and nonarthritic groups, respectively. Average age was higher in the RA and OA groups, compared to the nonarthritic group. The female-to-male ratio was higher in the RA and OA groups, compared with the control group. Indirect or nonmedical expenditures were incurred in 1992 by 82 (66.7%), 45 (38.8%), and 16 (17.0%) of RA, OA, and nonarthritic respondents, respectively. Excluding wage losses, the average indirect and nonmedical expenses in 1992 for respondents with RA, OA, and no arthritis were $889.54, $725.89, and $334.99, respectively. Residents with RA and OA required 3 times more days of medical care and incurred more than 5 times as many indirect and nonmedical expenditures in 1992 as their nonarthritic cohorts. Residents with RA incurred more expenditures than those with OA, but the indirect and nonmedical expenditures among residents with OA were more similar to those with RA than to controls. Fifteen percent of residents with RA, 9% of those with OA, and 5% of controls reported they were unable to get a job because of their medical condition. Residents with RA were 3 times more likely than those with OA or controls to have reduced household income. Functional status was significantly worse for residents with RA, compared with those with OA. Those residents with OA had worse functional status than controls.

Conclusion.—The indirect and nonmedical costs incurred by residents with OA were more similar to those of residents with RA than residents who did not have arthritis. This has social and financial significance, considering the high incidence of OA.

▶ The costs for patients with OA and RA as compared with those of control groups of individuals without arthritis is important information to justify the role of the rheumatologist to managed care organizations. In this very nice study from the Mayo Clinic, investigators determined the disease-specific costs including indirect and nonmedical costs for OA and rheumatoid disease. These are significant. This paper should be part of your library when dealing with managed care organizations to justify continuity of care with the rheumatologist.

M.E. Weinblatt, M.D.

Direct Medical Costs Unique to People With Arthritis

Gabriel SE, Crowson CS, Campion ME, et al (Mayo Clinic and Found, Rochester, Minn)

J Rheumatol 24:719–725, 1997 1–3

Introduction.—When estimating the cost of a medical condition, it is hard to determine whether to measure the total cost of caring for individuals with the disorder (total cost approach) or the cost of caring only for the particular condition being evaluated (attributable cost approach). Reported are findings of a population-based analysis of all health services used and charges incurred over a 1-year period in a community-based cohort of people with osteoarthritis (OA), RA, and people from the same community who never had a diagnosis of arthritis (NA). The purpose was to determine the attributable costs of arthritis.

Methods.—The unique data resources of the Rochester Epidemiology Project were used to identify patients with OA and RA and a population-based control cohort in Olmsted County. Information on health utilization and charges was obtained from the Olmsted County Health Care Utilization and Expenditure Database.

Results.—Age- and sex-adjusted average 1-year direct medical charges for cohorts in the RA, OA, and NA groups were $3,802.05, $2,654.51, and $1,387.83, respectively. Median charges were $1,050.00, $663.55, and $232.04, respectively. Charges for the RA and OA groups were significantly higher than for the NA group for musculoskeletal disease care and care of numerous other conditions including respiratory, cardiovascular, gastrointestinal, neurologic, psychiatric, and general medical care. Charges for diagnostic and therapeutic procedures, in-hospital care, imaging studies, physician services, equipment, and laboratory studies were higher for the RA and OA groups than for the NA group. Significantly more prescription drugs were used by the RA and OA cohorts than the NA cohort.

Conclusion.—Community-based cohorts of individuals with RA and OA had significantly higher charges for arthritis-related and non–arthritis-related medical care than individuals who did not have arthritis. All health service utilization should be evaluated, not just disease-related use, when ascertaining the economic impact of a chronic illness.

▶ This is the only study of complete economic burden based on a population. The importance of this kind of research is that, in a health care system that is increasingly capitated and managed, costly diseases or groups of diseases will be targeted for cost reduction. What shows up on the radar screen of managers nowadays is crude billing information based on billing codes. The idea that a person can have more than 1 condition at a time sometimes gets lost in projections.

M.H. Liang, M.D., M.P.H.

Outcomes

Rheumatology Visit Frequency and Changes in Functional Disability and Pain in Patients With Rheumatoid Arthritis

Ward MM (Stanford Univ, Calif)

J Rheumatol 24:35–42, 1997 1–4

Background.—Patients with chronic illness require frequent physician visits, which compose a substantial part of their health care costs. To optimize the effectiveness of this care, it is necessary to determine the frequency of physician visits that are associated with improved patient outcome. The association between the number of visits to rheumatologists and changes in functional disability and pain was examined over 6-month periods in a cohort of patients participating in an RA study.

Study Design.—The study group was composed of participants in the Stanford Outcomes in Rheumatoid Arthritis Study, a prospective, longitudinal study of health status, treatment, health care utilization, and outcome in patients with RA. Study participation consisted of answering a Health Assessment Questionnaire (HAQ) that was completed every 6 months. From the original 330 patients, 25 with juvenile arthritis, 23 with less than 18 months of follow-up, and 155 who had not seen a rheumatologist for at least a year were excluded. This left 127 participants. The 155 excluded patients did not differ from the study group in age, sex, race, education level, marital status, or comorbidity, but they had a lower average HAQ score and pain score and a longer average RA duration.

Results.—The participants were predominantly middle aged, female, white, married, and well educated. The mean HAQ Disability Index and pain score at study entry indicated moderate levels of functional disability and pain. The average frequency of rheumatology visits for these patients was 8 each year. There was a significant association between number of rheumatology visits and change in the Disability Index during the next 6-month period. Each visit was associated with a decrease in the Disability Index of 0.007 points. There was also an association between rheumatology visits and concurrent decreases in pain. Each visit was associated with a decrease in the pain score of 0.02 points. There was a U-shaped relationship between the rate of functional disability progression and the mean annual frequency of rheumatology visits, such that the minimal rate of progression was associated with 7 to 11 visits each year. Patients were divided into those who visited a rheumatologist less than 7 times each year, 7 to 11 times, and more than 11 times each year. There were no differences between these groups in age, sex, education, marital status, or duration of RA. Univariate analysis indicated that age, longer RA duration, white race, and use of a primary care physician were associated with a higher rate of progression. Long-term treatment with a second-line antirheumatic medication was associated with a lower rate of progresssion.

Conclusion.—This prospective, longitudinal study of patients with RA has shown improvement in functional disability and pain associated with the number of visits these patients made to rheumatologists. The lowest rate of disease progression was associated with a frequency of 7 to 11 rheumatology visits per year. The results of this study indicate that continued rheumatology subspecialty care is associated with improved outcomes in patients with RA.

▶ Investigators from Stanford University using the American Rheumatism Association Medical Information System database reported that patients who have more frequent visits to rheumatologists have greater improvement in pain and functional status than those who do not. This important article should be kept in the growing file of information to be presented to managed care organizations to justify why patients continue to need to see us for management of their RA. Continued rheumatology care is associated with improved outcome in RA!

M.E. Weinblatt, M.D.

Health Outcomes of Two Telephone Interventions for Patients With Rheumatoid Arthritis or Osteoarthritis

Maisiak R, Austin J, Heck L (Univ of Alabama at Birmingham)

Arthritis Rheum 39:1391–1399, 1996 1–5

Introduction.—Current guidelines identify routine telephone contact as an effective nondrug therapy for osteoarthritis (OA). Some form of counseling or educational intervention is important for patients with arthritis and other rheumatic diseases who require extensive communication with their physician but do not always retain or accurately understand what they are told. Previous studies have shown that telephone contact is effective in patients with OA. Two different telephone contact strategies were evaluated in patients with OA or RA.

Methods.—The randomized, controlled trial included 405 patients, 186 with primary OA of the hip or knee and 219 with primary RA. The patients were assigned into 2 telephone-contact groups and 1 usual-care group. One telephone-contact group received a symptom-monitoring strategy, in which the patients' symptoms were reviewed in detail but no advice was offered. The other group received a treatment-counseling strategy. This strategy used a reality therapy approach to improve patient interactions with the medical care system and to improve patients' ability to care for themselves through symptom review, self-care, and stress control. This intervention was based on a structured protocol and designed for quick adoption by a counselor with little additional training. The study continued for 9 months. The outcomes of the 3 groups were compared on the Arthritis Impact Measurement Scales (AIMS2).

Results.—The AIMS2 scores of the treatment-counseling group were consistently and significantly lower than those of the other 2 groups. This strategy brought significant improvement in both the RA and OA patients. The symptom-monitoring approach brought no significant improvement, compared with usual care. The specific benefits of treatment counseling differed for the OA and RA patients, with the OA group showing greater improvement in pain scores and the RA group showing greater improvement in physical and affect scores. Osteoarthritis patients receiving treatment counseling had a significant reduction in the number of medical visits.

Conclusions.—Routine telephone contact using a treatment-counseling strategy produces significant benefits for patients with arthritis. Patients with RA become less disabled and are better able to cope with chronic pain; those with OA have improved physical function and reduced pain. Telephone interventions have several advantages that make them a useful addition to the spectrum of arthritis care.

▶ A series of studies from Indiana and Alabama extended the interesting observation that simple telephone contact can improve health status and even decrease health resource utilization. This paper is important in that the nature of the telephone contact was studied for both RA and OA. One intervention was simply advice on treatment, and the other one was the monitoring of symptoms. Getting additional information on treatment helped both RA and OA patients improve their overall health status. The results were not explained by the telephone interactions increasing visits to physicians. These observations have many interpretations: one is affirming, showing that human interactions have power above and beyond providing specific information and that organized approaches that are patient centered result in tangible economic and health benefits. For special populations who cannot travel to see their providers, outreach on the phone can be an effective tool.

M.H. Liang, M.D., M.P.H.

Variation in Rheumatologists' and Family Physicians' Perceptions of the Indications for and Outcomes of Knee Replacement Surgery

Coyte PC, Hawker G, Croxford R, et al (Univ of Toronto; Women's College Hosp, Toronto; Hosp for Sick Children, Toronto)

J Rheumatol 23:730–738, 1996 1–6

Purpose.—Knee replacement (KR) is an effective treatment for arthritis patients for whom medical treatment has failed to offer sufficient disease control. As rates of KR rise, there is little information on how it is used by rheumatologists and family physicians. These 2 specialties were surveyed to determine how well they agreed about the use and outcomes of KR for patients with severe osteoarthritis (OA) of the knee.

Methods.—A survey was sent to 98 rheumatologists and 250 family practitioners in Ontario, Canada. Response rates were 70% for rheumatologists and 52% for family practitioners. The members of the 2 groups were asked about their indications for referral for KR, their use of nonsurgical management options, and their perceptions of the outcomes of KR. The physicians were also asked how many patients they saw with severe OA of the knee, and this was compared with their opinions regarding KR.

Results.—Of 32 factors possibly affecting the decision to refer for KR, family physicians disagreed about 28 and rheumatologists disagreed about 26. When presented with 10 treatments for knee OA, the 2 specialties consistently disagreed about 8. The 2 groups stated similar outcomes of KR, though agreement was lower for the family practitioners. Compared to data previously obtained from orthopedic surgeons, the family physicians showed greater disagreement as to the indications for and outcomes of KR. Rheumatologists disagreed more about the indications for KR than did orthopedic surgeons. However, they were similar in their perceptions of the outcomes.

Conclusions.—Different groups of referring physicians have varying opinions about the indications for KR referral and the treatments for arthritis of the knee. Family practitioners have higher rates of disagreement in this area than rheumatologists, who are more likely to disagree than orthopedic surgeons. Future studies should look at the reasons for the differing perceptions of these 3 groups. The various specialties may need specific guidelines to address the problem of clinical uncertainty.

▶ You ask 4 doctors and you get 5 opinions! A central observation in the study of health resource utilization is the striking variation observed. The greatest variation is seen in the procedures or treatments with the greatest uncertainty. This study shows that the indications for KR and nonsurgical treatment options showed are not agreed on by clinicians, family practitioners, and rheumatologists. One can see the glass half-full or half-empty. I am struck by the fact that there is relatively good agreement among the physicians. Assessing physician behavior by asking them is not the same as behavior observed. More studies would have to be done to nail this down as an important cause of variation.

M.H. Liang, M.D., M.P.H.

Impact of Patient With Patient Interaction on Perceived Rheumatoid Arthritis Overall Disease Status

Baker PR, Groh JD, Kraag GR, et al (Univ of Ottawa, Canada)

Scand J Rheumatol 25:207–212, 1996 1–7

Introduction.—A chronic illness that affects approximately 1.5% of the population, RA is multifaceted. Management focuses on reducing pain and inflammation; however, it is also acknowledged that the psychosocial aspects of this disease are devastating. Quality-of-life measures should also be used in clinical trial protocols in RA. Whether patient-with-patient interaction has an effect on perceived disease severity and ability to cope with RA was investigated.

Methods.—Forty patients with RA were assessed using clinical global assessment, a visual analogue pain scale, joint counts, patient global assessment, and the Stanford Health Assessment Questionnaire. Most of the patients were women (88%), with a mean age of 58.5 years and an average disease duration of 12.7 years. All the participants took part in 6 one-on-one conversations with other patients with RA about their disease activity on the effect that their disease had on their lives. Conversations were limited to 10 minutes. After these conversations, the participants were asked to fill out a follow-up questionnaire, which asked them to compare their perception of the disease before and after the conversations.

Results.—After the conversations, the scores of the participants' patient global assessment improved, showing a statistically significant difference before the conversation and after the conversation. As a result of this interaction, 60% of the participants said their ability to cope with their disease had improved.

Conclusion.—Patients were very enthusiastic about discussing their arthritis symptoms with other patients. In the short term and long term, patient education and self-management programs are integral parts of patient management, and they can help to reduce health care costs. Patient-with-patient interaction is endorsed to improve perceived well-being among this group.

▶ Patient and health professional interaction is important in the patient's perception of disease activity. An improvement in patient global assessments occurred after a series of weekly conversations with other patients about disease activity and the impact of the disease on the patient's life. This observation supports the development of support groups and case managers to provide education and feedback for patients with chronic disease. Phone intervention can reduce physician visits and physician telephone calls and improve patients' perception of disease activity. This presents a new opportunity for educational programs. This increased interaction with health care professionals may be a reason for the beneficial heightened response noted in patients enrolled in clinical trials in RA.

M.E. Weinblatt, M.D.

Predicting Length of Stay After Hip or Knee Replacement for Rheumatoid Arthritis

Escalante A, Beardmore TD (Univ of Texas, San Antonio; Rancho Los Amigos Med Ctr, Downey, Calif)

J Rheumatol 24:146–152, 1997 1–8

Introduction.—To control costs, it is important to identify factors affecting length of stay (LOS) in patients with RA who undergo total arthroplasties of the hip (THA) or knee (TKA). Clinical, demographic, and surgical procedure characteristics were evaluated to identify predictors of postoperative LOS after THA or TKA in patients with RA.

Methods.—Records of all patients with RA who underwent reconstructive joint surgery from 1987 to 1991 were reviewed retrospectively. One hundred thirty-seven patients with RA underwent 119 TKAs and 105 THAs. All patients evaluated participated in an inpatient rehabilitation program that discharged patients to home after they became functionally independent. The relationship between postoperative LOS and demographics, clinical characteristics, medications, and postoperative course was analyzed.

Results.—A single joint was implanted in 148 surgeries, and 2 joints were implanted simultaneously in the remaining 38 surgeries. The average LOS after THA was 16.9 days and after TKA 19.5 days (Fig 1). Although there is a national trend toward shorter hospital stays after THA and TKA, this trend was not observed in patients with RA who underwent THA or TKA. On a national level, only a small number of THA and TKA procedures are performed on patients with RA. Significant preoperative patient characteristics related to longer LOS were age older than 55 years, female sex, nonwhite ethnicity, known positive rheumatoid factor, and poor functional status (Steinbrocker functional class 3 or 4). Surgical characteristics associated with longer LOS were use of bone cement, operating

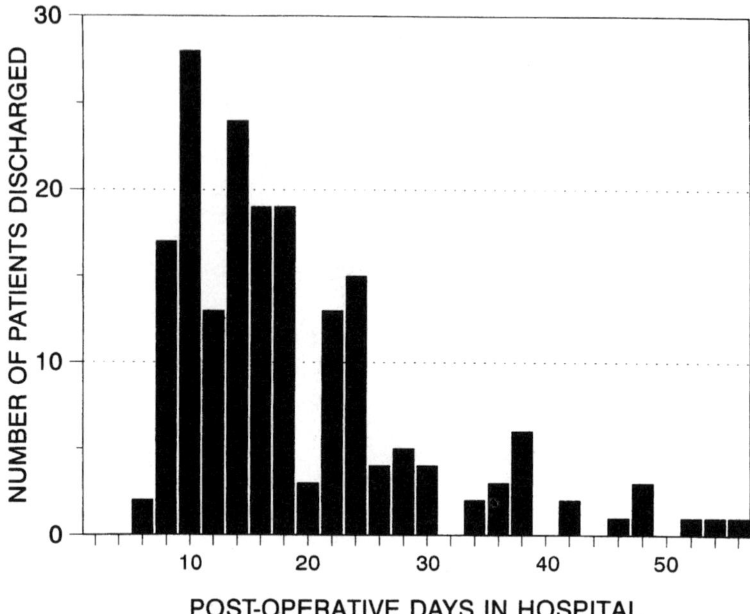

FIGURE 1.—Distribution of the number of days of LOS after 186 surgical encounters totaling 119 total knee arthroplasties and 105 total hiparthroplasties. Average LOS ± 1 SD = 18.2 ± 10.2 days, median 15, range 5 to 56. *Abbreviation: LOS,* length of stay. (Courtesy of Escalante A, Beardmore TD: Predicting length of stay after hip or knee replacement for rheumatoid arthritis. *J Rheumatol* 24:146–152, 1997.)

time longer than 6 hours, postoperative wound infection, and performance of more than 1 operation at a time.

Conclusion.—Health status was an important determinant of the rate of postoperative recovery. Postoperative LOS was significantly related to known positive rheumatoid factor, prolonged operating time, use of bone cement, and postoperative wound infection. Total hospital days could have been reduced by 29% if patients had received surgery before reaching Steinbrocker functional status class 3 or 4.

▶ Preoperative functional status was an important determinant of the rate of recovery of functional independence after surgery. This suggests that we should try to maximize the functional status of patients before total joint replacement. The major deficiency of this study is the average LOS after THA at this center was 17 days and 20 days after TKA. In Boston, the average LOS is less than 5 days for a hip replacement in the acute-care setting. With the more rapid discharges from institutions, preoperative functional status becomes even more important.

M.E. Weinblatt, M.D.

Healthcare

Do Physician-Payment Mechanisms Affect Hospital Utilization? A Study of Health Service Organizations in Ontario

Hutchison B, Birch S, Hurley J, et al (McMaster Univ, Hamilton, Ont)

Can Med Assoc J 154:653–661, 1996 1–9

Background.—Ontario's Health Service Organizations (HSOs), introduced in 1975, are the only capitation-based practices in Canada. A major objective of the HSO program is to reduce hospitalization through more preventive and ambulatory care. Initial reports indicated that hospitalization rates were 20% lower among patients enrolled in HSOs than in those attending fee-for-service practices, but it is possible that factors other than method of payment accounted for the difference in rates.

Methods.—A retrospective cohort study was designed to examine the effect of physician-payment method on hospital utilization rates. These rates were compared for 39 physicians who converted from fee-for-service to capitation and 77 physicians who remained in fee-for-service practice during the study period (June 1985 to January 1989). Periods examined were 3 years and 1 year before and 3 years after the transition to capitation-based payment, together with the corresponding years for physicians remaining in fee-for-service practice. Two hospital-utilization rates were determined: hospital separations and hospital-days per 1,000 patients in each practice.

Results.—With adjustments for patient age, sex, and social-program-recipient status, the mean annual rate of hospital-days used in capitation-based practices fell from 1,085 per 1,000 patients in the 3 years before conversion to 1,030 in the year before conversion and to 984 after 3 years. Corresponding annual rates for matched physicians in fee-for-service practices were 1,085, 1,035, and 956 hospital-days per 1,000 patients. Rates of hospital separations showed a similar pattern (Table 5). Neither rates of hospitalization nor changes in rates differed significantly between capitation-based and fee-for-service practices for the 3 periods reviewed.

Discussion.—Primary health care provided on a capitation basis did not reduce patient hospitalization rates when the rates were compared with those of fee-for-service practices. Hospitalization rates may have fallen in both groups because of a reduction in the number of acute care beds available, a shift in the hospital admission decision from primary care physicians to secondary or tertiary care physicians, or other factors.

▶ Canada's one payor health care system looks increasingly attractive to U.S. physicians beleagured by a system that is undergoing a sea change. Conventional wisdom has it that capitation and risk sharing will contain health care costs, and primary care physicians will control access to expensive surgery, specialty services, and hospitalizations.

TABLE 5.—Hospital Utilization (Hospital Separations or Hospital-Days Used), Adjusted for Age, Sex, and Social-Program-Recipient Status

	Measure of hospital utilization					
	Hospital separations mean annual rate per 1000 patients (and 95% CL*)			Hospital days used, mean annual rate per 1000 patients (and 95% CL)		
Period, in relation to the transition to capitation-based practice	Capitation-based practice $n = 39$	Fee-for-service practice $n = 77$	p value	Capitation-based practice $n = 39$	Fee-for-service practice $n = 77$	p value
3 yr before	164.3 (160, 169)	166.0 (163, 169)	0.543	1084.6 (1019, 1151)	1085.4 (1025, 1146)	0.988
1 yr before	155.1 (150, 161)	156.0 (152, 160)	0.795	1029.8 (962, 1097)	1034.8 (976, 1094)	0.917
3 yr after	105.5 (100, 111)	106.6 (103, 111)	0.743	954.3 (892, 1017)	956.4 (898, 1015)	0.965
Change from 3 yr to 1 yr before	−9.2 (−2.2, −16.2)	−10.0 (−4.8, −15.2)	0.710	−54.9 (−149.0, 39.3)	−50.6 (−134.0, 33.2)	0.568
Change from 1 yr before to 3 yr after	−49.6 (−42.0, −57.2)	−49.4 (−43.7, −55.1)	0.312	−75.4 (−167.0, 16.5)	−78.4 (−161.0, 4.37)	0.774

*CL, confidence limits.

(Reprinted by permission of the publisher from Hutchison B, Birch S, Hurley J, et al: Do physician-payment mechanisms affect hospital utilization? A study of Health Service Organizations in Ontario. *Can Med Assoc J* 154:653–661, 1996.)

This report suggests that when beds are tight and controlled largely by specialists, hospitalization rates are unaffected by the payment system. The business paradigm that drives much of U.S. health reform doesn't always hold, and this should be an affirmation to those who still believe that medical care is a calling, not a product line.

M.H. Liang, M.D., M.P.H.

2 Rheumatoid Arthritis

Introduction

This year's selections present a potpourri from the worlds of clinical and basic research. The basic science articles highlight our increasing knowledge of the immunogenetics and immunopathology of RA. They include articles on apoptosis, interleukins involved in the disease process, genetics, and gene products. In the therapeutic area, selections include evaluation of the "sawtooth" strategy, several articles on methotrexate, studies of sulfasalazine, corticosteroids, cyclosporin A, intravenous gammaglobulin, and an initial study with soluble TNF receptor. Others relate to the acute-phase response HLA as predictors of certain outcomes in RA.

While the understanding of the disease process increases slowly and the appreciation of our better therapies becomes keener, we remain a long way from knowing how to consistently intervene effectively for patients with RA.

I had an opportunity to present my own approach to the therapy of RA at the 1996 American College of Rheumatology meeting. I intervene early. The issue then is whether to use single-drug or combination-drug therapy. In making this decision, it is important to consider the effects of the disease as visualized in a progression of radiographs over time. Erosions develop in patients early in the disease, and the curve of development is very steep in the first 24 months. This suggests that if the course of RA is to be modified, drug therapy must be started early. I use disease-modifying antirheumatic drugs (DMARDs) as soon as I make the diagnosis of RA. All newly diagnosed patients have been receiving nonsteroidal anti-inflammatory drugs (NSAIDs), and the particular DMARD I prescribe first depends on the patient's functional status. Can the patient afford to wait 4 to 6 months for the drug to take effect? Is the patient working? Has the patient missed work or school because of RA? Does the patient's RA have a malignant presentation? Does the patient want to become pregnant? The answers to such questions will determine the choice of drugs. If the disease is mild and the patient can afford to wait, I prescribe hydroxychloroquine (HCQ) or sulfasalazine (SSA). If the patient has aggressive disease, I prescribe methotrexate (MTX). Corticosteroids may serve as a bridge from NSAIDs to DMARDs. Ted Pincus has shown that over 60% of RA patients around the country are taking corticosteroids. As patients start DMARD regimens, their doses of corticosteroids may be stepped down. For patients with refractory RA, I first increase the dosage of MTX to 20 mg/week. If the patient does not respond, I switch the treatment to 25 mg/week of subcutaneous MTX. If the patient still does not respond, I start my first combination of MTX, SSA, and HCQ. My second combination is MTX and cyclosporine. While there are encouraging results with the biologic-response modifier (as reflected in my selections), their clinical application is several years away. Until then, rheumatologists must consider combination therapy for their patients who are not responding to traditional therapy.

Michael E. Weinblatt, M.D.

Immunogenetics and Pathophysiology

Further Evidence for Genetic Anticipation in Familial Rheumatoid Arthritis

McDermott E, Khan MA, Deighton C (City Hosp, Nottingham, England; Case Western Reserve Univ, Cleveland, Ohio; Manchester Univ, England)
Ann Rheum Dis 55:475–477, 1996 2–1

Objective.—Some familial diseases may become more severe and occur at earlier ages in each subsequent generation. This phenomenon, called "genetic anticipation," has been linked to unstable trinucleotide repeat sequences. Recent evidence suggests that genetic anticipation may occur in familial RA. A larger, independent sample of families with RA was studied to see if it showed features of genetic anticipation.

Methods.—The study included 59 multicase families from the National Repository of RA pedigrees of the British Arthritis and Rheumatism Council, 65 multicase families from Cleveland, and 253 consecutive RA patients seen at rheumatology clinics in Nottingham, England. The 3 groups were analyzed to see if they had the same features of genetic anticipation as seen in preliminary studies.

Results.—In all 3 groups, the mean age at disease onset was significantly lower in probands with RA than in their affected parents. The mean difference in age between mother and proband pairs was 16.0 years in the Arthritis and Rheumatism Council group, 7.8 years in the Cleveland group, and 10.4 years in the Nottingham group. The results were similar in father-proband pairs, though there were relatively few such pairs. Proband age at onset was not correlated with the parent's age at the proband's conception; there was such a correlation in the preliminary study.

Conclusions.—Findings in larger, independent samples support the preliminary evidence of genetic anticipation in familial RA. Molecular research is needed to study the phenomenon of genetic anticipation in families with 2 successive generations affected by RA. In other familial multifactorial diseases, the "Repeat Expansion Detection" system is being used to seek expanded trinucleotide repeats.

► A resident and colleagues recently emphasized this concept to me when we observed genetic anticipation in 3 generations of a family with giant cell arteritis.[1] My colleague Dr. Peter Zauber reminded me that certain other explanations must be considered—and excluded—for genetic anticipation to explain these observations. The observations include better detection or heightened awareness of disease leading to earlier diagnosis, or stronger environmental influences on subsequent generations causing earlier illness. Also, comparison of mean ages of familial with nonfamilial probands would have strengthened these authors' observations. I hadn't appreciated that the basis for genetic anticipation seems to be unstable, expanded trinucleotide repeat sequences. If genetic anticipation is not uncommon in rheumatic disease, further study of this at a molecular level may be of interest.

R.S. Panush, M.D.

Reference

1. Zauber NP, Zhang L, Berman E: Familial occurrence of temporal arteritis. *J Rheumatol* 24:611–612, 1997.

HLA-DRB1 Genes and Disease Severity in Rheumatoid Arthritis
Reveille JD, for the MIRA Trial Group (Univ of Texas Health Sciences Ctr, Houston; et al)
Arthritis Rheum 39:1802–1807, 1996 2–2

Introduction.—A sequence homology is shared in HLA-DRB1 alleles associated with RA within the third hypervariable region of the DR β chain encompassing amino acids 70–74. The concept of a shared epitope has emerged because this sequence may be encoded by certain HLA-DR4 or non-DR4 alleles. A more severe and destructive form of RA is exhibited by individuals homozygous for HLA-DRB1*0401. The role of the presence and dose of HLA-DR4 and non-DR4 alleles encoding the rheumatoid epitope in the severity of RA was examined.

Methods.—There were 169 patients with RA participating in a 48-week trial who had their blood typed for HLA-DRB1 and HLA-DQB1. There were 104 caucasians, 52 blacks, 10 Hispanics, and 3 from other ethnic groups. To assess disease severity, baseline erosions and new erosions at the last visit were measured as a proxy for progression.

Results.—There was no association between the specific alleles identified, the presence of erosive disease or rheumatoid factor status, and the dose of rheumatoid epitope (homozygous, heterozygous, none). Among the caucasian placebo-treated patients, there was a gradient observed for the 3 allelic subgroups and their gene doses in the occurrence of new erosions at the final visit; however, this was not observed in the minocyline-treated patients. In multivariate analysis, a treatment group/ HLA-DR4 epitope interaction was demonstrated. The rheumatoid epitope was not seen in approximately two thirds of black patients. Those who were typed and not typed had similar features—56% were seropositive, 13% had subcutaneous nodules, 28% had joint deformities, 5% had reconstructive joint surgery, and approximately 50% had taken disease-modifying antirheumatic drugs.

Conclusion.—In predicting the progression of disease in some caucasian patients, HLA-DRB1 oligotyping may be useful. Among black patients with RA, this epitope was infrequent. There was an increased frequency of HLA-DRB1*0401 among minocyline-treated patients compared with healthy North American controls; however, the minocyline-treated patients had shorter disease duration and less severe RA than those described in another study.

HLA Markers and Prediction of Clinical Course and Outcome in Rheumatoid Arthritis

Wagner U, Kaltenhäuser S, Sauer H, et al (Univ of Leipzig, Germany; Univ of Erlangen-Nuremberg, Erlangen, Germany)

Arthritis Rheum 40:341–351, 1997 2–3

Introduction.—The association of HLA-DR4 and RA has been studied. The association of different DR alleles with RA is accounted for by a shared motif within the third hypervariable region, located in the α-helical region of the first domain. Polymerase chain reaction-dependent HLA genotyping was used to assess the implication of HLA markers on the diagnosis and clinical course of RA in a comparative retrospective and prospective manner.

Methods.—Eighty-seven healthy blood donors were compared with 121 patients with RA. There were 66 patients who had RA for at least 5 years. In the retrospective study, HLA genotyping was performed on 66 patients. In the prospective study, methotrexate or sulfasalazine combined with steroids if necessary was the treatment. The prospective study included 76 healthy controls and 55 patients with RA who were measured for HLA-DRB1 specificities, DR4 alleles and their linked DQB1 alleles, as well as HLA-B27, using polymerase chain reaction-based methods. Epidemiologic means and multiple regression analysis were used to evaluate the impact of HLA markers.

Results.—In long-standing and recent onset RA, there was an association between shared epitope-positive (HVR3+) DR4 alleles and the HVR3 amino acid cassette QKRAA. In HVR3 shared epitope-positive patients, radiologic evidence of severe joint destruction was seen in long-standing RA. When expressed on a DR4 allele, there was a significantly higher ranking for the presence of the RA-associated HVR3 cassettes according to rank sum analysis of Larsen indices. There was a significantly increased risk of developing bony erosion among DR4-positive patients in the prospective study. There were significantly higher Larsen indices among HVR3 epitope-positive DR4-positive individuals than among those who were epitope-negative. There was an increased a posteriori likelihood of developing early erosive disease with the presence of the HVR3 epitope on DR4.

Conclusion.—For the prognosis of joint destruction in RA, HLA-DR genotyping and DR4 subtype determination provide valuable markers, although the contribution of HLA typing to establishing the diagnosis of RA is limited.

► The importance of the rheumatoid epitope still remains to be defined. The first of these two articles (Abstract 2–2), a study of patients enrolled in the minocycline trial in RA, confirmed the infrequency of the epitope among black patients with RA. Some of the caucasian patients with the epitope had increased erosions (a marker of severity).

This second selection (Abstract 2–3) also addressed the contribution of the shared epitope on the prognosis of joint disease and erosion formation. However, it is still premature to use this technology for therapeutic recommendations in day-to-day clinical practice. We don't yet have enough data—it may be premature to extrapolate information from isolated, selected populations and from animal studies. We await the results of broad population studies (which are in press).

M.E. Weinblatt, M.D.

The Presence of Interleukin-13 in Rheumatoid Synovium and Its Anti-inflammatory Effects on Synovial Fluid Macrophages From Patients With Rheumatoid Arthritis

Isomäki P, Luukkainen R, Toivanen P, et al (Turku Univ, Finland; Satalinna Hosp, Harjavalta, Finland; DNAX Research Inst, Palo Alto, Calif)

Arthritis Rheum 39:1693–1702, 1996 2–4

Introduction.—Several lines of evidence suggest that the Th2 cytokine interleukin (IL)-4 may attenuate the inflammatory process in rheumatoid synovium. Interleukin-13 has many of the same functional properties of IL-4, including downregulation of proinflammatory cytokine production and suppression of monocyte/macrophage cytotoxic function. The presence of IL-13 in rheumatoid synovium was evaluated, including an analysis of its effects on synovial fluid (SF) macrophages and T cells from patients with RA.

Methods and Findings.—The study included 47 patients with RA, median age 61 years and median duration of disease 18 years. Cytokine-specific enzyme-linked immunosorbent assays detected IL-13 in 96% of SF samples, compared with 64% of samples for IL-4. The mean IL-13 level was greater than the mean IL-4 level. The IL levels were unrelated to the patients' erythrocyte sedimentation rate, C-reactive protein level, age, duration of disease, or RA treatment. Reverse transcriptase-polymerase chain reaction and Southern hybridization detected IL-13 mRNA in 87.5% of SF mononuclear cell (SFMC) samples.

Further studies were performed to determine the effects of IL-13 on production of the proinflammatory cytokines IL-1β and tumor necrosis factor-α. Lipopolysaccharide was added to the SFMC samples to enhance macrophage activation. Production of these cytokines was significantly inhibited by both IL-4 and IL-13. They were not as potent as IL-10 in this regard. When added to IL-10–treated cultures, IL-4 and IL-13 produced further downregulation in production of IL-1β, although not TNFα.

Conclusions.—Interleukin-13 is consistently present in the joints of patients with RA. Not all patients with RA coexpress IL-4 and IL-13, suggesting that they may play separate roles in controlling the synovial immune response. Exogenous IL-13 can inhibit production of proinflammatory cytokines in SFMC. The results suggest a possible treatment role of IL-13 in patients with RA.

▶ We now need to add another cytokine to our list of potential players in RA. In this case, IL-13 appears to have similar activity to IL-4, which in RA might be beneficial. As for IL-4 and IL-10, which downregulate promoter inflammatory cytokines such as TNFα and IL-1, IL-13 appears to have a similar effect. Both IL-4 and IL-10 are under phase II clinical development and I would imagine that IL-13 is not far behind. I can envision a day when there may be several of these cytokines combined in clinical studies.

M.E. Weinblatt, M.D.

Accumulation of Soluble Fas in Inflamed Joints of Patients With Rheumatoid Arthritis

Hasunuma T, Kayagaki N, Asahara H, et al (St Marianna Univ, Kawasaki, Japan; Juntendo Univ, Tokyo; Nagasaki Chuo Hosp, Nagasaki, Japan)

Arthritis Rheum 40:80–86, 1997 2–5

Introduction.—Apoptic signals are transmitted to several types of cells by the Fas antigen. For elimination of cells that may cause imbalance of the host defense system, Fas-dependent apoptosis is essential in the immune system. A characteristic feature in the rheumatoid synovium in situ is apoptosis of synoviocytes. In the serum and synovial fluid of patients with RA and osteoarthritis, the concentration of the soluble form of the Fas molecule (sFas) was examined.

Methods.—There were 15 normal subjects, 13 patients with osteoarthritis, and 45 patients with RA in whom concentration of sFas was determined. Measurements were also taken of the level of several cytokines in serum and synovial fluid, the erythrocyte sedimentation rate, and the C-reactive protein level.

Results.—In the patients with RA, the synovial fluid concentration of sFas was higher than in the patients with osteoarthritis. There was a weak correlation between the serum levels of C-reactive protein, the erythrocyte sedimentation rate, and the synovial fluid levels of interleukin-2 receptor and intercellular adhesion molecule 1. Synovial cells and infiltrating mononuclear cells expressed sFas messenger RNA in the patients with RA according to reverse transcription-polymerase chain reaction analysis.

Conclusion.—In the inflamed joints of patients with RA, sFas accumulates, but it does not accumulate in patients with osteoarthritis. The activity of RA correlates with the level of sFas. In inflamed RA joints, sFas may inhibit apoptosis of synovial stromal cells in situ.

▶ The concentration of the Fas molecule is increased in the synovial fluid of patients with RA as compared with osteoarthritis. Fas-dependent apoptosis is a feature of rheumatoid synovitis. This paper suggests that high levels of Fas may be indicative of an impairment of the counter-regulatory mechanisms that terminate abnormal immune response.

M.E. Weinblatt, M.D.

Apoptosis in Rheumatoid Arthritis: p53 Overexpression in Rheumatoid Arthritis Synovium

Firestein GS, Nguyen K, Aupperle KR, et al (Univ of California, San Diego)

Am J Pathol 149:2143–2151, 1996 2–6

Introduction.—The p53 tumor suppressor is a nuclear phosphoprotein that functions as a key regulator of cell survival and cell replication. It acts as a transcriptional activator or gene that obstructs progression from G1 to S phase in mammalian cells, restricts angiogenesis, and regulates a variety of DNA repair mechanisms. The expression of p53 increases in response to DNA damage. The subsequent cell cycle prolongation allows DNA repair or apoptosis in severe instances. The expression of p53 as a key regulator of DNA repair and apoptosis was evaluated in the RA joint.

Methods.—Synovial tissues were obtained from 9 patients with RA at the time of joint replacement surgery. The monoclonal antibody Pab 1801 was used in immunohistochemical analysis. Tissues were analyzed using immunoperoxidase assays, flow cytometry, and western blot analysis. Findings were compared with those of fixed, permeabilized sections of osteoarthritis (OA) and other noninflammatory synovial tissues (STs).

Results.—The p53 protein was observed in both the cytoplasm and nuclei of lining cells. Nearly all RA tissues stained intensely in the synovial intimal lining. Cytoplasmic staining was more pronounced in the intimal lining and nuclear staining was seen more often in the sublining layer of RA ST. Some immunoreactive p53 was observed in OA ST, but the amount of staining was significantly less, compared to RA. Minimal or no staining was detected in 3 noninflammatory STs (normal, posttraumatic arthritis, and avascular necrosis). The p53 was constitutively expressed by fibroblast-like synoviocytes (FLS) using flow cytometry on permeabilized cells. Western blot analysis indicated that RA FLS expressed significantly more p53 than either OA FLS or dermal fibroblasts.

Conclusion.—The nuclear phosphoprotein p53 in RA is abnormally expressed in synovium, particularly the intimal lining where abundant

DNA strand breaks occur. If it is possible to target apoptosis defects in RA resulting from a specific gene defect, novel and exciting therapeutic approaches may be forthcoming.

► In a very elegant paper, results of study of p53 tumor suppressor gene expression are presented. Prominent staining of p53 was noted in the synovial lining cells and was more intense in RA but also was observed in OA. The study suggests that there is an overexpression of this gene in the synovial lining of patients with RA, and this leads to transformed synovial fibroblasts and joint disruption in RA. Stay tuned for the significance of this observation. [Dr. Firestein presented some of these exciting data and his interpretation of them in a lecture on "Synovial autoimmunity and anatomy: new concepts in rheumatoid arthritis" at the 1996 American College of Rheumatology meeting....R.S. Panush, M.D.]

M.E. Weinblatt, M.D.

Clinical Aspects

Rheumatoid Arthritis Lung Disease: Determinants of Radiographic and Physiologic Abnormalities

Saag KG, Kolluri S, Koehnke RK, et al (Univ of Iowa, Iowa City)

Arthritis Rheum 39:1711–1719, 1996 2–7

Introduction.—In RA, pulmonary disease may appear as pleural lesions, interstitial lung disease, and lung nodules. The prevalence of interstitial lung disease in RA is as high as 40%. Risk factors for this condition have been found to be the presence of serum rheumatoid factor, subcutaneous nodules, antirheumatic therapies, immunogenetic disease severity markers, and cigarette smoking, but these have not been confirmed. In a representative population of patients with RA, the frequency and risk factors for interstitial lung disease were determined.

Methods.—An evaluation of RA disease activity and severity was conducted on 336 patients with RA and lung disease. Outcome measures included chest radiographic findings of interstitial infiltrates, pulmonary function tests of forced vital capacity, and diffusion capacity for carbon monoxide. To determine the independent significance of cigarette smoking and other RA specific factors on the pulmonary abnormalities of interest, multivariable statistical modeling was used. Some of the characteristics of the patients were: 70.2% were females; the median age was 57.9 years; 98% were white; and they had a mean of 7.7 swollen joints (Table 1).

Results.—In 32.4% of all patients, at least 1 of 3 abnormal findings was identified. The abnormal findings included evidence of radiographic interstitial infiltrates in 40 patients, diffusion capacity for carbon monoxide of less than an 80% of predicted in 64 patients, and forced vital capacity of less than 80% predicted in 42 patients. A significant predictor of low diffusion capacity for carbon monoxide, low forced vital capacity, and interstitial abnormalities on chest radiograph was 25 or more pack-years of cigarette smoking (Fig 1). Another important risk factor for the decline

TABLE 1.—Disease Characteristics of Patients With Rheumatoid Arthritis

Characteristic	
Demographics	
Sex, % female	70.2
Age, years	57.9 ± 13.5
Race, % white	98.0
Current ACR criteria for RA, % patients	61.0
RA activity	
Swollen joint count (range 0–66)	7.7 ± 7.6
Tender joint count (range 0–69)	10.1 ± 12.9
Morning stiffness, hours	1.6 ± 3.4
HAQ DI (range 0–3)	1.0 ± 0.70
Patient assessment of pain by VAS (range 0–100)	37.6 ± 25.4
Patient assessment of global severity by VAS (range 0–100)	35.5 ± 23.3
Physician assessment of global severity by VAS (range 0–100)	25.1 ± 22.0
ESR, mm/hour	36.0 ± 26.0
RA severity	
Hand radiographic evidence of RA, % patients	71.7
Rheumatoid factor positive, % patients	63.4
Rheumatoid nodules, % patients	34.2
Mean disease duration, years	13.9 ± 11.2
Prior joint surgery, % patients	51.5
Current medication use	
NSAIDs, % patients	73.5
Second-line drugs, % patients	61.9
Corticosteroids, % patients	37.5

Note: Total number of patients = 336. Unless otherwise indicated, values are the mean ± SD.

Abbreviations: ACR, American College of Rheumatology; *HAQ*, Health Assessment Questionnaire; *DI*, Disability Index; *VAS*, visual analogue scale; *ESR*, erythrocyte sedimentation rate; *NSAIDs*, nonsteroidal anti-inflammatory drugs.

(Courtesy of Saag KG, Kolluri S, Loehnke RK, et al: Rheumatoid arthritis lung disease: Determinants of radiographic and physiologic abnormalities. *Arthritis Rheum* 39:1711–1719, 1996. Copyright American College of Rheumatology.)

in diffusion capacity for carbon monoxide and forced vital capacity was the health assessment questionnaire disability index, a measure of disease activity and poor long-term prognosis. Current methotrexate use seemed to have a deleterious effect on the forced vital capacity; however, it was not significantly associated with any pulmonary abnormalities.

Conclusion.—Smoking was the most consistent independent predictor of radiographic and physiologic abnormalities suggestive of interstitial lung disease in RA, but RA disease activity/severity was also important. Further studies to evaluate the other effects of cigarette smoking on RA would be beneficial.

▶ This is an extremely timely article in light of the popularity of methotrexate and that drug's pulmonary toxicity. Salient points include the frequency of pulmonary abnormalities in an unselected cohort of patients with RA, the strong association of lung disease with cigarette smoking, and the poor disability score as measured by a health assessment questionnaire. This study supports the observation that methotrexate has little impact on routine pulmonary function testing and that methotrexate lung disease is an infrequent event. The most important conclusion is that we should urge all our

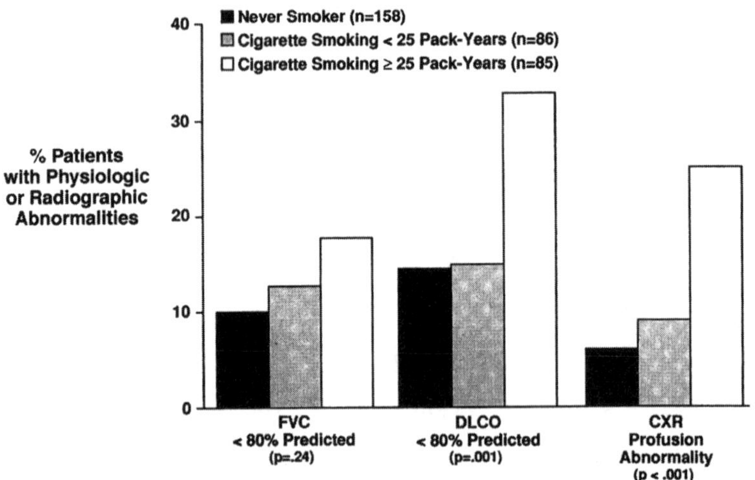

FIGURE 1.—Bar graph histogram demonstrating the univariate associations of smoking (expressed in pack-years) with abnormalities on pulmonary function studies (diffusion capacity for carbon monoxide [*DLCO*] and forced vital capacity [*FVC*]), and with chest radiograph (*CXR*) perfusion abnormalities (interstitial infiltrates). *P* values determined by chi-square trend test. (Courtesy of Saag KG, Kolluri S, Loehnke RK, et al: Rheumatoid arthritis lung disease: Determinants of radiographic and physiologic abnormalities. *Arthritis Rheum* 39:1711–1719, 1996. Copyright American College of Rheumatology.)

patients, including patients with RA, to stop smoking. This will have positive impact on overall health status and possibly reduce the risk of rheumatoid lung disease.

M.E. Weinblatt, M.D.

Rheumatoid Arthritis and Cancer Risk

Mellemkjær L, Linet MS, Gridley G, et al (Danish Cancer Society, Copenhagen; Natl Cancer Inst, Bethesda, Md; Danish Epidemiology Centre, Copenhagen; et al)

Eur J Cancer 32A:1753–1757, 1996 2–8

Introduction.—Rheumatoid arthritis has been linked to lymphatic and hematopoietic cancers. The best available evidence suggests an increased risk of non-Hodgkin's lymphoma, Hodgkin's disease, multiple myeloma, and leukemia in patients with RA. Danish registry data were used to evaluate the incidence of cancer among patients with RA.

Methods.—Data were obtained from the comprehensive Danish Hospital Discharge Register. All patients receiving diagnoses of juvenile RA, Felty's syndrome, palindromic arthritis, other and unspecified RA, or RA with chronic nodules from 1977 to 1987 were included in the study. Their data were linked to death and cancer registries, excluding the first year of cancer follow-up. A total of 20,699 patients were studied from first diagnosis of RA to death or through 1991. Cancer rates were compared with the expected population rates (Table 2).

TABLE 2.—Observed (Obs) Numbers and Relative Risk (RR) for Lymphatic and Haematopoietic Cancers Among 20,699 Patients Followed 1–15 Years After Hospitalization With RA

	Total				Men		Women	
Cancer site	Obs	Exp	RR	95% CI	Obs	RR	Obs	RR
All lymphatic and haematopoietic cancer	171	99.6	1.7	1.5–2.0	61	1.7†	110	1.7†
Non-Hodgkin's lymphoma	85	35.9	2.4	1.9–2.9	33	2.9†	52	2.1†
Hodgkin's disease	14	4.2	3.4	1.8–5.6	4	2.4	10	4.1†
Multiple myeloma	21	19.0	1.1	0.7–1.7	4	0.6	17	1.4
Leukaemia	50	39.8	1.3	0.9–1.7	19	1.2	31	1.3
Acute lymphocytic leukaemia	2	1.3	1.6	0.2–5.7	1	2.3	1	1.2
Chronic lymphocytic leukaemia	14	18.5	0.8	0.4–1.3	6	0.8	8	0.7
Acute non-lymphocytic leukaemia	25	13.1	1.9	1.2–2.8	11	2.4†	14	1.7
Chronic myeloid leukaemia	5	4.9	1.0	0.3–2.4	1	0.5	4	1.3
Other and unspecified leukaemia	4*	2.0	2.0	0.5–5.0	0	—	4	3.3
Mycosis fungoides	1	0.8	1.3	0.0–7.4	1	2.6	0	—

*One case of hairy cell leukemia, 1 case of megakaryocytic leukemia, 1 case of acute leukemia not otherwise specified, and 1 case of leukemia not otherwise specified.
†$P < 0.05$.
(Reprinted from Mellemkjær L, Linet MS, Gridley G, et al: Rheumatoid arthritis and cancer risk. *Eur J Cancer* 32A:1753–1757, copyright 1996, with kind permission from Elsevier Science Ltd, the Boulevard, Langford Lane, Kidlington OX5 1GB, UK.)

Results.—Patients with RA had a twofold elevation in risk of non-Hodgkin's lymphoma. The increase was noted in both sexes, including 84% nodal cases. For patients with secondary Sjögren's syndrome, the relative risk of non-Hodgkin's lymphoma was 9.8. The increased risk of Hodgkin's disease was significant in females. The risk of acute nonlymphocytic leukemia was doubled. There was no increased risk of multiple myeloma or chronic lymphocytic leukemia. One woman had Kaposi's sarcoma. The risks of colorectal carcinoma and breast cancer were reduced.

Conclusions.—This and previous studies suggest that patients with RA are at increased risk of non-Hodgkin's lymphoma, Hodgkin's disease, and lung cancer. All studies to date are from Nordic countries. Some of these studies show a reduction in colorectal and breast cancer risk. The same factor that increases the risk of RA in women could reduce the risk of breast cancer This was a large study with a high degree of ascertainment for cancer cases, and it offered some insight into the histologic subtypes of some malignancies.

▶ This study is consistent with other large data sets regarding the increased risk of lymphoproliferative diseases with RA. The very large population is from Denmark and also reports an increase of lymphoproliferative malignancies with non-Hodgkin's lymphoma. Information about background disease-modifying anti-rheumatic drugs therapy was, unfortunately, lacking and would have been of interest. A decreased risk of colon cancer possibly attributable to nonsteroidal antiinflammatory drug use is reassuring. These data are important when evaluating the risk of drugs like methotrexate, azathioprine, cyclosporin A, and the potential risk for the development of lymphoproliferative illness in the context of the underlying disease.

M.E. Weinblatt, M.D.

Epstein-Barr Virus Clonality in Lymphomas Occurring in Patients With Rheumatoid Arthritis

van de Rijn M, Cleary ML, Variakojis D, et al (Univ of Pennsylvania, Philadelphia; Stanford Univ, Calif; Northwestern Univ, Chicago)

Arthritis Rheum 39:638–642, 1996 2–9

Background.—Prior studies have reported that some patients with rheumatic disease have lymphomas that are similar to Epstein-Barr virus (EBV)–positive posttransplant lymphoproliferative disorders. Two new patients with RA and EBV-positive lymphomas were described, and the results of analysis of frozen tissue sections were included.

Methods.—Two patients with RA and lymphomas were studied. Southern blotting was performed to detect immunoglobulin gene rearrangements, terminal repeat analysis was performed to evaluate the clonality of the EBV genome, and the lymphoma cells were double-labeled by in situ hybridization and immunoperoxidase staining to confirm the presence of EBV in these cells.

Results.—The first patient was a woman with a 12-year history of RA, which had been treated by nonsteroidal anti-inflammatory drugs and gold. In 1989, a regimen of methotrexate (MTX) and prednisone was initiated. In 1993, she was seen for the presence of 2 soft-tissue masses. A biopsy revealed diffuse large-cell lymphoma. Methotrexate was halted, and chemotherapy was started. The patient responded completely. The second patient was a woman with a 20-year history of RA. In 1977, she began gold therapy; in 1980, this was changed to penicillamine and prednisone; and in 1984, it was changed to hydroxychloroquine. In 1993, she was told that she had cervical adenopathy. A biopsy revealed a lymphoma. She died several weeks later. Histologic sections from lesions in both patients revealed a diffuse malignant proliferation of lymphoid cells with large irregular nuclei containing obvious nucleoli. Both large-cell lymphomas had a B phenotype. The majority of cells were positive for the EBV EBER 1 gene. Double-labeling demonstrated that the EBV signal was localized to the malignant B cells. Both lymphomas had clonal Ig gene rearrangements.

Conclusions.—Patients with RA can have lymphomas that resemble EBV-positive posttransplant lymphomas develop. All lymphomas detected in patients with RA should be tested for the presence of EBV. Withdrawal of antirheumatic therapy should be considered as a first approach to controlling lymphomas in those patients with EBV-positive lymphomas.

▶ This study extends observations on EBV and lymphomas in patients receiving MTX. The authors report 2 patients who had lymphomas; the first was treated with MTX, and the second patient had a lymphoma but had only been treated with gold, penicillamine, and hydroxychloroquine. The authors, using some elegant molecular biology techniques, demonstrated that both of these B-cell lymphomas showed a positive reaction by in situ hybridization for the EBV genome and that EBV was localized to the malignant B cells. These results suggest a role for EBV in the development of lymphomas in these patients. The study is important in that the association of EBV with the lymphomas in RA is not entirely dependent on treatment with MTX or other immunosuppressive agents. The authors recommend that patients with RA who have lymphomas develop should have the tissue tested for EBV by in situ hybridization techniques. In those patients in whom there is evidence of EBV, withdrawal of antirheumatic therapy is recommended first rather than just institution of chemotherapy. It is intriguing that cases similar to this have not been reported in psoriasis, in which there has been long-term administration of similar immunosuppressive drugs including MTX, azathioprine, and cyclosporin A. This suggests that it is not only the drugs but also the underlying disease that may be important in the development of the syndrome.

M.E. Weinblatt, M.D.

The Validity of Self-reported Diagnosis of Rheumatoid Arthritis: Results From a Population Survey Followed by Clinical Examinations

Kvien TK, Glennås A, Knudsrød OG, et al (Diakonhjemmet Hosp, Oslo, Norway)

J Rheumatol 23:1866–1871, 1996 2–10

Objective.—Patient self-reports of health status have proved valid for use in epidemiologic studies of RA. These studies often use self-reported diagnoses as well, sometimes under such broad terms as "arthritis" or "arthritis and rheumatism." The validity of self-reported diagnoses has not been proved in patients with RA. This issue was addressed in a population survey, including whether self-reported symptoms or health status can correctly predict the diagnosis of RA.

Methods.—A questionnaire was mailed to 10,000 randomly selected adults. The participants were asked to report any musculoskeletal pain, stiffness, rheumatic diagnoses, disability, and mental distress. One hundred fifty-eight patients reported having RA, 30 of whom were identified in a local registry of patients with RA. The rest were invited for rheumatologic evaluation, including routine blood tests and additional tests as needed to make a diagnosis.

Results.—The survey response rate was 59%. Sixty-two percent of patients reported musculoskeletal pain, stiffness, or both during the preceding month. Of the 158 patients who reported having RA, 107 had been given this diagnosis from a physician and 142 self-reported it. However, the diagnosis of RA was confirmed in only 35 patients: 30 from the register and 5 by clinical and laboratory evaluations. Self-reported swollen joints and disability scores differed for patients with perceived and actual RA.

However, no set of useful predictors was identified on multivariate analysis.

Conclusions.—Only one fourth of patients who report having RA actually have the disease, this study suggests. Thus, self-reported RA appears to be unreliable for clinical or research purposes. The findings are consistent with previous studies showing disagreement in the diagnosis of specific rheumatic conditions by general practitioners and rheumatologists alike. Most patients who report having RA have various other rheumatic conditions.

Validity of Self-reported Rheumatoid Athritis in Elderly Women

Star VL, Scott JC, Sherwin R, et al (Univ of Maryland, Baltimore; Univ of California, San Francisco)

J Rheumatol 23:1862–1865, 1996 2–11

Purpose.—Questionnaires used for epidemiologic research often elicit information on self-reported medical diagnoses. The accuracy of a patient self-report of physician-diagnosed RA is unclear. The validity of self-reported diagnoses of RA in elderly women was evaluated.

Methods.—The analysis included 2,424 women enrolled in the Study of Osteoporotic Fractures, a multicenter, prospective cohort study of factors associated with fractures. All participants were Caucasian women aged 65 years or older. As part of a questionnaire administered during entry to the study, the women were asked whether a doctor had ever told them that they had any kind of arthritis or rheumatism. If the answer was yes, they were asked to specify which kind of arthritis the doctor said they had. If a participant reported receiving a diagnosis of RA, her physician was sent a questionnaire asking for information on the condition. The presence of RA was classified on the basis of the 1987 revised American College of Rheumatology (ACR) criteria. In addition, posteroanterior radiographs of the hand were obtained at baseline in each participant. These films were reviewed for evidence of RA, including erosions, juxta-articular osteopenia, and joint space narrowing.

Results.—Five percent of the women reported a physician diagnosis of RA. Women with and without self-reported RA were similar in terms of age and current marital status. Those reporting RA were more likely to have taken steroids and had more years of formal education. Of the 127 women reporting RA, 10 died, 6 could not be contacted, and 15 refused permission for physician contact. Eighty-seven of 96 questionnaires sent to physicians were completed and returned. Of these, only 11 (12.6%) indicated that the patient met the ACR criteria for a diagnosis of RA. Overall, the self-reported physician diagnosis of RA was confirmed in just 26 of 127 women. Assuming that all women with a physician diagnosis of RA reported it, the positive predictive value of the self-reported diagnosis was 20.5%.

Conclusions.—Only about one fifth of women reporting a physician diagnosis of RA met the criteria for this disease on review. The absence of such a self-report is a valid indicator that the disease does not exist. Epidemiologic studies using self-reported diagnoses of RA, particularly for case-definition purposes, should be interpreted with caution.

► Two studies, 1 from Norway (Abstract 2–10) and 1 from the United States (Abstract 2–9), report that there is very little value in questionnaires of self-reported diagnoses of RA. Self-reported diagnoses of RA in both studies were unreliable. This has implications with regard to health services research and epidemiology in which self-reporting questionnaries are used to determine the incidence and frequency of RA in the population. Confirmation of the diagnosis of this rheumatic illness is required for studies that use patient self-reported diagnoses.

M.E. Weinblatt, M.D.

Prediction of Articular Destruction in Rheumatoid Arthritis: Disease Activity Markers Revisited

Coste J, Spira A, Clerc D, et al (Hôpital Cochin, Paris; Hôpital de Bicêtre, Paris; Hôpital Ambroise Paré, Boulogne, France)

J Rheumatol 24:28–34, 1997 2–12

Introduction.—It would be helpful in both clinical research and practice to be able to predict joint damage progression in RA, but there is no agreement regarding which markers are the best. The predictive value for joint damage progression was assessed via commonly used disease activity or process measures in 72 patients with RA.

Methods.—Patients underwent clinical, laboratory, and radiographic assessments twice yearly for 2 years. Clinical assessment included: duration of morning stiffness, number of swollen joints, the Ritchie index, visual analogue scale (VAS), and a health assessment questionnaire. The primary outcome variable was progression of articular destruction.

Results.—Predictors of 6-month radiographic joint damage progression were (in order of decreasing significance) iron, C-reactive protein, erythrocyte sedimentation rate, and α_1-acid glycoprotein. There were no predictive markers for 12- and 18-month progression. Consistent with other reports, there were no clinical markers predictive of joint damage progression.

Conclusion.—Only a few laboratory markers (iron, C-reactive protein, erythrocyte sedimentation rate, and α_1-acid glycoprotein) were predictive of joint damage. No assessed marker was able to predict outcome past 6-month joint damage progression. There were no significant correlations between clinical and laboratory markers of disease progression. These findings add to the growing evidence of lack of association between clinical, laboratory, radiographic, and functional assessments of RA.

Individual Relationship Between Progression of Radiological Damage and the Acute Phase Response in Early Rheumatoid Arthritis: Towards Development of a Decision Support System

van Leeuwen MA, van Rijswijk MH, Sluiter WJ, et al (Univ Hosp, Groningen, The Netherlands; Univ Hosp, Nijmegen, The Netherlands; Hammersmith Hosp, London)

J Rheumatol 24:20–27, 1997 2–13

Introduction.—As irreversible joint destruction begins during the first months of RA, there is a trend to start aggressive therapy early. During the first years of the disease, there may be an association between serum C-reactive protein concentration or erythrocyte sedimentation rate and the extent of synovial inflammation, as seen on radiologic studies. A model was developed to describe the individual relationship between C-reactive protein concentration and radiologic progression of RA during the first years.

Methods.—The prospective study of 149 patients with early RA included monthly C-reactive protein assays and Sharp scores of radiographs taken of the hands and feet every 6 months. Adjustments were made mathematically for discontinuity in the radiographic scoring system and for clustering in the occurrence of score points in the initial phase.

Results.—In each patient, time-integrated C-reactive protein values correlated closely with radiologic progression. However, between individuals with similar radiographic scores, there was considerable variation. The individual relationship between C-reactive protein and radiologic damage was reflected by a k value for each patient that was based on C-reactive protein measurements and radiographic scores. The model accurately predicted the extent of radiologic progression that was observed by using the k value combined with actual C-reactive protein levels over 3 and 6 years. The k value from 6- or 12-month observational data provided the best results to obtain a prediction. A software program that indicates the levels to which C-reactive protein should fall to prevent further joint damage has been created to incorporate this model for routine clinical use.

Conclusion.—Rheumatoid disease activity is strongly associated with the individual relationship between time-integrated C-reactive protein and erythrocyte sedimentation rate, and this has been used to create a model for a software program. Outcome can be predicted from 6 months after presentation and can be used as a practical decision support system.

The Acute Phase and Function in Early Rheumatoid Arthritis: C-Reactive Protein Levels Correlate With Functional Outcome

Devlin J, Gough A, Huissoon A, et al (Univ of Leeds, England)

J Rheumatol 24:9–13, 1997 2–14

Background.—The primary therapeutic goal of treatment for patients with RA is the prevention of functional deterioration. The level of C-

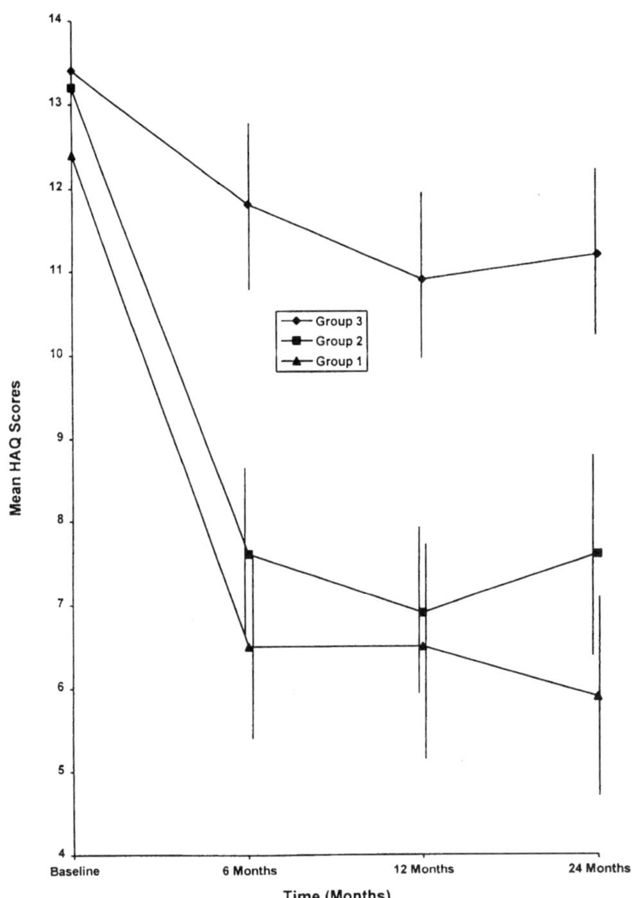

FIGURE 1.—Health Assessment Questionnaire (*HAQ*) scores relative to C-reactive protein (CRP) response in the first 6 months. At 6 months, patients were divided on the basis of their CRP response. In group 1, CRP normalized; in group 2, there was a 50% reduction in CRP; in group 3, there was a less than 50% reduction in CRP (*error bars* = lower to upper quartiles). (Courtesy of Devlin J, Gough A, Huissoon A, et al: The acute phase and function early in rheumatoid arthritis: C-reactive protein levels correlate with functional outcome *J Rheumatol* 24:9–13, 1997.)

reactive protein (CRP) is often monitored as a marker of acute disease, but its correlation with disease outcome is not well understood. An investigation was undertaken to determine whether normalization of the CRP level is associated with stabilization of functional state and whether this can be used as a predictor of outcome in patients with RA. The relationship between CRP and the Health Assessment Questionnaire (HAQ) was evaluated over the 24 months of the study.

Methods.—A prospective study was performed of 109 patients who met the American Rheumatism Association's 1987 criteria for RA, had elevated CRP level before steroid or second-line therapy, and were referred to the early synovitis clinic at Selly Oak Hospital. These patients had had symptoms for less than 1 year and had not previously been treated for this condition. Patients received treatment according to standard protocols. The patients were examined at baseline and at 3, 6, and 12 months, and then annually. Levels of CRP and the HAQ score were determined at each visit. Patients were divided into 3 groups based on CRP suppression within the first 6 months: group 1, CRP suppressed to normal levels; group 2, CRP suppressed 50%; and group 3, CRP not reduced by 50%.

Findings.—There were 34 patients in group 1, 31 patients in group 2, and 44 patients in group 3. There was no difference between the 3 groups in initial HAQ or proportion of patients with disease epitopes. During the initial 6-month period, HAQ score improved in all 3 groups. Patients in groups 1 and 2 had significantly lower HAQ scores after 6 months than the patients in group 3. This correlation between HAQ and CRP levels was also present at 12 and 24 months (Fig 1). Among the 34 patients in group 1, 28 maintained their CRP levels in the normal range at 12 months, and this was associated with a further decrease in HAQ score. The 6 group 1 patients who had a re-elevation of CRP levels had a slight increase in HAQ score. Worsening HAQ scores were only observed among patients with re-elevation of CRP. Among the entire group of 109 patients, increased HAQ score was observed in 18 patients during the first 12 months. Levels of CRP had increased from baseline in all of these patients.

Conclusion.—This study of 109 patients with early RA and elevated C-reactive protein levels has demonstrated that CRP is a good indicator of disease activity, and correlates with short- and medium-term functional outcome. Elevation of CRP was associated with functional deterioration, whereas suppression of CRP levels was associated with functional stabilization or improvement. Changes in CRP were also correlated with changes in the HAQ score. The HAQ score appears to be a sensitive indicator of functional change in the early phases of rheumatoid disease.

▶ These three selections (Abstracts 2–12, 2–13, and 2–14) focus on the importance of surrogate markers for disease and the progression of radiographic damage in RA. The first paper found that clinical variables such as baseline swollen joint counts and painful joint counts were not predictive of further joint damage, but levels of C-reactive protein were associated with radiographic progression at 6 months but not at 12 months or longer.

Investigators from Europe have for years written about the relationship between elevated C-reactive protein (CRP) and radiographic progression (Abstract 2–12); they have argued that normalization of the CRP should be a goal, as the CRP may be a surrogate marker for radiographic damage. Authors from Holland (Abstract 2–13) demonstrate that time-integrated CRP values correlated closely with radiographic progression. A computer model was developed for clinical use. This software program indicates the reduction in CRP required in individual patients to prevent further damage. This is extremely intriguing, and I look forward to further studies in this area.

The third article (Abstract 2–14) is from the early synovitis clinic at the University of Leeds, a tremendous resource because of the ability to recruit patients with early RA. These investigators looked at the correlation between CRP values and functional assessments. In patients in whom the CRP was suppressed to normal, there was a significant improvement in functional activity levels as measured by the HAQ. There was also improvement in patients with 50% improvement in CRP. In those patients who had a persistently elevated CRP and those in whom a re-elevation occurred, a deterioration in functional status was observed. There has been increasing interest not only in measuring CRP in clinical studies but also in guiding therapy toward decreasing CRP levels. This study suggests that CRP is a surrogate marker of functional outcome.

As we develop better treatments for RA, we should pay greater attention to this easy-to-measure parameter. CRP has emerged as an important outcome marker in clinical trials. However it does not supplant clinical observations (i.e. swollen joints) in following individual patients.

M.E. Weinblatt, M.D.

The Effect of Progressive Resistance Training in Rheumatoid Arthritis

Rall LC, Meydani SN, Kehayias JJ, et al (Tufts Univ, Boston; New England Med Ctr, Boston)

Arthritis Rheum 39:415–426, 1996 2–15

Purpose.—Loss of body cell mass, or "rheumatoid cachexia," is an important problem in patients with RA. One contributing factor may be the decreased physical activity observed in RA patients. Exercise has been shown to improve physical performance capacity, cardiorespiratory fitness, muscle strength, and activities of daily living for RA patients. Few studies have evaluated the use of total body dynamic resistive strength training in patients with RA. The effects of high-intensity progressive resistance training were compared in RA patients vs. healthy control subjects.

Methods.—The study included 8 untrained subjects with RA, ranging in age from 25 to 65 years, as well as 8 untrained healthy young adults and 14 untrained healthy elderly subjects. The healthy young subjects and the RA patients underwent a 12-week strength training program. Subjects in the healthy elderly group were randomized to receive either strength training or warmup exercise only. The progressive-resistance strength training program consisted of dynamic exercise, including concentric and eccentric contractions, of all major muscle groups. Strength training sessions were held twice weekly, and strength testing was performed every 2 weeks. The various groups were compared at baseline and follow-up for fitness, body composition, energy expenditure, function, disease activity, pain, and fatigue.

Results.—Strength increased in all 3 strength training groups: 57% in the RA patients, 44% in the young healthy subjects, and 36% in the elderly healthy subjects. Self-reported pain and fatigue scores decreased significantly in the RA patients, with no change in the number of painful or swollen joints. The RA patients also had significant improvement in 50-foot walking scores and in balance and gait scores. No group showed significant changes in body composition.

Conclusions.—High-intensity strength training can significantly increase strength and reduce pain and fatigue in selected patients with RA. The benefits accrue with no exacerbation of disease activity or joint pain. Strength training not only improves the reduced muscle strength of RA patients but brings them up to the level of healthy subjects. Resistance training may be considered for all patients with RA, as long as their disease is under control and there are no contraindications.

Protein Metabolism in Rheumatoid Arthritis and Aging

Rall LC, Rosen CJ, Dolnikowski G, et al (Tufts Univ, Boston; St Joseph Hosp, Bangor, Maine; New England Med Ctr, Boston)

Arthritis Rheum 39:1115–1124, 1996 2–16

Purpose.—Little is known about how the inflammation of RA affects metabolism and body composition. Patients with RA are hypermetabolic, with a resting energy expenditure of more than 10% predicted, in association with doubled production of tumor necrosis factor α(TNFα) and interleukin-1β. Cytokine-related loss of lean body mass—or rheumatoid cachexia—may play an important role in the morbidity and mortality of RA. It is important to identify the factors mediating the decline in body cell and protein mass in RA. The effects of RA on whole-body protein metabolism were assessed. The study also evaluated the impact of progressive resistance exercise, the only physiologic stimulus known to improve catabolism.

Methods.—The study included 8 untrained patients with RA, age range 25 to 65 years; 8 untrained healthy young adults; and 14 untrained healthy elderly subjects. The RA patients and the healthy young subjects underwent a 12-week muscle strength training program, while the healthy elderly subjects were randomized into strength-training and non–strength-training control groups. Indicators of protein metabolism and its hormonal and cytokine mediators were measured before and after the study interventions.

Results.—Protein breakdown rate was 80 μmole/g total body potassium/hr in the RA group, compared with 60 and 64 μmole/g total body potassium/hr, respectively, in the young and elderly healthy subjects. Age had no significant effect on protein breakdown. Within the RA group, protein breakdown rates were normal in those receiving methotrexate. After 12 weeks of strength training, the RA-associated increase in protein catabolism was no longer present. Multiple regression analysis showed that TNFα and growth hormone levels were significantly associated with protein breakdown. Plasma glucagon level was inversely correlated with protein synthesis, and growth hormone and glucagon were significantly associated with protein oxidation. Resistance training significantly improved the strength and functional status of RA patients.

Conclusions.—Patients with RA have higher than normal protein breakdown rates. Growth hormone, glucagon, and tumor necrosis factor-α are important factors involved in protein metabolism, and the relationships between these factors are disturbed in patients with RA. Though resistance training improves strength and function in RA patients, it does not produce any change in protein metabolism or hormone levels.

▶ Rheumatoid cachexia has had little study but appears to be like cachexia seen in some cancers and to be cytokine associated. Patients with RA have been shown to be hypermetabolic and this has been shown to be directly associated with the production of tumor necrosis factor-α and interleukin-1 from peripheral mononuclear cells.

These studies (Abstracts 2–15 and 2–16) demonstrate that adults with RA have increased protein breakdown rates compared with control subjects. Endogenous growth hormone, glucagon, and tumor necrosis factor-α can be modulated by resistance training. But in multivariable analyses, even though progressive resistance training led to improved strength and functional status, there were no changes in protein metabolism or hormone levels as a result of the training intervention.

M.H. Liang, M.D., M.P.H.

Are Both Genetic and Reproductive Associations With Rheumatoid Arthritis Linked to Prolactin?

Brennan P, Ollier B, Worthington J, et al (Univ of Manchester, England)

Lancet 348:106–109, 1996 2–17

Introduction.—Given the higher rates of RA in women vs. men, considerable research has focused on the possible role of the female hormones, particularly sex hormones, and reproductive history. Rheumatoid arthritis risk has been linked with breastfeeding and with reduced fecundity. These apparently contradictory risk factors have one thing in common: high levels of prolactin. The authors propose prolactin as the mechanism behind these 2 reproductive risk factors for RA.

Prolactin Link?—The authors suggest that infertility and breastfeeding may be linked to RA through an interaction between high prolactin concentrations and the immune system. Genetic research has found that the only consistent genetic association with RA is for genes encoded in the HLA complex, particularly HLA-DR4. Recent research has suggested that HLA-DR4 status has a significant impact on the effects of both breastfeeding and nulliparity. Thus, some interaction between genetic and reproductive risk factors could be involved in the underlying cause of RA. The prolactin gene is located close to the HLA region on the short arm of chromosome 6. This suggests that the link between DR4 and reproductive risk factors in RA may result from linkage disequilibrium between the HLA loci and polymorphisms of the prolactin gene.

Discussion.—Prolactin may account for the observed genetic and reproductive associations with RA. More study is needed to look for prolactin gene polymorphisms in linkage disequilibrium with HLA-DRB1 alleles. The development of RA could be related to some conserved, extended HLA haplotype that encodes the potential for high levels of prolactin production.

► Women destined to have RA appear to have underlying infertility. The increased risk of RA postpartum may be due to breastfeeding, with the risk increasing more than fivefold in the year after the episode of the breastfeeding. These investigators posit an explanation relating to high prolactin concentration. The hypothesis goes that the associations between DR-4 (which is the most consistent genetic association with RA) and reproductive risk factors in RA are due to linkage disequilibrium between DR-4 and an abnormally regulated prolactin gene polymorphism. The prolactin gene is in close proximity to the HLA region on the short arm of chromosome 6, which makes it a possibility.

M.H. Liang, M.D., M.P.H.

Therapy

Famotidine for the Prevention of Gastric and Duodenal Ulcers Caused by Nonsteroidal Antiinflammatory Drugs

Taha AS, Hudson N, Hawkey CJ, et al (Glasgow Royal Infirmary, Scotland; Univ Hosp, Nottingham, England; Merck Sharp & Dohme, Hoddesdon, England; et al)

N Engl J Med 334:1435–1439, 1996 2–18

Introduction.—The H_2-receptor antagonist famotidine can protect against gastric mucosal injury in normal patients receiving short-course therapy with aspirin or naproxen. However, the safety and effectiveness of famotidine in patients receiving long-term nonsteroidal anti-inflammatory drugs (NSAIDs) are unknown. Famotidine was evaluated for its ability to prevent NSAID-related gastric and duodenal ulcers in patients with arthritis.

Methods.—The randomized, placebo-controlled study included 285 patients who were receiving long-term NSAID therapy for RA or osteoarthritis. All were free of peptic ulcers at the start of the study. The patients were assigned to receive oral famotidine in a 20-mg or 40-mg twice-daily dose or placebo. Clinical and endoscopic evaluations were performed in blinded fashion using standardized criteria at baseline and after 4, 12, and 24 weeks of treatment. The 24-week cumulative incidence of gastric and duodenal ulcers was compared between groups.

Results.—Gastric ulcers developed in 20% of the placebo group, 13% of the famotidine 20-mg group, and 8% of the famotidine 40-mg group. Duodenal ulcers developed in 13%, 4%, and 2% of these groups, respectively. The higher dose of famotidine significantly reduced the incidence of ulcers at both sites, although the lower dose only reduced the rate of duodenal ulcers. Factors associated with an increased risk of ulcers were an increased peripheral white-cell count and duodenal erosions with submucosal hemorrhage. Both famotidine doses were well tolerated.

Conclusion.—Famotidine, in a dose of 40 mg twice daily, can safely reduce the incidence of gastric and duodenal ulcers in patients with arthritis who are receiving long-term NSAID therapy. A lower dose of famotidine may not reduce the incidence of gastric ulcers. Famotidine may also reduce dyspepsia, which is not always present in patients with NSAID-induced ulcers.

▶ Nearly all patients treated with NSAIDs are highly likely to have gastric mucosal irritation (and to a far lesser extent, irritation elsewhere in the gastrointestinal tract) develop. The endoscopic appearance of this irritation, called "stomach rash" by some, ranges from erythema to shallow erosions. This is a benign lesion in most individuals, with notable exceptions: the elderly (particularly elderly women), patients with exogenous Cushing's disease, those taking anticoagulants, and those exposed to other mucosal toxins such as alcohol. For all others, treating the NSAID-related gastric mucosal rash is a testimony to marketing, not to clinical judgment.

With that background, let us examine yet another such trial. A total of 570 patients, most with RA, were invited and 389 accepted an invitation to undergo serial endoscopies to evaluate the effectiveness of famotidine, an H_2-receptor antagonist, in abrogating the more impressive form of the rash: the 3-mm shallow ulcer. Of the 389, 104 already had such lesions and were excluded; the remaining 285 were randomized to placebo or 2 doses of famotidine. The cumulative incidences (and confidence intervals) of these 3-mm shallow ulcers were 28 (19–38) in those receiving placebo, 16 (9–24) in those receiving low-dose famotidine, and 11 (4–17) in those receiving the high-dose famotidine regimens.

So what?

By the way, for the subsets at risk for clinically important gastrointestinal events while taking NSAIDs (the elderly, those taking steroids or anticoagulants, the alcoholic), the more defensible therapeutic posture is to stop the NSAIDs rather than introduce another putatively protective agent. Who must have an NSAID anyway?

N.M. Hadler, M.D.

Outcome in Patients With Early Rheumatoid Arthritis Treated According to the "Sawtooth" Strategy

Möttönen T, Paimela L, Ahonen J, et al (Turku Univ, Finland; Malmi Hosp, Helsinki; Jyäskylä Central Hosp, Finland)

Arthritis Rheum 39:996–1005, 1996 2–19

Background.—The "sawtooth" strategy has recently been proposed for the treatment of RA. This strategy involves early initiation of slow-acting antirheumatic drugs (SAARDs) before joint damage appears; continual, serial use of 1 or many SAARDs; and careful follow-up. The results of this approach were documented.

Methods.—One hundred forty-two patients with early RA were enrolled in a prospective study. The patients were treated actively with SAARDs for a mean of 6.2 years and were closely clinically monitored.

Findings.—The average cumulative number of SAARDs used was 3.3. Lack of treatment efficacy necessitated changes in treatment more often than did adverse effects. The proportion of patients entering remission increased with time to 32%. However, the condition of 24% deteriorated to Steinbrocker functional class III or IV.

Conclusions.—The "sawtooth" treatment approach appears to improve the outcome of early RA. "Sawtooth" therapy remained beneficial in most of the patients in the current study for at least 6 years. However, one fourth of the patients did not respond to treatment.

▶ This open study from our colleagues in Finland uses the "sawtooth strategy" in patients with early RA. Patients had RA for less than 2 years and never received a slow-acting anti-rheumatic drug (SAARD), or as we call them in the United States, DMARD. The sawtooth strategy as described by Jim Fries includes early DMARD therapy, the use of one or more multiple DMARDs, and, after every 3–6 months if there is no response, replacing the DMARD with another or use in combination. In this study IM gold, sulfasalazine, and hydroxychloroquine were used first. There was very low utilization of methotrexate, which may have affected the results. It is possible that because of this low use, this study may not be applicable to the U.S. population. Remission was achieved in 20% of patients; however, remission was temporary. The number of patients receiving IM gold decreased in contrast to the number of patients on methotrexate but only 24% of patients had a deterioration in functional status to class III or class IV. This study suggests that early institution of SAARD therapy with adjustments for clinical response may be important in maintaining functional status but its effects on the radiographs may be variable.

This study confirms my clinical impression regarding treatment of RA. I do believe that early institution of DMARDs can stabilize clinical symptoms and functional status, but to date we do not have any definite therapy that halts radiographic progression. The challenge for the future is development of new drugs or combinations of existing drugs that may affect other mechanisms of disease activity and thereby reduce erosion and cartilage narrowing. Classes of drugs that inhibit metalloproteinases will be essential if we are to achieve our goal of halting radiographic progression. Our available armamentarium is good but not great for RA.

M.E. Weinblatt, M.D.

Sulfasalazine Has a Better Efficacy/Toxicity Profile Than Auranofin: Evidence From a 5 Year Prospective, Randomized Trial

McEntegart A, Porter D, Capell HA, et al (Gartnavel Gen Hosp, Glasgow, Scotland)

J Rheumatol 23:1887–1890, 1996 2–20

Background.—The disease-modifying antirheumatic drugs sulfasalazine and auranofin have been shown to produce both laboratory and clinical improvement in patients with RA. An open, prospective trial comparing these 2 drugs for efficacy and toxicity found no significant difference at 12 months. The 5-year results of that trial were reported.

Methods.—The trial included 200 patients with classic RA who had active synovitis or prolonged morning stiffness requiring second-line drug therapy. Patients who had previously taken sulfasalazine (25 patients) or auranofin (4 patients) were assigned to the opposite drug. Those who had received IM gold but who had stopped taking it because of lack of effect or major side effects (26 patients) were assigned to sulfasalazine. The rest were randomized to sulfasalazine, starting at 500 mg/day and increasing to a target dose of 40 mg/kg/day, depending on side effects, or auranofin, starting at 3 mg twice a day and increasing to 3 mg three times a day if needed for response. Clinical and laboratory follow-up continued for 5 years.

Results.—The 2 treatment groups were similar in terms of age, disease duration, and rheumatoid factor positivity. At 5 years, 31% of patients were still taking sulfasalazine and 15% were still taking auranofin (Table 2). The proportion of patients taking sulfasalazine was still greater even after exclusion of patients previously treated with IM gold. The number of patients discontinuing treatment because of loss or lack of effect was 34 in the sulfasalazine group and 26 in the auranofin group. Side effects were the reason for discontinuation in 24 patients, in the sulfasalazine group and in 49 patients in the auranofin group. The major side effects were diarrhea in the auranofin group and upper gastrointesinal symptoms and rashes in the sulfasalazine group. Leukopenia developed in 6 patients taking sulfasalazine and in 3 patients taking auranofin; thrombocytopenia occurred in 1 patient taking auranofin. These complications resolved when treatment with the offending drug was stopped. There were no drug-related deaths, but all deaths occurred during treatment with 1 of the 2 drugs.

Conclusions.—A 5-year prospective follow-up study shows poor results with auranofin in the treatment of active RA. Patients are more likely to

TABLE 2.—Percentage of Patients Continuing Treatment During the 5-Year Period

Year	1	2	3	4	5
Sulfasalazine	65	56	41	35	31
Auranofin	48	38	29	19	15

(Courtesy of McEntegart A, Porter D, Capell HA, et al: Sulfasalazine has a better efficacy/toxicity profile than auranofin: Evidence from a 5 year prospective, randomized trial. *J Rheumatol* 23:1887–1890, 1996.)

continue taking sulfasalazine during follow-up, which suggests that it is better tolerated, more effective, or both. Auranofin should not be used in patients who have stopped gold therapy because of inefficacy or minor toxic effects.

► This 5-year randomized, open study confirms what we have known for some time, that is, that auranofin is not a terribly effective drug for the treatment of RA. In this study, sulfasalazine was continued for 5 years by 31% of the patients compared with 15% who continued with auranofin. If one extrapolates retention rates for clinical response, one can assume that sulfasalazine is twice as effective as auranofin, which is probably correct. This study illustrates the need, however, for additional therapies for this disease because retention rates of 30% at 5 years are still not acceptable if we expect to control the disease process.

M.E. Weinblatt, M.D.

Oral Administration of an Easily Prepared Solution of Injectable Methotrexate Diluted in Water: A Comparison of Serum Concentrations vs Methotrexate Tablets and Clinical Utility

Marshall PS, Gertner E (Univ of Minnesota, St Paul)

J Rheumatol 23:455–458, 1996 2–21

Background.—Methotrexate (MTX) is a common antirheumatic medication that is frequently used in the treatment of RA. It is available as a tablet and in a cheaper, injectable formulation. Oral ingestion of the injectable form of MTX might provide a cheaper, easier alternative to patients who take the tablet form of MTX. The bioavailability of an oral solution of MTX in comparison with MTX tablets was assessed.

Methods.—Six patients with RA participated. The oral form of MTX was prepared by diluting 0.4 mL of the injectable form in 8 oz of water. Participants first received the oral formulation and then received the tablet formulation 1–2 weeks later. A fluorescence polarization immunoassay was used to determine MTX serum concentrations at 0, 0.5, 1, 1.5, 2, 5, and 8 hours after MTX administration. The area under the curve, maximum concentration, and time to reach maximum concentration, were calculated.

Results.—There were no significant differences between the 2 MTX formulations in any of the variables analyzed. Patients found the oral MTX formulation easier to use than the injectable form and cheaper than the tablet form of MTX.

Conclusions.—The use of an oral formulation prepared from the injectable form of MTX provides a convenient and inexpensive alternative method for the administration of MTX. This may be of particular benefit to those patients for whom the purchase of MTX tablets is a financial hardship.

► This is an extremely practical article that demonstrates that the parenteral solution, when administered orally, achieves the same pharmacokinetics as the tablet. In this study, the injectable formulation was prepared by the pharmacist and diluted in water. The shelf life of MTX is stable up to 8 months. The authors recommend that the syringes be prepared by a pharmacist in a vertical flow hood, which is consistent with Occupational Safety and Health Administration guidelines. Pharmacists could prefill an order so that patients could take home a prescribed number of syringes with MTX and administer the MTX in 8 oz of water. The importance of this article is that it confirms that the pharmacokinetics of the parenteral solution are equivalent to the tablet. There is a significant cost savings with the parenteral solution when administered orally as compared with the tablet. This method of administration is one that I am using in my practice for patients who cannot afford oral MTX tablets, and it is one that I recommend to the readers.

M.E. Weinblatt, M.D.

Survival and Drug Discontinuation Analyses in a Large Cohort of Methotrexate Treated Rheumatoid Arthritis Patients

Alarcón GS, Tracy IC, Strand GM, et al (Univ of Alabama, Birmingham)

Ann Rheum Dis 54:708–712, 1995 2–22

Background.—Methotrexate (MTX) is now considered a standard option in the treatment of RA. In a previous cohort study of patients with RA given MTX, the probability of continuing MTX at 5 years was approximately 50%. The reasons for discontinuing MTX in this cohort were reported, as were overall survival and causes of death.

Methods.—One hundred fifty-two patients with RA began MTX treatment between 1981 and 1986. The patients underwent annual follow-up assessment.

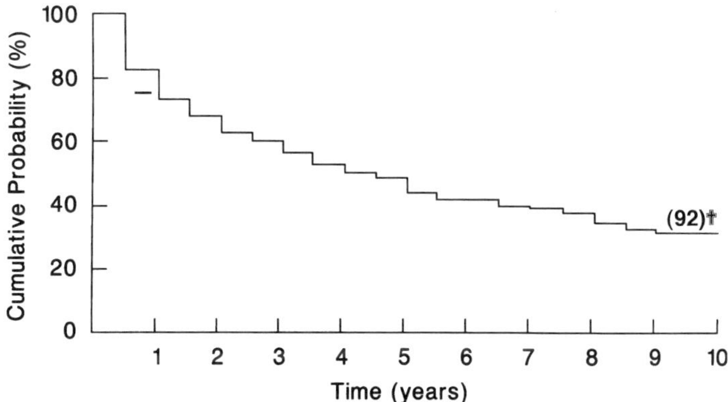

FIGURE 1.—Cumulative probability of continuing to take methotrexate in a cohort of 152 patients with RA. *Dagger* indicates the number of patients remaining in the cohort. (Courtesy of Alarcón GS, Tracy IC, Strand GM, et al: Survival and drug discontinuation analyses in a large cohort of methotrexate treated rheumatoid arthritis patients. *Ann Rheum Dis* 54:708–712, 1995.)

Findings.—Among the first subjects to enter the cohort, the probability of continuing MTX at 10 years was 30% (Fig 1). The most common reason for discontinuing therapy was toxicity (and its severity). The cumulative probabilities of survival for women and men were 85% and 45%, respectively. The number of deaths from infection was greater than expected. However, the numbers of deaths from cancer and cardiovascular diseases were in the expected range.

Conclusion.—In this cohort, the most common reason for quitting MTX treatment was toxicity. Survival was comparable to that for RA reported in other cohorts. However, MTX may have been an associated factor in deaths from infection.

▶ After a slow start, MTX has come to dominate all other second-line agents for RA in the Americas. The zeal rests less firmly on clinical trial data than on the observation that patients seem less inclined to discontinue MTX usage compared with other agents.

However, that is no reason for complacency on the part of the treating physicians. Witness the experience at the University of Alabama described in this paper. Of 152 RA patients given MTX, only 30% were still taking the agent 10 years later (Fig 1). That is not what is so disturbing. What is disturbing is that 50 patients were withdrawn from MTX because of toxic events, including excess infectious deaths. Some argue that MTX is the best we have; I am not so certain. But I am certain that its risk:benefit ratio is so marginal that we must all hope for better agents.

N.M. Hadler, M.D.

Spontaneous Regression of Lymphoproliferative Disorders in Patients Treated With Methotrexate for Rheumatoid Arthritis and Other Rheumatic Diseases

Salloum E, Cooper DL, Howe G, et al (Yale Univ, New Haven, Conn)
J Clin Oncol 14:1943–1949, 1996 2–23

Background.—Patients with RA have a somewhat increased risk for having lymphomas develop. This may be a result of a reduction in the ability to control Epstein–Barr virus (EBV) infection. Twenty-eight cases from the literature and 9 new cases of lymphomas occurring in patients with RA who were treated with methotrexate (MTX) were described.

Methods.—A Medical Literature Analysis and Retrieval System On-Line search was conducted to identify 28 patients with RA who had lymphomas develop while receiving MTX. Nine new cases were assayed for the presence of EBV by in situ hybridization.

Results.—In addition to MTX, 19 patients received corticosteroids, 3 received azathioprine, and one received cyclosporine immunosuppressive therapy. Extranodal disease was detected in 16 of the 37 patients in this study. There were 5 cases of Hodgkin's disease and 7 low-grade lymphomas, and the rest were aggressive lymphomas. In situ hybridization studies

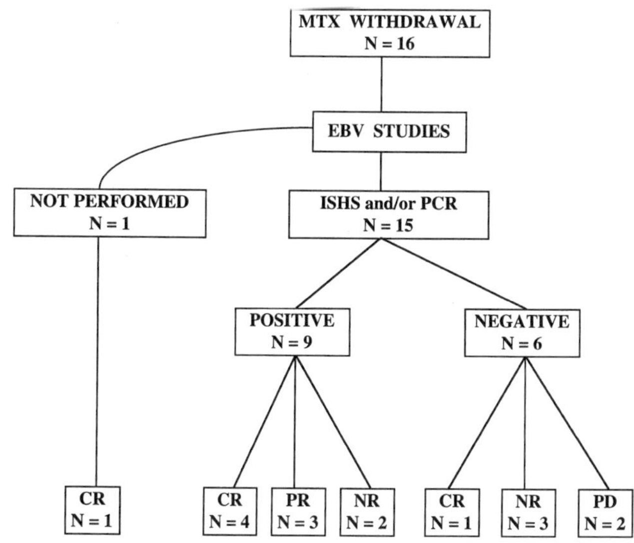

FIGURE 2.—Correlation between response to MTX withdrawal and results of EBV studies in patients with rheumatic diseases. *Abbreviations: NR,* no response; *PD,* progressive disease; *CR,* complete remission; *PR,* partial regression; *MTX,* methotrexate; *EBV,* Epstein–Barr virus; *ISHS,* in situ hybridization studies; *PCR,* polymerase chain reaction. (Courtesy of Salloum E, Cooper DL, Howe G, et al: Spontaneous regression of lymphoproliferative disorders in patients treated with methotrexate for rheumatoid arthritis and other rheumatic diseases *J Clin Oncol* 14:1943–1949, 1996.)

were positive for EBV in 12 of 27 patients. Sixteen patients were initially treated by MTX withdrawal only. Of these 16, 6 achieved complete remission, 3 had a partial remission, and one had a minimal response, yielding an overall response rate of 62%. Among these 10 patients who responded to MTX withdrawal, EBV was detected by in situ hybridization in 6 and by PCR in 2. One patient had a complete response but was not assayed for the virus, and another achieved a complete response despite the inability to detect EBV DNA (Fig 2).

Conclusions.—These results confirm that patients with RA who have lymphomas develop while receiving MTX therapy may show disease regression if MTX is withdrawn. Therefore, MTX withdrawal should be considered as a part of the initial management of lymphoma in patients with RA. In those with low-grade lymphomas, this may be all that is necessary to achieve complete remission. Further studies are necessary to determine the role of EBV in tumor development and as a prognostic factor in the response of the lymphoma to MTX withdrawal. The role of MTX withdrawal in disease regression also requires further study. It is suggested that a registry be established to report all cases of patients with RA who have lymphomas while receiving MTX.

▶ This paper is both a review of the literature of 28 patients plus a study of 9 additional patients who had lymphoproliferative disorders develop in the setting of MTX therapy. Non-Hodgkin's lymphoma (B cell) was confirmed in

27 of these patients. The Epstein-Barr virus was identified in 12 of 27 patients (44%). Withdrawal of MTX led to improvement in the lymphomas in 62% of patients, including 6 complete remissions, 3 partial responses, and 1 minimal response. It is important that rheumatologists be aware of the association of lymphoproliferative disorders associated with treatments for RA. Similar lymphomas have been seen now with cyclosporin A and azathioprine in patients who have received transplants. All had some association with EBV, but whether the virus is directly responsible for the lymphomas is unknown. As with the patients who received transplants, extranodal involvement is common. Regression in the tumor without chemotherapy may occur if the immunosuppressive or MTX therapy is discontinued. This has occurred most commonly in patients who have evidence of EBV in the tumor. Before starting chemotherapy, physicians should withdraw MTX or other immunosuppressive therapies and allow a short period of observation before administering chemotherapy. The development of a registry is also a worthwhile idea and is one that I enthusiastically support. With increasing use of MTX and other immunosuppressive therapies for systemic rheumatic disease, this is an area of further research and clinical observations.

M.E. Weinblatt, M.D.

Pulmonary Function in Patients Receiving Long-term Low-dose Methotrexate

Cottin V, Tébib J, Massonnet B, et al (Centre Hospitalier Lyon Sud, France)
Chest 109:933–938, 1996 2–24

Background.—The main pulmonary side effect in patients taking methotrexate (MTX) for RA is acute interstitial pneumonitis. The current prospective study of patients receiving low-dose MTX therapy for chronic arthritis determined the incidence of MTX-induced pneumonitis during low-dose long-term treatment; the value of periodic pulmonary function tests in detecting MTX pneumonitis before clinical symptoms; and whether subclinical abnormalities of pulmonary function were present in asymptomatic patients taking MTX.

Methods and Findings.—One hundred twenty-four patients underwent pulmonary function testing, including measures of diffusing capacity for carbon monoxide, at treatment initiation, 3 months, 6 months, and every 6 months thereafter. The mean treatment duration was 23 months. In 6 patients, MTX therapy was interrupted for acute onset of clinical symptoms. Four patients met diagnostic criteria for MTX pneumonitis, for an incidence of 3.2%. No risk factors were identified. There was no significant reduction in pulmonary function parameters before the onset of clinical symptoms of MTX pneumonitis. Periodic function tests could not predict this adverse effect. There was a significant reduction in forced vital capacity, forced expiratory volume in 1 sec, and diffusing capacity per alveolar volume, but not in diffusing capacity for carbon monoxide in 118 other asymptomatic patients during MTX therapy.

Conclusions.—Minor subclinical changes were found in pulmonary function in asymptomatic patients receiving low-dose long-term MTX therapy. However, periodic pulmonary function tests did not enable the detection of MTX-induced pneumonitis before clinical symptoms.

▶ Methotrexate-induced pulmonary toxicity is of concern to all rheumatologists, in part because of the idiosyncratic and unpredictable nature of this toxicity. There have been discussions about the value of baseline and surveillance pulmonary function testings for identifying patients at risk for pneumonitis. This study by our colleagues in France shows that surveillance pulmonary function tests are of limited value and should not be done routinely. I totally agree with this recommendation. Surveillance pulmonary function testing is neither helpful nor cost-effective in monitoring for the development of acute pneumonitis.

M.E. Weinblatt, M.D.

Renal Biopsy Findings and Followup of Renal Function in Rheumatoid Arthritis Patients Treated With Cyclosporin A: An Update From the International Kidney Biopsy Registry

Rodríguez F, Krayenbühl JC, Harrison WB, et al (Las Matas, Madrid; Sandoz Pharma AG, Basel, Switzerland; Oslo Sanitetsforenings, Norway; et al)

Arthritis Rheum 39:1491–1498, 1996 2–25

Background.—The use of cyclosporin A (CsA) in the treatment of RA has been limited by concerns about its potential to induce nephropathy. However, the incidence of CsA-induced nephropathy is difficult to estimate, because the most common findings are nonspecific. Data from the International Kidney Biopsy registry were reviewed to better define the occurrence of CsA-induced nephropathy.

Methods and Findings.—The findings of 60 first and 14 second renal biopsies done in patients with RA and treated with CsA for up to 87 months were reviewed. The patients were 44 females and 16 males, aged 10–68 years. At the time of biopsy, the mean daily dose was 2.8 mg of CsA per kilogram. The mean duration of CsA treatment until the first biopsy was 19 months. Serum creatinine concentrations increased after treatment was begun, then declined until the first biopsy, when the relative increase was 18.5% higher than baseline values. First biopsies were graded as class I in 32 patients, class II in 23, and class III in 5. The mean patient age at the beginning of treatment and the initial, maximum, and mean daily CsA doses until biopsy were higher in the group with class III kidney biopsy changes. Nephropathy was very rare in patients given dosages of 5.5 mg CsA per kilogram per day or less. Nephropathy did not develop in any of the 22 patients who started treatment with less than 4 mg of CsA per kilogram per day and whose maximum dosage was 5 mg of CsA per kilogram per day or less. Baseline creatinine values were higher in patients with class III changes than in those with class I or II changes. Continued

TABLE 7.—Summary of Biopsy Findings in the Patients With RA Who Underwent 2 Renal Biopsies

Parameter (score)	First biopsy	Second biopsy
Arteriolopathy		
None (0)	11	12
Minimal (1)	3	0
Slight (2)	0	2
Moderate (3)	0	0
Severe (4)	0	0
Tubular atrophy		
None (0)	1	5
Minimal (1)	9	5
Slight (2)	3	2
Moderate (3)	0	2
Severe (4)	1	0
Interstitial fibrosis		
None (0)	2	4
Minimal (1)	9	7
Slight (2)	2	1
Moderate (3)	0	2
Severe (4)	1	0

(Courtesy of Rodríguez F, Krayenbühl JC, Harrison WB, et al: Renal biopsy findings and followup of renal function in rheumatoid arthritis patients treated with cyclosporin A: An update from the International Kidney Biopsy Registry. *Arthritis Rheum* 39:1491–1498, 1996. Copyright American College of Rheumatology.)

evaluation of renal function showed no evidence of deterioration over time in patients receiving low maintenance doses of CsA (Table 7).

Conclusions.—The risk of CsA-induced nephropathy in patients with RA treated according to current dosing recommendations is low. There was no trend toward progression of morphological lesions over time, despite the longer duration of therapy.

▶ This is a very important article for any rheumatologist who prescribes cyclosporin therapy. Despite the lack of baseline renal biopsies (an understandable weakness of the study), the authors report a low incidence of renal pathology when cyclosporin is used at low doses and the dose is adjusted so that the serum creatinine level does not increase 30% above baseline. Underlying renal dysfunction and hypertension (the most common side effects even with low-dose therapy) appear to be risk factors for renal pathology, which is intuitive and makes sense. The article is reassuring for those of us who use this immunosuppressive and supports the concept of "dose low and go slow." Close monitoring of blood pressure and creatinine levels with careful dose titrations is essential to avoid structural renal disease.

M.E. Weinblatt, M.D.

Intact Adrenocorticotropic Hormone Secretion but Impaired Cortisol Response in Patients With Active Rheumatoid Arthritis: Effect of Glucocorticoids

Gudbjörnsson B, Skogseid B, Öberg K, et al (Uppsala Univ, Sweden)

J Rheumatol 23:596–602, 1996 2–26

Introduction.—Endogenous cortisol secretion may have a disease-modifying effect in RA. It has been suggested that the surgery-related impairment of cortisol response in patients with RA may be related to defective hypothalamic-pituitary function, resulting in impaired production of adrenocorticotropic hormone (ACTH). The hypothalamic-pituitary axis was studied in patients with RA.

Methods.—The study included 18 consecutive patients with moderately high inflammatory activity, as reflected by laboratory values. Those receiving anti-inflammatory drugs were excluded because of potential confounding effects. A group of healthy control subjects was studied as well. The 2 groups were compared for their responses to IV corticotropin-releasing hormone (CRH), thyrotropin-releasing hormone, and luteinizing-releasing hormone. The patients were also studied after 1 week of treatment with prednisolone, 15 to 20 mg/day, to study the short-term effects of anti-inflammatory therapy.

Results.—At baseline, the RA patients had a lower ratio of cortisol to ACTH than the controls, 14 vs. 10×10^3. The RA patients had a normal ACTH response to CRH stimulation; however, their serum cortisol levels fell significantly during the later phases of the test. Levels of other hormones—luteinizing hormone, follicle-stimulating hormone, and thyroid-stimulating hormone—were normal before and after stimulating. Multiple releasing hormone stimulation produced an impaired prolactin response in the patients with RA. Prednisolone therapy reduced the absolute response of serum cortisol to CRH. The prolactin response to stimulation was normalized as well.

Conclusions.—This study demonstrates impaired cortisol secretion but intact ACTH secretion in patients with RA. The findings suggest that these patients have relative adrenal glucocorticoid insufficiency. The impaired cortisol secretion of RA is probably related to adrenal mechanisms, rather than to the hypothalamic-pituitary axis. Some patients with RA may have relative adrenal insufficiency.

▶ We know that adrenocorticoids are powerful anti-inflammatory agents and benefit patients with RA. Here is biological data on patients to show that the inflammatory disease may have direct effects on adrenal function that are not mediated by effects on the pituitary-hypothalamic axis. Interestingly, exogenous steroids seem to suppress disease activity and improve adrenal function. These observations underscore more similarities than dissimilarities between substances that are considered separately as inflammatory mediators, neurotransmitters, and endocrine factors.

M.H. Liang, M.D., M.P.H.

A Double-blind Study of Perioperative Steroid Requirements in Secondary Adrenal Insufficiency

Glowniak JV, Loriaux DL (Oregon Health Sciences Univ, Portland)

Surgery 121:123–129, 1997 2–27

Introduction.—The adrenal glands secrete increased amounts of cortisol during acute stress such as a major operation. To maintain hemodynamic stability under these circumstances, it is believed that increased steroids are necessary, but it is not known how much glucocorticoid is necessary to prevent hypotension. In patients having elective operations who had been clinically treated with glucocorticoids, how much glucocorticoid was necessary to prevent hypotension was determined.

Methods.—All patients took 7.5 mg of prednisone daily for at least 2 months and had secondary adrenal insufficiency that was defined by adrenocorticotropic hormone testing. There were 2 groups of patients, with 6 patients receiving perioperative saline solution and cortisol and 12 patients receiving perioperative injection of saline solution alone. The usual daily prednisone dose was administered to all patients throughout the study.

Results.—The operations were joint replacements, abdominal operations, and other procedures. One patient from each group had hypotension, which resolved with volume replacement. In both groups during the perioperative period, the average pulse rates and blood pressures were similar. Postoperative complications, none of which were serious, were seen in 3 patients from the placebo group, and the complications included 3 days of ileus, ileus and pneumonia, and 1 day of postoperative fever.

Conclusion.—When given only their daily dose of steroids for surgical procedures, patients with secondary adrenal insufficiency do not experience hypotension or tachycardia caused by inadequate glucocorticoid levels. Further supplementation is not required to prevent hemodynamic compromise in the perioperative period, as long as patients continue taking their usual daily dose of steroids. The small number of patients studied was a weakness in this study.

► For decades, we have ordered stress dose steroids in our steroid-dependent patients undergoing surgery. This small study suggests that patients receiving chronic low-dose steroids do not require anything besides fluids and their usual daily dose of steroids. This study needs to be validated in a larger population—its implications are obvious.

M.E. Weinblatt, M.D.

Corticosteroid Injection in Rheumatoid Arthritis Does Not Increase Rate of Total Joint Arthroplasty

Roberts WN, Babcock EA, Breitbach SA, et al (Med College of Virginia, Richmond; Univ of Florida, Gainesville; Univ of Virginia, Charlottesville)

J Rheumatol 23:1001–1004, 1996 2–28

Background.—Most authorities recommend limiting intra-articular corticosteroid injections in a given joint. The maximum safe dose of intra-articular corticosteroid for osteoarthritis (OA) and RA has been debated. Suppressing inflammation by intra-articular corticosteroid injection may slow cartilage degradation from active RA enough to compensate for any accelerated secondary OA that results from the corticosteroid preparation. In a bilateral pair of joints affected by RA, a strategy of intensive corticosteroid injections may produce enough protection from continuous severe RA to permit the most frequently injected joint to lose cartilage at a rate equal to or less than that of the contralateral joint.

Methods and Findings.—A 1987 database of patients with rheumatic diseases was reviewed, and patients with RA receiving 4 or more intra-articular injections in an asymmetric pattern in 1 year were identified. Thirteen patients followed up for a mean of 7.4 years were studied as the cohort of a prospective 5-year study. A total of 1,622 injections were given. However, joint replacement surgery was not significantly more frequent in the heavily injected joints of these patients.

Conclusions.—Frequent intra-articular steroid injection does not greatly increase the risk inherent in continued disease activity in patients with established RA. The patients in the current study did not have an increased risk of joint replacement in heavily injected joints. Frequent corticosteroid injection may confer some chondroprotection in joints that would otherwise have continuous disease activity.

▶ The question of whether repetitive steroid injection increases the risk of joint damage is of interest to the rheumatology community. To adequately address this question, a large prospective randomized trial would be required. Short of that, these investigators did a retrospective review of patients with RA who had received 4 or more intra-articular injections in a single joint for at least a year. The joints that were injected did not have an increased risk of requiring joint replacement surgery during a 5-year period. This small study suggests that there was no great increase of joint replacement after repetitive steroid injections. The study refutes the concept that frequent steroid injections (i.e., 4 in a year) predisposes the joint to acceleration in osteoarthritic changes, thereby requiring eventual joint replacement. Several investigational therapies are also being studied as potential intra-articular treatments. These include novel anti-inflammatory drugs, monoclonal antibodies directed against the T cell, and cytokine inhibitors. Direct visualization of cartilage and newer imaging studies including MRI may allow for a greater understanding of the effect not only of these newer therapies but also of the effects of corticosteroids.

M.E. Weinblatt, M.D.

Low-Dose Corticosteroids in Rheumatoid Arthritis: A Meta-analysis of Their Moderate-term Effectiveness

Saag KG, Criswell LA, Sems KM, et al (Univ of Iowa, Iowa City; Univ of California at San Francisco)

Arthritis Rheum 39:1818–1825, 1996 2–29

Background.—Although low-dose corticosteroids are commonly prescribed for patients with RA, there has been no quantitative analysis of the literature to evaluate the effectiveness of this treatment. Meta-analyses were performed to evaluate the effectiveness of low-dose corticosteroids in the treatment of RA.

Methods.—A computerized literature search of all English language clinical studies in MEDLINE through 1994 was conducted. Both *Arthritis and Rheumatism* and the *Scandinavian Journal of Rheumatology* were hand-searched up through 1994. The reference lists of all selected studies were examined for potential studies for this meta-analysis. Studies met the critereia for inclusion if they were either randomized, controlled, or crossover design trials lasting at least 3 months and using a corticosteroid, such as prednisone, at an average dosage of no more than 15 mg daily. Studies could be included if they contained placebo or active drug controls. Studies had to include at least 1 of the following outcome measurements: joint tenderness, joint swelling, grip strength, and erythrocyte sedimentation rate. The studies were rated for quality.

Findings.—Altogether, 34 studies were identified for the meta-analysis, but only 9 of these met the criteria for inclusion (Fig 1). Four of these studies were placebo-controlled, and 5 were active drug–controlled studies. Reasons for exclusion included lack of randomization, higher cortico-

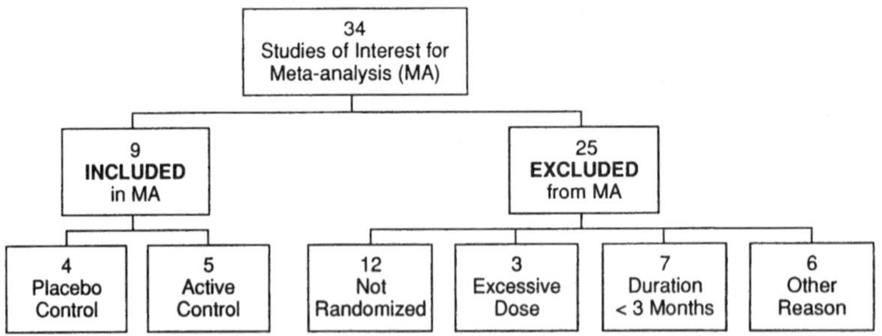

FIGURE 1.—Final disposition of each of the 34 studies identified from the structured literature search. (Courtesy of Saag KG, Criswell LA, Sems KM, et al: Low-dose corticosteroids in rheumatoid arthritis: A meta-analysis of their moderate-term effectiveness. *Arthritis Rheum* 39:1818–1825, 1996. Copyright American College of Rheumatology.)

TABLE 2.—Results of the Standard Meta-analysis

Outcome measure	Summary mean (95% CI)	Effect size (95% CI)	No. of evaluable studies
No. of tender joints			
Active drug and placebo controls	1.78 (0.12, 3.43)	0.60 (−0.31, 1.51)	6
Placebo controls only	2.43 (0.27, 4.58)	0.90 (−0.18, 2.00)	4
No. of swollen joints			
Active drug and placebo controls	2.08 (−0.60, 4.77)	0.71 (−0.41, 1.83)	4
Placebo controls only	3.09 (0.51, 5.66)	1.05 (−0.30, 2.38)	3
Erythrocyte sedimentation rate			
Active drug and placebo controls	8.02 (1.75, 14.3)	0.72 (−0.17, 1.61)	5
Placebo controls only	11.8 (4.28, 19.4)	1.20 (−0.26, 2.65)	3

*There were 9 active drug- and placebo-controlled studies evaluated; 4 of them used only placebo controls.
Abbreviation: CI, confidence interval.
(Courtesy of Saag KG, Criswell LA, Sems KM, et al: Low-dose corticosteroids in rheumatoid arthritis: A meta-analysis of their moderate-term effectiveness. *Arthritis Rheum* 39:1818–1825, 1996. Copyright American College of Rhematology.)

steroid dose, less than 3 months' duration, incompatible outcome measures, and continuations of reports that were already included in the meta-analysis. The results of the standard meta-analysis suggested that corticosteroid treatment was more effective than placebo and more effective than active drug controls in improving conventional outcome measures (Table 2). A second meta-analysis compared corticosteroids to second-line agents previously examined in the meta-analysis. In this meta-

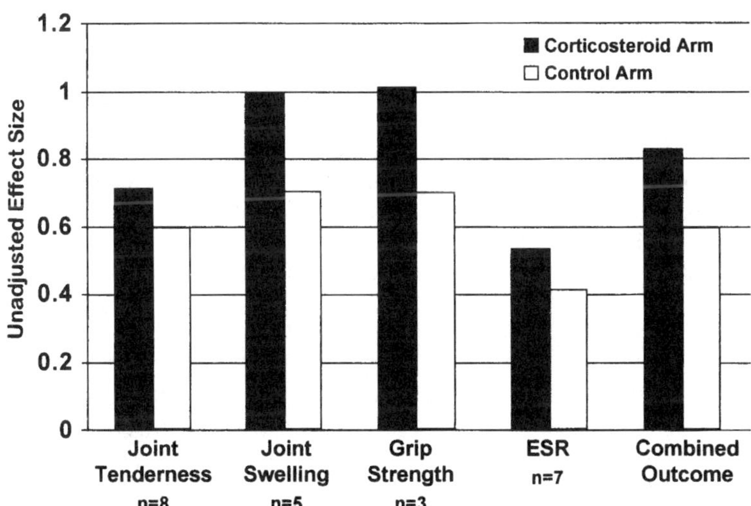

FIGURE 3.—Unadjusted effect size comparing the pooled corticosteroid treatment arms and the control treatment arms for each of the 4 outcome measures. The combined outcome effect size is the mean of the effect sizes for the 4 disease activity outcome measures. *Abbreviation: ESR*, erythrocyte sedimentation rate. (Courtesy of Saag KG, Criswell LA, Sems KM, et al: Low-dose corticosteroids in rheumatoid arthritis: A meta-analysis of their moderate-term effectiveness *Arthritis Rheum* 39:1818–1825, 1996. Copyright American College of Rheumatology.)

analysis, corticosteroids were almost as effective as second-line agents (Fig 3).

Conclusions.—The findings emphasize the limited data that are available to evaluate the moderate-term effectiveness of low-dose corticosteroids as a treatment for RA. The results of a standard meta-analysis suggested that corticosteroids are more effective than placebo or active drug controls in the treatment of RA, as assessed by conventional outcome measures. A second meta-analysis suggested that corticosteroids are similar in effectiveness to traditional second-line antirheumatic agents, as assessed by conventional outcome measures. These findings support the use of corticosteroids as treatment for RA for a period of approximately 6 months. Further investigation should focus on the trade-off between the beneficial effects of low-dose corticosteroid treatment and its toxicity.

▶ The authors performed a meta-analysis of the effectiveness of low-dose corticosteroids in RA. For a topic as widely debated as this, there is a paucity of well-done studies. In fact, the authors were only able to find 9 out of 34 studies that met their criteria for inclusion. Not unexpectedly, the meta-analysis indicated that steroids were more effective than placebo in conventional outcome measurements. It should be noted that methotrexate was not an active control in any of these studies. There were not a sufficient number of papers to investigate the radiographic effects, which are of critical interest. This paper highlights the need for further studies with steroids, particularly those that investigate long-term toxicity and radiographic changes. [See also discussion of this in "The effect of glucocorticoids on joint destruction in rheumatoid arthritis," 1997 YEAR BOOK OF RHEUMATOLOGY, pp 134–136....R.S. Panush, M.D.]

M.E. Weinblatt, M.D.

Calcium and Vitamin D_3 Supplementation Prevents Bone Loss in the Spine Secondary to Low-dose Corticosteroids in Patients With Rheumatoid Arthritis

Buckley LM, Leib ES, Cartularo KS, et al (Med College of Virginia, Richmond; Univ of Vermont, Burlington)

Ann Intern Med 125:961–968, 1996 2–30

Purpose.—Patients with allergic and autoimmune diseases are commonly treated with low-dose corticosteroids. Over time, this treatment can lead to reduced bone mineral density, with a corresponding increase in the risk of vertebral fracture. Supplemental calcium and vitamin D_3, which improves calcium absorption, have been suggested for use in reducing bone loss. However, there are few data to support the efficacy of this intervention. Patients receiving low-dose corticosteroids were studied to determine whether supplemental calcium and vitamin D_3 can prevent spinal bone loss.

Methods.—The randomized, controlled trial included 96 patients with RA, 65 of whom were being treated with corticosteroids. The mean corticosteroid dosage was 5.6 mg/day. The patients were randomly assigned to receive supplementation with calcium carbonate, 1,000 mg/day, and vitamin D_3, or placebo for 2 years. At 1 and 2 years, they underwent measurement of bone mineral density in the spine and femur.

Results.—The rate of bone mineral density loss in patients taking prednisone who were assigned to placebo was 2.0% per year in the lumbar spine and 0.9% per year in the trochanter. In contrast, patients taking prednisone who received supplemental calcium and vitamin D_3 had increasing bone mineral density: 0.72% per year in the lumbar spine and 0.85% per year in the trochanter (Fig). This group showed no increase in bone mineral density in the femoral neck or the Ward triangle, however. Patients who were not taking corticosteroids showed no improvement in bone mineral density with calcium and vitamin D_3 supplementation.

Conclusions.—In patients taking low-dose corticosteroids, supplementation with calcium carbonate and vitamin D_3 prevents declining bone mineral density in the spine and hip. These supplements are available over the counter and have few toxic effects. They may help to reduce the risk of vertebral fracture in patients who require long-term corticosteroid treatment.

► This is a very timely study examining the effects of calcium and vitamin D supplementation in patients with RA. In a double-blind, placebo-controlled trial, the authors have shown that the use of calcium, 1,000 mg/day, and vitamin D_3, 500 IU/day, reduces the loss of bone mineral density (lumbar spine and trochanter) in patients with RA treated with low-dose corticosteroids. There are a number of limitations to the study which are noted appropriately in the Discussion section of the original article. The study is important, and this regimen should be used in all our patients receiving steroid therapy. Whether additional therapy such as antiresorptive treatments, diuretics, or parathyroid hormone will be beneficial is under investigation. Within the next several years, we should have additional treatments for steroid-induced osteoporosis.

M.E. Weinblatt, M.D.

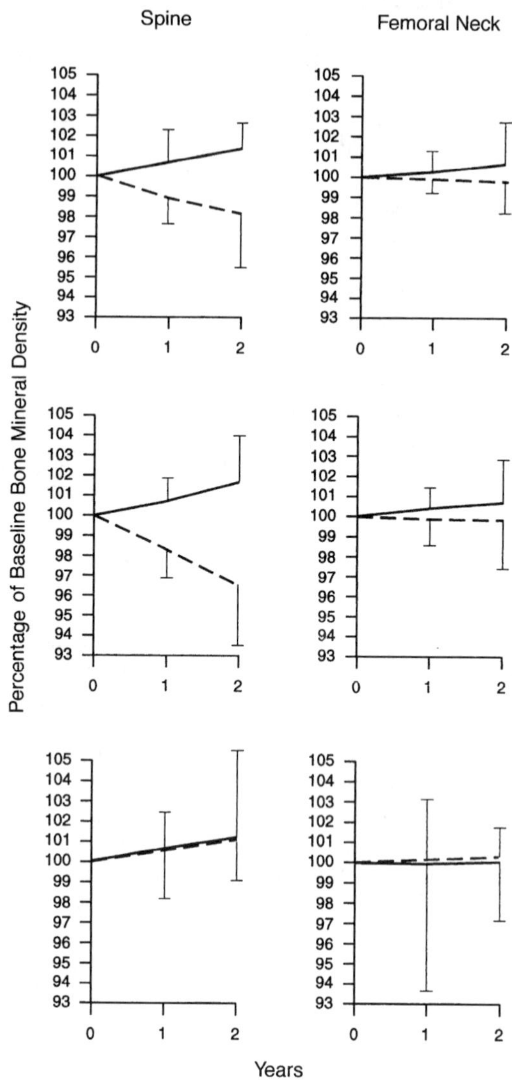

FIGURE.—Change in bone mineral density during the 2-year study period in patients with RA. **Top,** all patients; **middle,** patients receiving prednisone; **bottom,** patients not receiving prednisone. *Solid lines* indicate values for patients in the calcium and vitamin D_3 group; *dashed lines* indicate values for patients in the placebo group. *Bars* represent 95% confidence intervals. A significant difference was seen between the rate of change in bone mineral densities of the spine and trochanter over 2 years in all patients and in patients receiving prednisone. (Courtesy of Buckley LM, Leib ES, Cartularo KS, et al: Calcium and vitamin D_3 supplementation prevents bone loss in the spine secondary to low-dose corticosteroids in patients with rheumatoid arthritis. *Ann Intern Med* 125:961–968, 1996.)

(*Continued*)

FIGURE (cont.)

Ward Triangle
Trochanter
105
104
103
102
101
100
99
98
97
96
95
94
93
0
1
2
Years

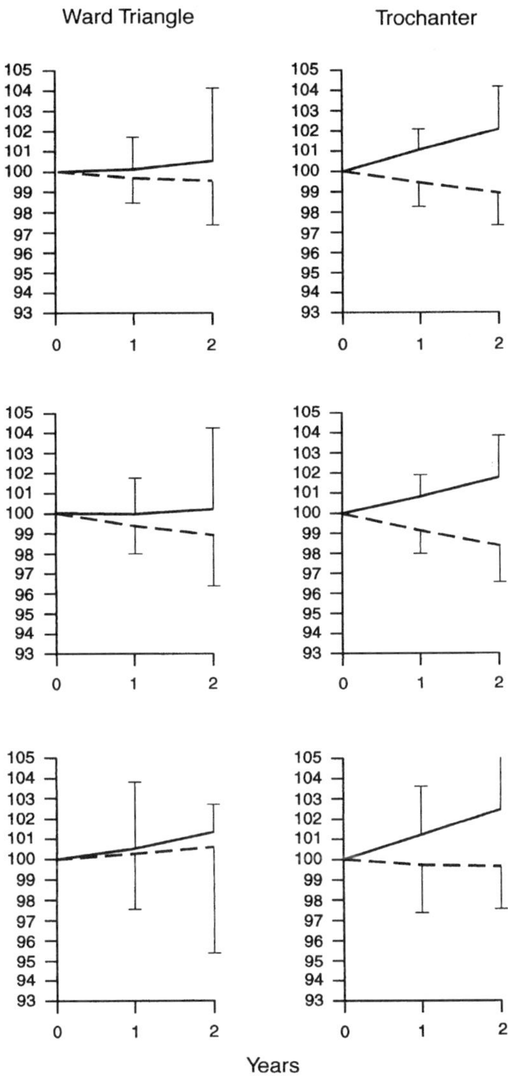

Increased Bone Mass With Pamidronate Treatment in Rheumatoid Arthritis: Results of a Three-year Randomized, Double-blind Trial

Eggelmeijer F, Papapoulos SE, van Paassen HC, et al (Univ Hosp, Leiden, The Netherlands; St Franciscus Hosp, Rotterdam, The Netherlands; Bronovo Hosp, The Hague, The Netherlands)

Arthritis Rheum 39:396–402, 1996 2–31

Background.—Patients with RA are at risk of generalized osteoporosis. It may be difficult to control the risk factors for demineralization, such as persistently active disease and immobility. Specific bone-sparing therapies may be needed, but studies of their effectiveness have been limited. The bisphosponate drug pamidronate was studied as a specific bone-sparing agent for patients with RA.

Methods.—The randomized, double-blind trial included 105 patients with RA. Their mean age was about 50 years, and they had had RA for a mean of about 4 years. The patients were assigned to 3 years of treatment with either oral pamidronate, 300 mg/day, or placebo. Every 12 months, bone mineral density (BMD) of the lumbar spine and hip (dual-x-ray absorptiometry) and forearm (single-photon absorptiometry) was measured.

Results.—Patients treated with pamidronate had a significant 8% increase in lumbar spine BMD and a 5% increase in forearm BMD. In contrast, the placebo-treated patients had no significant changes at either of these sites—an increase of less than 1% in the lumbar spine and a 1% decrease in the forearm. In the femoral neck, the pamidronate group had a significant 3% increase in femoral neck BMD, whereas the placebo group had a significant 4% decrease. At all 3 sites, the observed changes in BMD were significantly different between groups. There were no differences in radiographic evidence of joint damage or in disease activity, however.

Conclusions.—Long-term treatment with oral pamidronate can reduce bone loss and increase bone mass in patients with RA. More time is needed to tell if this specific bone-sparing treatment can reduce the rate of fractures and other complications related to bone loss. Pamidronate may be a useful treatment option for patients with RA.

► A long-term study showing the effects of a diphosophonate in increasing the femoral neck, lumbar, spine, and forearm bone mass. It would have been interesting to see what the agent did in juxta-articular osteoporosis seen in RA. Even though there was an objective improvement at 3 years, the long-term effects on clinical endpoints such as fracture would be interesting.

M.H. Liang, M.D., M.P.H.

Failure of Low-Dose Intravenous Immunoglobulin Therapy to Suppress Disease Activity in Patients With Treatment-Refractory Rheumatoid Arthritis

Kanik KS, Yarboro CH, Naparstek Y, et al (Natl Inst of Arthritis and Musculoskeletal and Skin Diseases, Bethesda, Md; Hadassah Univ, Jerusalem)

Arthritis Rheum 39:1027–1029, 1996 2–32

Background.—Treatment of autoimmune diseases with high doses of IV (IVIg) has been demonstrated to be a beneficial but expensive therapy. It has been shown that treatment with low-dose IVIg can be beneficial in a rat model of autoimmune disease. This randomized, double-blind, placebo-controlled pilot trial was performed to determine the effect of low dose IVIg on patients with refractory RA.

Methods.—Twenty adult patients with active, refractory RA were randomized to receive either 5 mg/kg IVIg or albumin every 3 weeks for 18 weeks. The participants were examined before the 1st, 2nd, and 6th dose and 3 weeks after the completion of the study.

Results.—There were no complications in either part of the study. Five patients dropped out before the study was completed. There were no significant differences between the 2 groups in any indices of disease activity. The trial ended prematurely because of possible hepatitis C contamination of IVIg. All participants who had received IVIg were tested for hepatitis C, but the results were negative.

Conclusions.—This pilot study of the treatment of patients with refractory RA with low-dose IVIg therapy did not demonstrate any therapeutic benefit. Therefore, this therapy cannot be recommended on the basis of these study results.

▶ This small pilot study performed at the National Institutes of Health examined the role of IVIg in patients with refractory RA. In this study of patients who had failed to respond to at least 2 disease-modifying antirheumatic drugs (the majority had failed to respond to or had been intolerant to methotrexate), there was no advantage to receiving IVIg. The study was halted prematurely because of the concern about possible hepatitis C contamination. Even with the small number of patients, there was no advantage noted with IVIg treatment. In a constrained financial environment there appears to be limited support for the use of this treatment in patients with this illness. There appears to be no rationale for the support of this expensive and potentially toxic treatment.

M.E. Weinblatt, M.D.

Recombinant Soluble Tumor Necrosis Factor Receptor (p80) Fusion Protein: Toxicity and Dose Finding Trial in Refractory Rheumatoid Arthritis

Moreland LW, Margolies G, Heck LW Jr, et al (Univ of Alabama at Birmingham; Lexington, Ky)

J Rheumatol 23:1849–1855, 1996 2–33

Introduction.—Several lines of evidence suggest that tumor necrosis factor-α (TNF-α) is involved in the pathogenesis of RA, probably through its proinflammatory actions. These actions are mediated by binding of TNF to its receptors. Soluble TNF receptors have been identified as arising from the shed, extracellular portion of membrane-bound molecules. Levels of these receptors are elevated in the sera and synovial fluid of patients with RA. A recombinant human soluble TNF receptor (sTNFR) fusion protein (p80) (rhTNFR:Fc) has been developed as a TNF-α antagonist. A phase I toxicity and dose-finding study of rhTNFR:Fc in patients with refractory RA was reported.

Methods.—The double-blind study included 16 patients with active, refractory RA. The patients were treated in 4 groups of 4 patients each, of whom 3 received rhTNFR:Fc in varying doses and 1 received placebo. Patients received a single IV loading dose (range, 4–32 mg/m^2) followed by 8 subcutaneous injections given twice weekly for 4 weeks (range, 2–16 mg/m^2). The IV dose was diluted in normal saline to a volume of 100 mL and given by infusion over 30 minutes. The subcutaneous injections were given in the morning at a volume of 0.5–3.0 mL. After 4 weeks, the patients given placebo were treated with rhTNFR:Fc. Each group completed its dose level without dose-limiting toxicity before the next group was entered into the trial. Another 6 patients were treated using the lowest or highest dose to obtain additional safety information.

Results.—The patients' mean age was 53 years, and their mean duration of disease was 8.5 years. Of 22 patients studied, none had serious adverse effects. Eight had mild rashes at the injection site, which did not interfere with treatment. There was no obvious dose–response relationship, so all patients were grouped together for analysis. The mean improvement in total painful joint, swollen joint, and total joint scores was 45% in patients receiving rhTNFR:Fc vs. 25% in patients receiving placebo. Treatment with rhTNFR:Fc produced a 58% reduction in average duration of morning stiffness and a 32% decline in Westergren erythrocyte sedimentation rate. No patient had antibodies to rhTNFR:Fc develop. The mean reduction in C-reactive protein levels was 30% with rhTNFR:Fc vs. 13% with placebo.

Conclusions.—Treatment with rhTNFR:Fc fusion protein warrants further evaluation in the treatment of RA. It produces a trend toward clinical improvement in clinical and biochemical variables and has no serious toxicity. There is no clear dose response, although the biochemical improvements tend to be greater at higher doses. The efficacy of rhTNFR:Fc treatment will be determined in a multicenter, phase II, randomized, controlled trial.

► [This experience with p75/80 TNF expands on observations previously discussed in the 1997 YEAR BOOK OF RHEUMATOLOGY, pp 70–71....R.S. Panush, M.D.] In this short-term study, the clinical response was noted, and there were no measurable antibodies to the receptor detected. The IV loading dose followed by subcutaneous dosing is no longer used because studies now use the subcutaneous dose only. The study did not measure autoantibody production (i.e., antinuclear antibody and anticardiolipin antibodies. There was no clear dose response, which is of some concern with any potential therapeutic agent. Several other inhibitors of TNF, including monoclonal antibodies, and the other soluble receptors (p55) also report short-term clinical responses in RA. Questions regarding long-term response and toxicity need to be further clarified.

M.E. Weinblatt, M.D.

Gamma-Linolenic Acid Treatment of Rheumatoid Arthritis: A Randomized, Placebo-controlled Trial

Zurier RB, Rossetti RG, Jacobson EW, et al (Univ of Massachusetts, Worcester; Massachusetts Gen Hosp, Boston)

Arthritis Rheum 39:1808–1817, 1996 2–34

Objective.—Gamma-linolenic acid (GLA), a fatty acid from plant seed oil, has been shown to significantly reduce synovitis in patients with RA at a dosage of 1.4 g/day. Efficacy and tolerability of GLA treatment (2.8 g/day) in patients with RA and synovitis were studied for 1 year.

Methods.—The participants were 56 patients with arthritis (7 male). Patients were randomly assigned in a double-blind fashion to receive either 2.8 g/day GLA as the free fatty acid (n = 28) or placebo (n = 28) for 6 months. For the next 6 months, all patients then received 2.8 g of GLA per

TABLE 5.—Overall Clinical Response to Treatment of RA With γ-Linolenic Acid (*GLA*)

	First 6 months		Second 6 months		
Overall response	GLA (n = 22)	Placebo (n = 19)	GLA (n = 21)	Placebo/GLA (n = 14)	GLA for 12 months (n = 21)
Remission	0	0	0	0	0
Meaningful improvement	14*	4	9	5	16
No meaningful change	8	9	10	8	3
Deterioration	0	6	2	1	2

Note: The placebo and GLA group took GLA only during months 6–12. Values are the number of patients.
**P* = 0.015 compared with placebo (chi-square test with Yates' correction).
(Courtesy of Zurier RB, Rossetti RG, Jacobson EW, et al: Gamma-linolenic acid treatment of rheumatoid arthritis: A randomized, placebo-controlled trial. *Arthritis Rheum* 39:1808–1817, 1996. Copyright American College of Rheumatology.)

day in a single-blind trial. Patients were evaluated at 3-month intervals during the study and 3 months after the end of the study.

Results.—Patients receiving GLA had moderate but significant improvement in swollen joint count and score, tender joint count and score, duration of morning stiffness, patient's global assessment and assessment of pain, and Health Assessment Questionnaire score at 6 months. Because not all measures improved with GLA vs. placebo, the 35% oleic acid content of the sunflower seed oil placebo may have relieved some symptoms. Doses of nonsteroidal anti-inflammatory drugs or prednisone were reduced during the trial in 7 patients receiving GLA. Gamma-linolenic acid is converted to dihomo-GLA, which suppresses 5-lipooxygenase and 12-lipooxygenase. Although some have considered that GLA can function as a nonsteroidal anti-inflammatory drug, the fact that patients with RA are better after 12 months than 6 months of treatment (Table 5) suggests that GLA acts more like a disease-modifying antirheumatic drug.

Conclusion.—The fatty acid GLA appears to regulate cell activation, immune responses, and inflammation in patients with RA. At 2.8 g/day, GLA had a modest but significant clinical effect on RA and is well tolerated. Additional controlled studies need to be conducted.

► Bob Zurier and colleagues carried out an exemplary study documenting modest clinical efficacy (see Table 5) and good tolerability of GLA at 2.8 g/day for patients with RA. This complements other similar and valuable work with marine fatty acids. What is the place of marine or botanical lipids in treating rheumatic diseases? I would not consider these as disease-modifying antirheumatic drugs, a possibility the authors suggest. In fact, I don't particularly like the terms we use to categorize our therapies—disease-modifying, remission-inducing, slow-acting, symptomatic, and palliative are all unsatisfying. They suggest characteristics that are not well founded on evidence, that reflect traditional (and probably outdated) views, that blur among therapies, and that constrain our thinking. Increasingly, I use the deliberately imprecise term "antirheumatic" therapies and avoid classifications that simplistically imply outcomes which have not been validated. Although I respect the contributions of researchers studying the therapeutic potential of polyunsaturated fatty acids, I don't often use them. I think about these for patients in several situations: (1) the patient who doesn't want to take medications, (2) the patient who can't take certain medications (those with gastrointestinal or ulcer disease, those with allergy to or intolerance of nonsteroidal anti-inflammatory drugs, the elderly, and women who are pregnant or lactating), and (3) the patient not doing well on other antirheumatic therapies for whom this could be adjunctive therapy.

R.S. Panush, M.D.

Comparison of High and Low Intensity Training in Well Controlled Rheumatoid Arthritis: Results of a Randomised Clinical Trial

van de Ende CHM, Hazes JMW, le Cessie S, et al (Univ Hosp Leiden, The Netherlands)

Ann Rheum Dis 55:798–805, 1996 2–35

Objective.—Exercise is recommended to improve strength and physical conditioning in patients with RA. Most studies recommend avoiding dynamic and weight-bearing exercises for fear of causing joint damage and worsening of disease activity. There is recent evidence that dynamic weight-bearing exercise is beneficial in RA. A randomized trial was performed to compare the effects of intensive dynamic exercise versus range of motion (ROM) and isometric exercise in patients with RA.

Methods.—The trial included 100 consecutive patients with RA who were on stable medication regimens. They were randomized into 4 different 12-week exercise programs. One group performed intensive, dynamic group exercises, including full–weight-bearing and condition exercise. These exercises were performed on a stationary bicycle at a heart rate of 70% to 85% of the age-predicted maximum. Another group performed group ROM and isometric exercises, while the third group was assigned to individual isometric and ROM exercises. The fourth group received instructions to perform isometric and ROM exercises at home. Before and 12 weeks after intervention, the subjects were assessed on physical conditioning, muscle strength, joint mobility, daily functioning, and disease activity. The results were analyzed by intention to treat.

Results.—Patients assigned to high-intensity group exercise had a 17% increase in aerobic capacity, a 17% increase in muscle strength, and a 16% increase in joint mobility. The other 3 groups had nonsignificant changes in these measurements. Throughout the period of high-intensity exercise, the patients showed no change in measures of disease activity. By 12 weeks after the end of the exercise program, exercise-related gains had disappeared.

Conclusions.—High-intensity training is beneficial for patients with well-controlled RA. This type of exercise offers greater improvement in aerobic capacity, joint mobility, and muscle strength than obtained by ROM exercise and isometric training. There are no adverse effects of high-intensity training, but the benefits disappear quickly when the exercise program is stopped. The long-term benefits of dynamic and weight-bearing exercises for patients with RA remain to be determined.

► "Use it or lose it" applies to RA and every disease it's been studied in. This one refines the axiom and specifies the regimen that is most effective. Just as training helps, stopping quickly brings one to baseline deconditioning. The message is "Don't stop."

M.H. Liang, M.D., M.P.H.

Experimental Models

Interleukin-10 Inhibition of the Progression of Established Collagen-induced Arthritis

Walmsley M, Katsikis PD, Abney E, et al (Kennedy Inst of Rheumatology, London)

Arthritis Rheum 39:495–503, 1996 2–36

Introduction.—Interleukin-10 (IL-10), a cytokine, is a powerful suppressor of monocyte/macrophage function. Because of its ability to inhibit production of tumor necrosis factor-α (TNF-α) and IL-1, pro-inflamma-

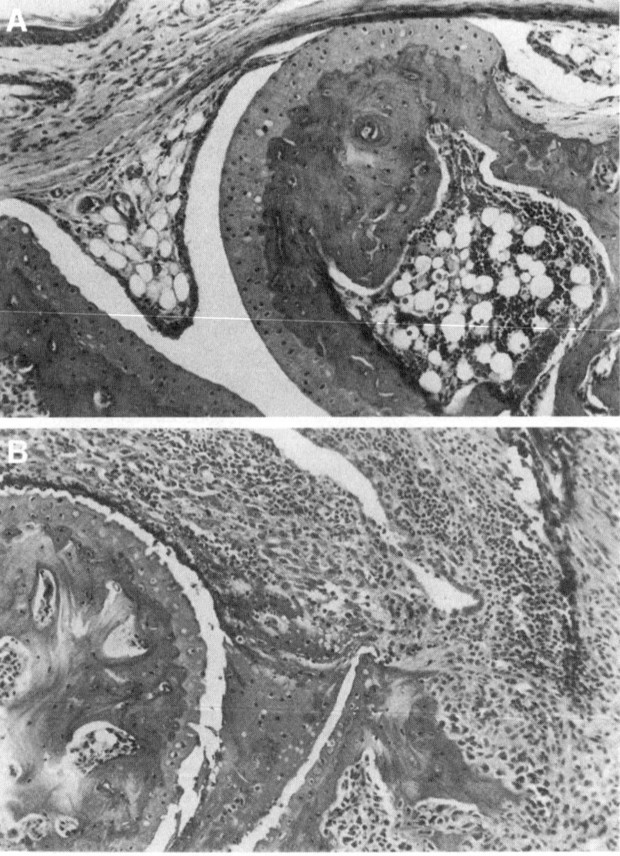

FIGURE 2.—Histologic assessment of arthritic joints 10 days after the clinical onset of arthritis. **A**, interphalangeal joint from a mouse treated with interleukin-10, 5 μg/day from the day of disease onset. Mild arthritis is seen (minimal synovitis without cartilage/bone erosions). **B**, interphalangeal joint from a control mouse treated with phosphate-buffered saline. Severe arthritis is seen (synovitis, erosions, and loss of joint integrity), (hematoxylin-eosin; original magnification, ×40). (Courtesy of Walmsley M, Katsikis PD, Abney E, et al: Interleukin-10 inhibition of the progression of established collagen-induced arthritis. *Arthritis Rheum* 39:495–503, 1996. Copyright American College of Rheumatology.)

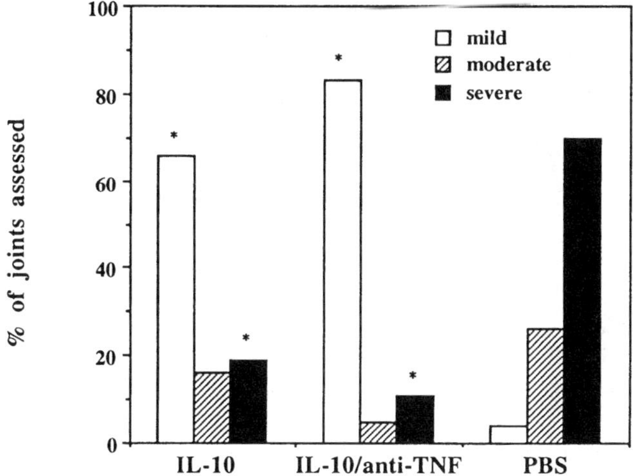

FIGURE 3.—Histologic findings after treatment with interleukin-10 (*IL-10*), combined IL-10/anti–tumor necrosis factor (*anti-TNF*) monoclonal antibody (*MAb*), or phosphate-buffered saline (*PBS*). Interleukin-10 was administered daily (5µg/day), starting on day 1 of clinical arthritis. Anti–TNF-α MAb (300 µg) was given as a single injection on day 1 of arthritis. Arthritis in interphalangeal joints from hindpaw sections was assessed histologically 10 days after the onset of clinical disease, and was scored as mild, moderate, or severe (IL-10 treatment: 12 paws, 32 joints assessed; IL-10/anti-TNF treatment: 7 paws, 18 joints assessed; PBS treatment: 10 paws, 27 joints assessed). * = $P < 0.01$ vs. PBS-treated group. (Courtesy of Walmsley M, Katsikis PD, Abney E, et al: Interleukin-10 inhibition of the progression of established collagen-induced arthritis. *Arthritis Rheum* 39:495–503, 1996. Copyright American College of Rheumatology.)

tory cytokines implicated in the pathogenesis of RA, the effects of IL-10 were studied in the collagen-induced arthritis model of RA.

Methods.—Male DBA/1 mice were immunized with bovine type II collagen in adjuvant. Animals showing erythema, paw swelling, or both were randomly assigned to a treatment or a control group. Treatments consisted of injections of recombinant murine IL-10 or anti-TNF. Arthritis was monitored during a 10-day period, with animals given a clinical score and graded for paw swelling. Arthritic hindpaws were removed post mortem for histopathologic assessment.

Results.—Compared with saline controls, mice treated with IL-10 showed significant reductions in paw swelling and in clinical score on day 10. Histologic examination of hindpaws also showed benefits of treatment with IL-10. Compared with control mice, the treated mice had significantly more joints that were only mildly affected and significantly fewer joints with changes classified as severe (Fig 2). The effectiveness of IL-10 was dose dependent. A single dose of 300 µg of anti-TNF did not result in a sustained benefit, but combining anti-TNF and IL-10 produced an additive therapeutic effect (Fig 3). This finding offers indirect evidence that IL-10 acts, at least in part, by means of suppression of TNF-α activity.

Conclusion.—Treatment with IL-10 was beneficial in a rodent model of arthritis, in which reductions in clinical parameters of disease severity were concordant with reductions in histopathologic severity. There may be a therapeutic role for IL-10 in RA and other chronic inflammatory diseases.

▶ Interleukin-10 is a potent inhibitor of the production of TNF-α and IL-1. In this study, when clinical disease was present, IL-10 blocked the inflammation and cartilage erosion of the type 2 collagen-induced arthritis in the mouse. It is proposed as a therapeutic modality in the treatment of human RA. [But beware extrapolating information from animal studies for application to human RA....R.S. Panush, M.D.]

E.C. LeRoy, M.D.

Synovial Fibroblasts of Patients With Rheumatoid Arthritis Attach to and Invade Normal Human Cartilage When Engrafted Into SCID Mice

Müller-Ladner U, Kriegsmann J, Franklin BN, et al (Univ of Alabama, Birmingham; Univ Hosp Zurich, Switzerland)

Am J Pathol 149:1607–1615, 1996 2–37

Background.—T-cell–dependent pathways are generally believed to play the most important role in the pathophysiology of RA. However, recent evidence suggests a role of T-cell–independent pathways. The interaction between isolated RA synovial fibroblasts and normal human cartilage engrafted into SCID mice was evaluated to determine the importance of T-cell–independent pathways.

Methods.—Human synovial RA, osteoarthritis (OA), and normal fibroblasts were obtained. Fibroblasts and normal human cartilage were implanted under the renal capsule of SCID mice, which lack T cells and other human cells. The various types of fibroblasts were compared for invasive growth into normal human cartilage. The appearance and extended activation of the RA fibroblasts were assessed as well.

Results.—Implanted RA fibroblasts showed intensive ingrowth into cartilage. Their appearance was transformed to large pale nuclei with prominent nucleoli and abundant cytoplasm. The OA fibroblasts showed only isolated ingrowth (Table 1). All RA implants had matrix-degrading enzymes (cathepsins) at or near the site of invasion. The pattern of location and distribution of the various cathepsins was similar between RA implants. Cathepsin L mRNA was detected in small clusters adjacent to the cartilage at pocket-shaped zones of invasion, whereas cathepsin B was produced by fibroblasts close to and attached to the cartilage. Cathepsin D was expressed by fewer fibroblasts, which were not in close contact with the cartilage. None of the control specimens exhibited detectable cathepsin production. Only single RA fibroblasts at the invasion site expressed VCAM-1 protein, which is normally abundantly present in the lining layer of RA synovial tissue.

Conclusions.—Synovial RA fibroblasts—unlike OA fibroblasts or other types of fibroblasts—invade normal human cartilage when engrafted into SCID mice. These cells exhibit persistently invasive and destructive behav-

TABLE 1.—Degree of Invasion Into Normal Human Cartilage by Different Types of Human Fibroblasts Engrafted Under the Renal Capsule of SCID Mice

Fibroblast origin	Grade of destruction of the adjacent cartilage in each of the single implants (1 to 5) 1	2	3	4	5	Mean ± SEM
RA synovium	3.5	1	3	2.5	2	2.4 ± 0.96*
OA synovium	0	0.25	0	0.25	0	0.1 ± 0.14
Normal skin	0	0	0			0 ± 0
Normal synovium	0	0				0 ± 0

Note: Scoring: 0, not visible; 1, <10%; 2, 11% to 20%; 3, 21% to 30%; 4, 31% to 40% destruction of the cartilage.
*$P < 0.01$ as compared with osteoarthritis fibroblasts.
(Courtesy of Müller-Ladner U, Kriegsmann J, Franklin BN, et al: Synovial fibroblasts of patients with rheumatoid arthritis attach to and invade normal human cartilage when engrafted into SCID mice. *Am J Pathol* 149:1607–1615, 1996. Permission granted; copyright American Society for Investigative Pathology.)

ior even in the absence of human T cells. The findings support the hypothesis that T-cell–independent pathways play a key pathogenetic role in RA. The synovial fibroblast appears to be the key cell involved in cartilage and bone destruction in RA.

▶ This is a very nice study using the SCID mouse model. When grafted to the SCID mouse, synovial fibroblasts from patients with RA can invade cartilage in the absence of T cells. This study supports the concept that a proportion of the destructive process of RA is T-cell–independent. This paper also highlights the importance of the fibroblast in the destructive process of RA.

M.E. Weinblatt, M.D.

Pristane-induced Arthritis in Rats: A New Model for Rheumatoid Arthritis With a Chronic Disease Course Influenced by Both Major Histocompatibility Complex and Non-major Histocompatibility Complex Genes

Vingsbo C, Sahlstrand P, Brun JG, et al (Lund Univ, Sweden; Univ of Bergen, Norway)

Am J Pathol 149:1675–1683, 1996 2–38

Purpose.—Avridine-induced arthritis in rats is a useful model of RA. However, it involves mixing of avridine with mineral oil, which is a complex mixture that has its own arthritis-inducing properties. Pristane is a well-defined synthetic mineral oil that induces arthritis in mice. Pristane-induced arthritis (PIA) in rats was investigated as a new model of RA.

Methods and Results.—Intradermal injection of pristane, 150 µL, at the base of the tail, produced arthritis in rats. Different strains showed varying susceptibility. In susceptible strains, severe arthritis developed within 2–3 weeks. It tended to begin in the hind ankles in LEW rats. In DA rats, it usually started in the interphalangeal or metatarsal joints before spreading to the ankles. Serum levels of interleukin-6 were elevated at day 14, corresponding with the onset of arthritis. Females tended to be more affected than males, particularly in LEW rats. Further experiments demonstrated that PIA was T-cell–dependent in both the acute and chronic phases. Histologically, PIA was associated with a prominent pannus tissue containing activated T cells, large macrophage-like cells, neutrophilic granulocytes, and class-II–expressing cells.

Conclusions.—Pristane-induced arthritis is a useful new model for study of the pathogenesis of RA. It causes erosion of the peripheral joints, is associated with major histocompatibility complex genes, and is more frequent in females. Also similar to RA, it has a pronounced chronic active phase. Pristane has no known immunogenic properties; its effects are probably based on nonspecific activity as an adjuvant.

▶ We read about another animal model of inflammatory arthritis, the pristane-induced arthritis model. There are some interesting aspects of this model including the fact that it does not require immunogenic adjuvants. However, I am not convinced that this will be any better a model than those seen with the other animal models including streptococcal cell wall or collagen. Suffice it to say that these are only models and do not completely reproduce the human disease. These models are of value in furthering our understanding of the pathology of arthritis, but they do not replace human disease in the therapeutic setting.

M.E. Weinblatt, M.D.

Juvenile Rheumatoid Arthritis

Serum p55 and p75 Tumour Necrosis Factor Receptors as Markers of Disease Activity in Juvenile Chronic Arthritis

Gattorno M, Picco P, Buoncompagni A, et al (Inst for Children, Genoa, Italy; Natl Inst for Cancer Research, Genoa, Italy)

Ann Rheum Dis 55:243–247, 1996 2–39

Objective.—Tumor necrosis factor-α (TNF-α) has been implicated in the development of RA. The TNF-α receptors p55 and p75 are thought to be associated with TNF-α production. The relation of these receptors and TNF-α in sera and synovial fluid from 45 patients with juvenile chronic arthritis (JCA) with characteristics of disease activity was studied.

Methods.—Sera from 45 patients (22 women) with JCA and 20 age-matched controls and synovial fluid from 5 patients with antinuclear antibody–positive JCA were tested retrospectively for TNF-α, receptors p55 and p75, and interleukin-6 . Disease activity was scored as physician global estimate of disease activity, fever and joint scores, erythrocyte sedimentation rate, Hb concentration, and C reactive protein values. Expression of sTNFαRp55 and sTNFαRp75 on mononuclear cells was determined by flow cytometry.

Results.—There was no difference in mean serum concentration of TNF-α between high disease activity, low disease activity, and control groups or among JCA types. There was no relationship between TNF-α and any disease activity measures. Both p55 and p75 were significantly correlated with several measures of disease activity. Expression of sTNFαRp75 was detected in synovial fluid from 4 of 5 patients with antinuclear antibody–positive JCA but not on macrophages.

Conclusion.—sTNFαRp55 and sTNFαRp75 are markers of disease activity in patients with JCA and appear to be indirect evidence for the role of TNF-α in the pathogenesis of JCA.

► One of the concomitants of cytokine activation of cells is shedding of the cognate receptor from the cell membrane. Thus, the presence of the 2 TNF receptors in the serum of patients with JCA and their positive correlation with more traditional measurements of disease activity can be taken as indirect evidence of a role for TNF-α in the pathogenesis of this disease. Even though it may be temporary, if monoclonal antibodies to TNF-α could reduce disease activity to permit the most severely affected of these children to grow, it would be a worthwhile benefit.

E.C. LeRoy, M.D.

Patterns of Expression of Tumor Necrosis Factor α, Tumor Necrosis Factor β, and Their Receptors in Synovia of Patients With Juvenile Rheumatoid Arthritis and Juvenile Spondylarthropathy

Grom AA, Murray KJ, Luyrink L, et al (Univ of Cincinnati, Ohio; Univ of California, San Francisco; Marion Merrell Dow Research Inst, Cincinnati, Ohio; et al)

Arthritis Rheum 39:1703–1710, 1996 2–40

Objective.—There are varying clinical forms of juvenile RA, including pauciarticular, polyarticular, and systemic-onset forms. However, all feature chronic joint inflammation and are probably influenced by tumor necrosis factor-α (TNFα). Tumor necrosis factor-β (TNFβ) is a closely related cytokine with the same tissue receptors that is produced by activated T lymphocytes. Expression of TNFα and of TNFβ was assessed in synovium from patients with juvenile RA (JRA), juvenile spondylarthropathy (JSpA), and adult RA.

Methods.—The study included synovial tissue samples from 28 patients with JRA, 6 patients with JSpA, and 6 patients with RA. Expression of TNFα, TNFβ, and their receptors was evaluated by reverse transcriptase-polymerase chain reaction and immunohistochemistry.

Findings.—Eighty-five percent of tissue samples expressed TNFα. The level of TNFα varied considerably, in association with the degree of synovial inflammatory infiltration. Levels of TNFα expression were high in the JSpA group. Some degree of TNFβ staining was observed in 85% of JRA specimens, 67% of JSpA specimens, and all RA specimens. Levels of TNFβ were relatively lower in patients with pauciarticular JRA. Most specimens showed greater expression of the p55 TNF receptor than the p75 receptor (Table 1).

TABLE 1.—Immunohistochemistry Results in Synovial Tissue From Patients With Juvenile RA, Juvenile Spondyloarthropathy, and RA

Patient	Disease onset type	Disease course	Infiltrate type	TNFα	TNFβ	p55 TNFR	p75 TNFR	CD68+	CD3+
1	Systemic	Poly JRA	Aggreg	+++	++	+++	+	+++	++++
2	Systemic	Poly JRA	Aggreg	+	++	+++	−	++	++
3	Systemic	Poly JRA	Aggreg	−	+	++++	+	++++	++++
4	Systemic	Poly JRA	Aggreg	++++	+	++++	+	++++	++++
5	Systemic	Poly JRA	Aggreg	−	ND	++	+	++	++
6	Systemic	Poly JRA	Aggreg	++	++	++	+	++++	++++
7	Systemic	Poly JRA	Aggreg	−	++	++	−	++++	++++
8	Systemic	Poly JRA	Aggreg	++	++	++	−	++	++
9	Poly	Poly JRA*	Aggreg	+	++	++	+	+	+++
10	Poly	Poly JRA*	Aggreg	++	++	++++	+	++++	+++
11	Poly	Poly JRA†	Aggreg	++	+	−	++	+	++++
12	Poly	Poly JRA*	Aggreg	+	++	+	+	++	+
13	Poly	Poly JRA‡	Aggreg	++	++	++++	++	++++	++++
14	Poly	Poly JRA*	Diffuse	+	+	+	+	++	+
15	Poly	Poly JRA*	Aggreg	+++	+	++++	+	++++	++++
16	Pauci	Poly JRA	Aggreg	++	+	++++	+	++++	++++
17	Unknown	Poly JRA	Aggreg	++++	++	++++	++++	++++	++++
18	Pauci	Poly JRA	Aggreg	++	++	++++	++	++++	++++
19	Pauci	Poly JRA	Diffuse	++	+	++	−	++	+
20	Pauci	Poly JRA	Aggreg	++	++	++++	+	++++	++++
21	Pauci	Pauci JRA	Diffuse	+++	ND	++	++	++	++
22	Pauci	Pauci JRA	Aggreg	++	−	++	−	++++	++
23	Pauci	Pauci JRA	Diffuse	−	−	++++	++	+	++
24	Pauci	Pauci JRA	Aggreg	+	+	++++	++	++	++
25	Pauci	Pauci JRA	Diffuse	+	−	++++	++	+	++
26	Pauci	Pauci JRA	Diffuse	++	+	++++	+	+	+++
27	Pauci	Pauci JRA	Aggreg	−	+	++++	+	++++	++++
28	Pauci	Pauci JRA	Diffuse	−	−	−	−	++	++
29	Pauci	JSpA	Diffuse	+++	−	++++	++	++++	+++
30	Pauci	JSpA	Aggreg	+++	++	++++	++++	++++	++++
31	Pauci	JSpA	Aggreg	+++	++	+	++++	++++	++++
32	Pauci	JSpA	Aggreg	+++	++	++++	++	++++	++++
33	Pauci	JSpA	Diffuse	++	−	+	++	++	++
34	Pauci	JSpA	Aggreg	++	+++	++++	++++	++++	+++
35	RA	NA	Aggreg	++	+	+	+	+	++
36	RA	NA	Aggreg	+	+	++++	−	++++	++
37	RA	NA	Aggreg	++	+	+++	+	+	+++
38	RA	NA	Aggreg	+	+	+++	+	++++	++
39	RA	NA	Aggreg	+++	+	++++	++	++++	++++
40	RA	NA	Aggreg	++	++	++++	++	++++	+++

Note: The scoring system was as follows: 0, <1 or no cells staining definitely positive/high power field (HPF); +, 1–5 positive cells/HPF; ++, 5–25 positive cells/HPF; +++, 25–50 positive cells/HPF; ++++, >50 positive cells/HPF. Fields examined were areas of prominent cellular infiltration or aggregation.

*Rheumatoid factor (RF) positive.

†RF status unknown.

‡RF negative.

Abbreviations: TNFR, tumor necrosis factor receptor; *Poly*, polyarticular; *Aggreg*, aggregates and diffuse infiltrates; *ND*, not done (insufficient tissue for complete study); *Diffuse*, diffuse infiltrates alone; *Pauci*, pauciarticular; *NA*, not applicable; *JRA*, juvenile RA; *JSpA*, juvenile spondylarthropathy.

(Courtesy of Grom AA, Murray KJ, Luyrink L, et al: Patterns of expression of tumor necrosis factor α, tumor necrosis factor β and their receptors in synovia of patients with juvenile rheumatoid arthritis and juvenile spondylarthropathy. *Arthritis Rheum* 39:1703–1710, 1996. Copyright American College of Rheumatology.)

Conclusions.—The pattern of synovial TNFα expression in patients with polyarticular JRA and JSpA is similar to that seen in patients with adult RA. Staining for TNFβ is more prominent in patients with polyarticular JRA and JSpA than in those with pauciarticular JRA and RA. Prominent synovial TNFβ expression may be a distinct finding in JRA and JSpA.

► The role of TNFα as an important mediator in adult RA has been described in animal models and in patients in many papers. Therapeutic intervention directed against TNFα in JRA is the focus of this paper. Tumor necrosis factor-α and TNFβ, in the synovium and cells expressed with TNF receptors, are reported in JRA. There appears to be a difference in the expression of TNFα among the various subsets of JRA. This may have implications in the design of therapeutic studies. Selective responses may be seen based upon clinical classification of the disease.

M.E. Weinblatt, M.D.

Autoreactivity to Human Heat-Shock Protein 60 Predicts Disease Remission in Oligoarticular Juvenile Rheumatoid Arthritis

Prakken ABJ, van Eden W, Rijkers GT, et al (Univ Hosp for Children and Youth, Utrecht, The Netherlands; Univ of Utrecht, The Netherlands)

Arthritis Rheum 39:1826–1832, 1996 2–41

Background.—T-lymphocyte reactivity to endogenous human heat shock protein 60 (hsp60) may play a regulatory role in the course of oligoarticular juvenile RA (JRA). This hypothesis was tested in a prospective, longitudinal study of patients with newly diagnosed histocompatibility leukocyte antigen (HLA)-B27 negative oligoarticular JRA.

Methods.—Fifteen patients with newly diagnosed HLA-B27 negative oligoarticular JRA were enrolled in the study. Findings in this group were compared with those from a group of 20 patients with newly diagnosed polyarticular or systemic JRA or with acute arthritis caused by other systemic diseases or viral infections and from a group of 9 healthy individuals.

Findings.—Significant T-lymphocyte proliferative responses to hsp60 were observed in the peripheral blood mononuclear cells or synovial fluid mononuclear cells or both in 86% of the patients with oligoarticular JRA within 3 months after disease onset. Such positivity was apparent in only 5% of the patients in the rheumatologic disease control group. In all patients with oligoarticular JRA and positive responses to human hsp60, the disease remitted within 12 weeks. Serum samples obtained from 8 patients during this period showed significantly lower and even negative responses to hsp60 compared with active disease, when all 8 patients showed good responses.

Conclusions.—Significant proliferative responses to human hsp60 can occur early in the course of oligoarticular JRA. These responses were associated with disease activity, and T-cell reactivity to human hsp60 was apparently correlated with disease remission.

▶ Autoimmune reactions that predict outcome generate excitement for several reasons. First, they are clinically useful in the practical management of patients. Second, they may provide insights into pathogenesis. Finally, they suggest maneuvers for therapeutic intervention. Such is the stuff of this article wherein T-cell proliferative responses to human hsp60 were associated with remission in JRA. These reactions are of interest in the patients exhibiting them, and equally interesting are why other patients fail to make this response and whether they can be induced to do so (e.g., by appropriate immunization).

M. Reichlin, M.D.

Juvenile Rheumatoid Arthritis in Rochester, Minnesota 1960-1993: Is the Epidemiology Changing?

Peterson LS, Mason T, Nelson AM, et al (Mayo Clinic, Rochester, Minn)

Arthritis Rheum 39:1385–1390, 1996 2–42

Objective.—Two data sets were combined to describe trends in the incidence and long-term outcome of juvenile RA (JRA) in Rochester, Minnesota. Findings indicate that the incidence of JRA in Rochester has decreased in the past decade.

Methods.—The medical records of all Rochester residents with any potential diagnoses of JRA were screened, using the diagnostic retrieval

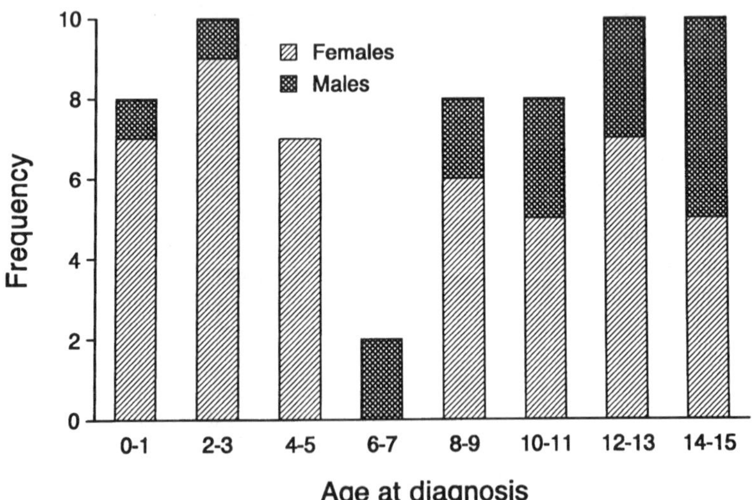

FIGURE 1.—Age at diagnosis in Rochester, Minnesota residents with juvenile RA, by sex. (Courtesy of Peterson LS, Mason T, Nelson AM, et al: Juvenile rheumatoid arthritis in Rochester, Minnesota 1960–1993: Is the epidemiology changing? *Arthritis Rheum* 39:1385–1390, 1996, copyright American College of Rheumatology.)

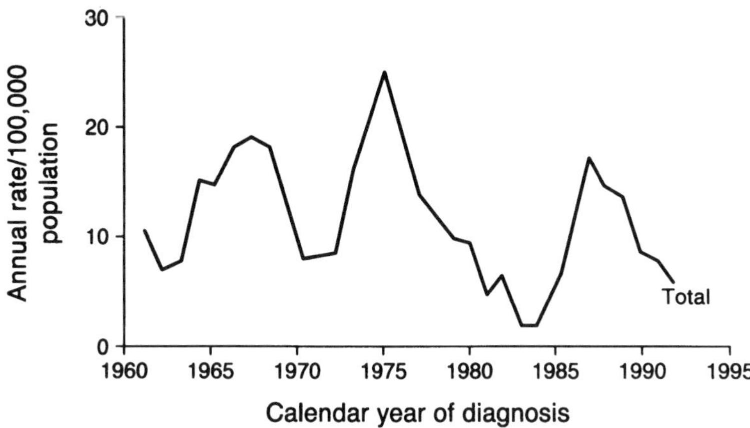

FIGURE 2.—Annual incidence of juvenile RA in Rochester, Minnesota residents, 1960–1993 (estimated using a 3-year moving average). (Courtesy of Peterson LS, Mason T, Nelson AM, et al: Juvenile rheumatoid arthritis in Rochester, Minnesota 1960–1993: Is the epidemiology changing? *Arthritis Rheum* 39:1385–1390, 1996, copyright American College of Rheumatology.)

system of the Rochester Epidemiology Project for the years 1978–1993. Using the same data collection instrument, a group of 49 patients with JRA identified in a previously published study was reviewed. These patients were diagnosed between January 1, 1960 and December 31, 1978. All cases fulfilled the American College of Rheumatology 1977 revised criteria.

Results.—Sixty-five cases of JRA diagnosed between 1960 and 1993 were identified in a screening of 1,240 medical records. The patients were 48 girls and 17 boys with a mean age of 7.8 years at diagnosis; the average follow-up was 12.7 years. Patients with pauciarticular onset (less than or equal to 4 joints involved) were given diagnoses at an older age (mean, 8.4 years) than those with polyarticular onset (greater than or equal to 5 joints involved; mean, 5.8 years) or systemic onset (extra-articular features; mean, 6.4 years). Overall, the 2 peak ages for diagnosis were 0–4 years and 9–15 years (Fig 1). Disease onset was pauciarticular in 72% of children, polyarticular in 17%, and systemic in 11%. The overall age- and sex-adjusted incidence rate of JRA was 11.7 per 100,000 population. Incidence rates declined in the community during the years reviewed; rates per 100,000 population for the years 1960–1969, 1970–1979, and 1980–1993 were 15.0, 14.1, and 7.8, respectively. A cyclical pattern was also identified; peaks occurred in 1967, 1975, and 1987 (Fig 2). In the polyarticular group, however, no significant change in incidence rate was observed during the 33-year period. The survival rate for patients with JRA was not significantly different from that of the Minnesota white population.

Discussion.—The decrease in the incidence of JRA during the past decade may have resulted from more precise diagnostic criteria and serologic tests or from a cyclical trough. Cyclical variations suggest that environmental factors may play a role in the pathogenesis and etiology of JRA.

▶ This is a very intriguing study from the Mayo Clinic in which the incidence and prevalence of JRA were examined during 33 years. The Mayo Clinic has a superb data bank that contains information on virtually all residents of Olmsted County. In this study, there was a decrease in the incidence of all types of JRA during the past decade. This might be partially explained by the greater abilites to exclude patients who previously might have been given a diagnosis of JRA but who now fall into other categories of rheumatic illnesses, such as Lyme disease. They also observed a seasonal variation in the onset of illness in the patients with systemic onset JRA. These observations suggest that there may be an environmental factor in systemic onset JRA. If the trends continue for the decreasing incidence of JRA, this will have an impact on health care planners and, more importantly, on fellowship program directors. Similar studies of the same quality are needed in adult rheumatic disease.

M.E. Weinblatt, M.D.

Bone Mineralization and Bone Mineral Metabolism in Children With Juvenile Rheumatoid Arthritis

Pepmueller PH, Cassidy JT, Allen SH, et al (Univ of Missouri, Columbia)
Arthritis Rheum 39:746–757, 1996 2–43

Background.—Because children with juvenile RA (JRA) have been found to have poor linear and skeletal growth, an increased number of fractures, and osteopenia, JRA is suspected of affecting bone mineralization. However, there have been few comprehensive studies of bone metabolism. To identify the specific mechanisms of osteopenia, bone mineral metabolism in children with JRA was investigated.

Methods.—Forty-one children with JRA and 62 healthy children were studied. Bone mineral content and density were measured by dual x-ray absorptiometry. Serum samples also were analyzed.

Findings.—The children with JRA had reduced bone mineral density at all sites. After adjustment for age, height, weight, and bone area, bone mineral density was reduced at cortical bone sites. Concentrations of osteocalcin and bone-specific alkaline phosphatase were low, suggesting decreased bone formation. Low levels of tartrate-resistant acid phosphatase suggested reduced resorption. Clinical disease severity scales were correlated negatively with measures of bone mass. Laboratory markers of disease severity were strongly associated with reductions in bone formation markers but not with those of resorption. Laboratory findings were similar in children with oligoarticular and with polyarticular disease. However, differences in bone mass were greater in children with polyarticular disease.

Conclusions.—Reduced bone mineralization in JRA appears to be associated with low bone formation that is related to disease severity. Thus, efforts to stimulate bone formation should be considered in prepubertal children with active JRA.

▶ The effects of chronic disease on physiologic status are important in all ages; however, even more in children. The effects of JRA on bone mineralization and metabolism were well studied in this article from Jim Cassidy's group. The bottom line is children with JRA have decreased bone mineralization; this is known. However, the interesting aspect of the study was that the decrease in bone density appears to result from decreased bone formation and not increased resorption. If this study is correct, strategies to increase bone formation are needed.

M.E. Weinblatt, M.D.

Intravenous Immunoglobulin Therapy in Systemic Onset Juvenile Rheumatoid Arthritis: A Followup Study

Uziel Y, Laxer RM, Schneider R, et al (Univ of Toronto)

J Rheumatol 23:910–918, 1996 2–44

Background.—Up to 30% of patients with juvenile RA (JRA) have systemic onset JRA (SOJRA). New treatment alternatives for SOJRA with active, prolonged systemic features are needed. Intravenous immunoglobulin (IVIg) is an effective treatment for several different autoimmune diseases. A previous study reported its short-term benefits in SOJRA. The long-term benefits of IVIg treatment for patients with SOJRA were assessed.

Methods.—The retrospective study included 27 patients treated with IVIg for SOJRA. Indications for treatment were persistent spiking "JRA" fever, active arthritis with multiple point effusions, lack of response to first-line therapy, or steroid dependency. There were 14 boys and 13 girls included, and their average age at disease onset was 6 years. The average duration of disease at the start of IVIg treatment was 22 months. Active systemic disease was present in 24 of 27 patients. Eighteen patients with active arthritis had more than 10 active joints.

Patients treated in the first 2 years of the experience received a 5% solution of IVIg by infusion at a dose of 1 g/kg/day for 2 consecutive days. Thereafter, 1 g/kg/day was given in a single dose. Treatment was given 2 days per month for at least 6 months in the early part of the experience. Later, the first 5 doses were given in a single infusion every 2 weeks, with subsequent doses given once every 4 weeks for at least 6 months. Treatment was discontinued or tapered if the disease was in remission after 6 months. Response was defined as at least a 50% reduction in the number of days of fever, the dose of prednisone, or the number of active joints. At final follow-up, patients were classified as in remission (no arthritis or systemic symptoms and not taking prednisone), improved (at least a 50%

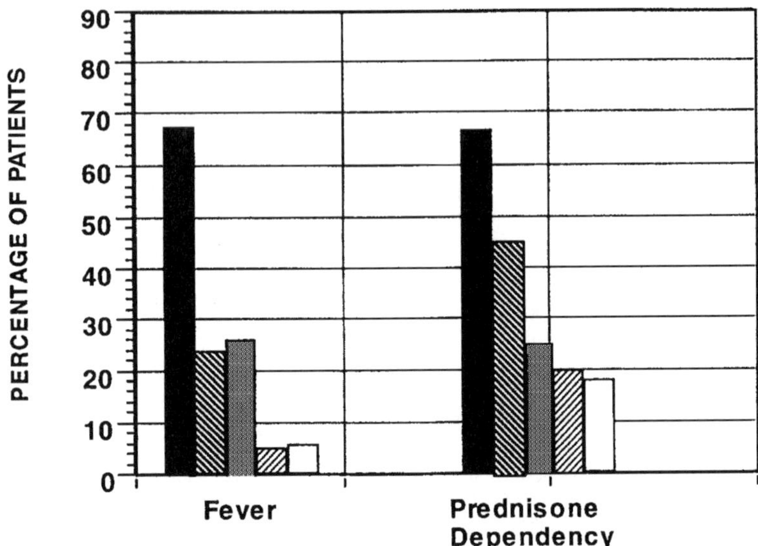

FIGURE 1.—Systemic disease activity during the study period. The *y* axis shows percentage of patients who had the individual clinical findings. The *x* axis shows patients with fever and patients who were prednisone dependent. The ■ indicates 25 patients assessed at study entry; ▧ 25 patients assessed at 6 months; ▩ 24 patients assessed at 1 year; ▨ 20 patients assessed at 2 years, and □ 17 patients assessed at greater than 2 years. (Courtesy of Uziel Y, Laxer RM, Schneider R, et al: Intravenous immunoglobulin therapy in systemic onset juvenile rheumatoid arthritis: A followup study. *J Rheumatol* 23:910–918, 1996.)

reduction in number of active joints and not taking prednisone), or treatment failures (active disease or taking prednisone).

Results.—Of 25 patients evaluated at 6 months, 20 were responders, though most still had some feature of active systemic disease. Of the 13 responders who were steroid dependent at the start of treatment, only 6 were still so at 6 months. Six of the responders received methotrexate therapy throughout the first 6 months, and others received other treatments. All 5 nonresponders started receiving methotrexate. Of 24 patients evaluated at 1 year, 21 were responders, including all 5 who were nonresponders at 6 months. Of 20 patients evaluated at 2 years, 19 were responders (Fig 1).

At a final follow-up of 38 months, 44% of patients were classified as being in remission. Six of these patients were receiving no treatment; the rest were taking nonsteroidal anti-inflammatory drugs, with or without IVIg. Sixteen percent of patients were improved and 40% were classified as treatment failures. However, 8 of these patients were still receiving IVIg, because their condition worsened when treatment was stopped. There were no serious side effects of infusion. Three patients had a second autoimmune or renal disease that may or may not have been related to IVIg.

Conclusions.—In patients with SOJRA, IVIg may be able to control systemic features while avoiding the need for steroids. Its effects on the natural long-term course of destructive arthritis are unclear. In combination, methotrexate and IVIg may be able to control systemic inflammation and prevent chronic destructive arthritis. Intravenous immunoglobulin may be considered for patients with SOJRA severe, steroid-dependent disease that does not respond to other treatments.

► The authors report the use of IVIg in an open study of systemic JRA. The use of IVIg in systemic JRA has a checkered past. Despite encouraging open studies, a randomized, placebo-controlled trial performed by the Clinical Centers of the Pediatric Rheumatology Collaborative Study Group (Dr. Silverman and his colleagues were involved) was unable to demonstrate a difference compared with placebo in a small trial.[1] In this retrospective study, IVIg administered monthly decreased fever and prednisone dose in patients with systemic onset JRA. It was not a controlled study and many patients received additional second-line therapies including methotrexate. Intravenous gammaglobulin did not impact on the arthritis in 40% of the patients. Whether the improvement in fever and prednisone dose reduction was attributable to the natural history of systemic onset JRA vs. the multiple therapies cannot be determined. The other interesting observation is the development of 3 other systemic autoimmune diseases including membranoproliferative glomerulonephritis, systemic lupus erythematosus, and vasculitis. There remains limited support for the use of IVIg to treat the arthritis associated with systemic onset JRA.

M.E. Weinblatt, M.D.

Reference

1. Silverman ED, Cakwell GD, Lovell JD, et al: IVIg in the treatment of systemic JRA: A randomized placebo controlled trial. *J Rheumatol* 21:2353–2358, 1994.

Intravenous Immunoglobulin in the Treatment of Polyarticular Juvenile Rheumatoid Arthritis: A Phase I/II Study

Giannini EH, for the Pediatric Rheumatology Collaborative Study Group (Univ of Cincinnati, Ohio; Univ of Toronto; Children's Hosp Med Ctr, Boston; et al)

J Rheumatol 23:919–924, 1996 2–45

Background.—None of the drug treatments used for the treatment of polyarticular juvenile RA (poly-JRA) is entirely satisfactory. Intravenous immunoglobulin (IVIg), initially used for the treatment of congenital and acquired immunodeficiencies, may also be useful in patients with other immunopathologic diseases. This pilot study assessed the safety and efficacy of IVIg for the treatment of poly-JRA.

Methods.—The phase I/II, multicenter trial included 25 children with poly-JRA that had not responded to other treatments. In the initial, open phase of the trial, all patients received IVIg, 1.5 to 2.0 g/kg/infusion, to a maximum of 100 g. Infusions were given bimonthly for the first 2 months, then monthly for up to 6 months. At 3 months, patients with clinically important improvement entered a randomized, double-blind (DB) phase, in which they received monthly infusions of either placebo or IVIg for 4 months. The patients were allowed to receive certain concomitant treatments: nonsteroidal anti-inflammatory drugs, slow-acting antirheumatic drugs, and prednisone at a constant dose of less than 10 mg/day. For patients who had clinically important worsening in the DB phase, an escape provision permitted a switch to IVIg for those taking placebo or to high-dose IVIg for those taking low-dose IVIg.

Results.—Nineteen of the 25 children had clinically important improvement during the open phase and progressed to the DB phase. The remaining 6 derived no benefit from IVIg treatment. In the responders, the magnitude of improvement was rated as moderate to large. Patients with a shorter duration of disease—less than 3 years—were more likely to respond. Patients who received IVIg in the DB phase showed continued improvement beyond that in the open phase. In contrast, those given placebo showed a rapid loss of benefit. Five of 9 patients randomized to placebo either "escaped" back to IVIg or dropped out of the study. There were no dropouts related to adverse drug reactions during either phase of the study. Most side effects were mild and related to the infusion process.

Conclusions.—Preliminary results suggest that patients with refractory poly-JRA show substantial clinical improvement while receiving IVIg therapy. About three fourths of patients respond; the benefits quickly disappear once IVIg treatment is stopped. No serious or unexpected adverse effects are reported in the short-term. The authors call for a larger, double-blind trial of IVIg for patients with poly-JRA.

▶ IVIg has been used in polyarticular JRA and seems to be effective, at least by anecdotal reports. This study, done by a consortium of pediatric rheumatologists, tested IVIg in children who could not be controlled with first- and second-line drugs. This effort reflects the rarity of this problem and the difficulties inherent in critically evaluating drugs in children with rheumatic diseases. It took 7 centers 3 years to amass 25 patients for this phase I/II withdrawal design with stratified entry. Three quarters of the children, especially those with less than 3 years of illness, were more likely to respond than those who had the condition for more than 5 years, and little in the way of toxicity was noted. However, the duration of the beneficial effects is short-lived after discontinuation. A larger double-blind pivotal study is needed in this subset of children and for a longer period, but it will take years before we will know definitively how effective IVIg is for these patients. [For more information on this topic, see Prieur A-M.[1]...R.S. Panush, M.D.]

M.H. Liang, M.D., M.P.H.

Reference

1. Prieur A-M: Intravenous immunoglobulins in Still's disease: Still conversial, still unproven (editorial). *J Rheumatol* 23: 797–800, 1996.

3 Systemic Lupus Erythematosus and Related Disorders

Introduction

The selection of articles this year—in the areas of systemic lupus erythematosus, antiphospholipids, Sjögren's syndrome, and immunological aspects of systemic rheumatic diseases—seems to have produced an array of papers that emphasize clinical diagnosis and pathogenesis, with only a few papers on the therapy of these disorders. I assure the readers that this is not because I have any lack of interest in therapy but because there were few papers concerning therapy. I remain optimistic that our ever increasing knowledge and understanding of immunopathogenesis in these disorders will soon yield important and interesting approaches to more specific and nontoxic therapy for our patients.

Morris Reichlin, M.D.

Lead Article

▶ Several articles have shown that both mouse and human autoantibodies to native or double-stranded (ds) DNA bind and enter cells in culture.[1, 2] There is also a report that this happens in vivo in murine lupus.[3] The ability of autoantibodies to intracellular antigens to bind and enter live cells opens up a new concept of pathogenesis. These autoantibodies can function much as do organ-specific autoantibodies such as anti-red cell antibodies in hemolytic anemia or anti-platelet antibodies in thrombocytopenic purpura. We do not have envision immune complex formation and trapping of these on vascular structures, and so on to understand their pathogenic role.

Moreover, among lupus autoantibodies to ubiquitous intracellular antigenic targets this property of anti-dsDNA (binding and penetration of live cells) is shared only with autoantibodies to ribosomal P proteins.[4] Interestingly, these are the two specific autoantibodies whose titer correlates with disease activity, especially nephritis. This property of autoantibody penetration of cells in culture is not shared by autoantibodies to Ro/SSA, La/SSB, U_1RNP, or Sm antigens.

This article describes an antibody that is kidney specific and yet binds DNA and a molecular surrogate for DNA (HP8/HEVIN) binding, which mediates binding to cells and subsequent penetration. Antibody binding to DNA or its surrogate is essential because mutations that affect DNA binding also block the ability to bind and penetrate cells.

Studies such as these are showing us new ways of looking at pathogenesis and provide ever-increasing reasons to understand why anti-dsDNA titers in patients with systemic lupus erythematosus usually correlate with disease activity.

M. Reichlin, M.D.

References

1. Yanase K, Smith RM, Cizman B, et al: A subgroup of murine monoclonal anti-deoxyribonucleic acid antibodies traverse the cytoplasm and enter the nucleus in a time and temperature-dependent manner. *Lab Invest* 71:52–60, 1994.
2. Koren E, Koscec M, Wolfson-Reichlin M, et al: Murine and human antibodies to native DNA that cross-react with the A and D SnRNP polypeptides cause direct injury of cultured kidney cells. *J Immunol* 154:4857–4864, 1995.
3. Vlahakos D, Foster MH, Ucci AA, et al: Murine monoclonal anti-DNA antibodies penetrate cells, bind to nuclei and induce glomerular proliferation and proteinuria *in vivo*. *J Am Soc Nephrol* 2:1345–1354, 1992.
4. Koscec M, Koren E, Wolfson-Reichlin M, et al: Autoantibodies to ribosomal P proteins penetrate into live hepatocytes and cause cellular dysfunction in culture. *J Immunol* 159:2033–2041, 1997.

Immunogenetics and Pathophysiology

Mechanisms of Cellular Penetration and Nuclear Localization of an Anti-double Strand DNA Autoantibody

Zack DJ, Stempniak M, Wong AL, et al (Veterans Affairs Med Ctr, Sepulveda, Calif; Olive View-Univ of Sylmar, California; Univ of Southern California, Los Angeles)

J Immunol 157:2082–2088, 1996 3–1

Background.—Autoantibodies to double-stranded (ds) DNA are thought to play a role in the pathogenesis of systemic lupus erythematosus. Monoclonal antibody (mAb) 3E10 is an anti-dsDNA antibody, localized in the cell nucleus, that can bind membranes of fixed human renal tubular cells and penetrate live murine renal tubular cells in vivo. In addition to dsDNA, mAb 3E10 binds the extracellular matrix protein HP8/HEVIN, which is expressed in high endothelial venules. Previous mutagenesis studies of mAb 3E10 have shown that although DNA and HP8 share some binding sites, separate and distinct binding sites also exist.

Objectives.—Site-directed mutants of mAb 3E10 were used to determine which binding characteristics were associated with cellular penetration of nuclear localization of this antibody. Further experiments evaluated the role of antibody (Ab) Fc in cellular penetration and the role of cytoplasmic proteins in nuclear localization.

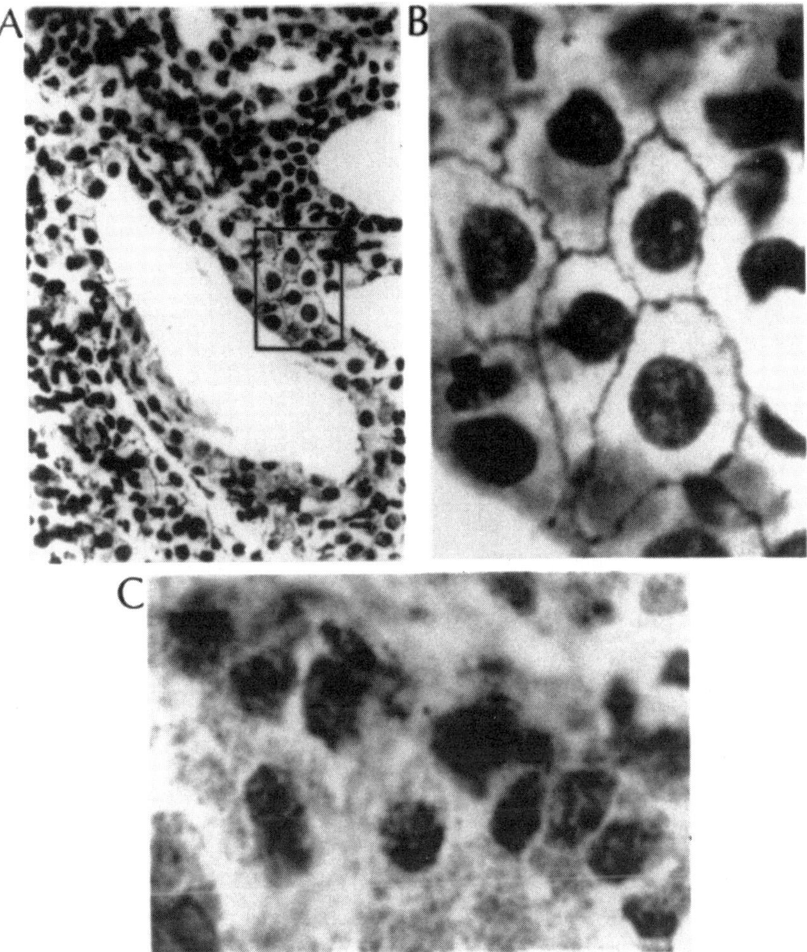

FIGURE 1.—Monoclonal antibody (*mAb*) 3E10 binds membranes of human renal tubular cells in vitro. **A**, low magnification of renal tubular cells incubated with mAb 3E10 shows reactivity with renal tubular cell membranes and nuclei. **B**, higher magnification of the inset (**A**) emphasizes linear binding of mAb 3E10 to membranes of renal tubular cells. **C**, incubation of another anti-DNA antibody, mAb 5C6, shows binding to nuclei, but absence of binding to tubular cell membranes. (Courtesy of Zack DJ, Stempniak M, Wong AL, et al: Mechanisms of cellular penetration and nuclear localization of an anti-double strand DNA autoantibody. *J Immunol* 157:2082–2088. Copyright 1996, the American Association of Immunologists.)

Methods and Results.—In vitro studies suggested that mAb 3E10 was the only anti-dsDNA Ab to bind to the cell surface of human renal tubular cells (Fig 1). Only the residues necessary for binding DNA were required for Ab penetration. The HP8/HEVIN binding residues were not essential for cell penetration, suggesting that DNA or Ab binding to a membrane determinant precisely resembling DNA was required for cellular penetration. Cellular penetration did not require Fc or multivalent Ab binding;

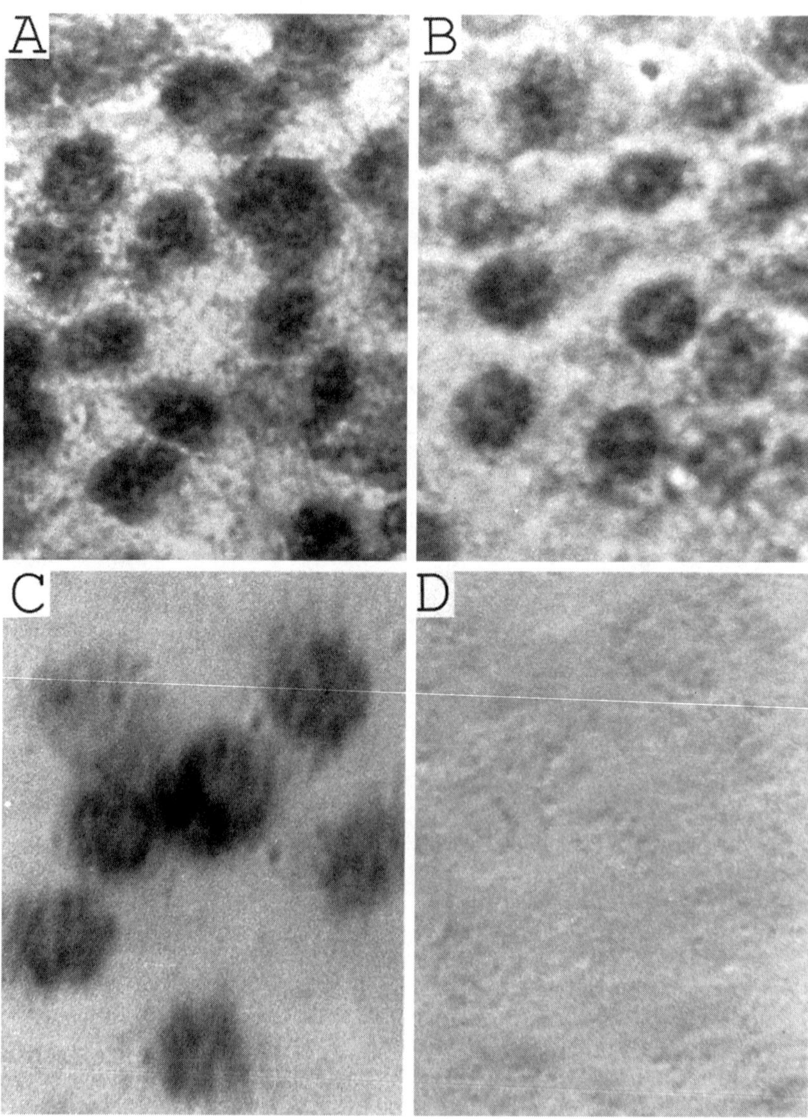

FIGURE 3.—Internalization of transport of monoclonal antibody 3E10 to the nucleus in human 293 kidney cells (**A**), monkey COS-7 kidney cells (**B**), and dog MDCK kidney cells (**C**), but not in colon cancer LS174T cells (**D**). (Courtesy of Zack DJ, Stempniak M, Wong AL, et al: Mechanisms of cellular penetration and nuclear localization of an anti-double strand DNA autoantibody. *J Immunol* 157:2082–2088. Copyright 1996, the American Association of Immunologists.)

evidence for this was that Ab Fab penetrated cells. Nuclear translocation did not occur for Ab synthesized in the cytoplasm by deletion of heavy- and light-chain signal peptides (Fig 3). Thus, some mechanism different from the usual protein nuclear localization signals appeared to be operative, such as a membrane-mediated pathway or posttranslational modification of the Ab.

Discussion.—Cellular penetration of the anti-dsDNA Ab mAb 3E10 appears to occur through the formation of Ab/DNA complexes, a mechanism that does not necessarily reflect the specific binding and internalization of mAb 3E10 to renal tubular cells. The mechanism of nuclear localization may differ from that used by most cytoplasmic proteins. Creating molecular mutants of autoantibodies is a valuable aid to studies of the cellular pathways of autoantibody penetration and nuclear localization.

▶ Several articles have shown that both mouse and human autoantibodies to native or ds DNA bind and enter cells in culture.[1, 2] There is also a report that this happens in vivo in murine lupus.[3] The ability of autoantibodies to intracellular antigens to bind and enter live cells opens up a new concept of pathogenesis. These autoantibodies can function much as do organ-specific autoantibodies such as anti-Red cell antibodies in hemolytic anemia or anti-platelet antibodies in thrombocytopenic purpura. We do not have to envision immune complex formation and trapping of these on vascular structures, and so on to understand their pathogenic role.

This article describes an antibody that is kidney specific and yet binds DNA and a molecular surrogate for DNA (HP8/HEVIN) binding, which mediates binding to cells and subsequent penetration. Antibody binding to DNA or its surrogate is essential because mutations that affect DNA binding also block the ability to bind and penetrate cells.

Studies such as these are showing us new ways of looking at pathogenesis and provide ever-increasing reasons to understand why anti-dsDNA titers in patients with systemic lupus erythematosus usually correlate with disease activity.

M. Reichlin, M.D.

References

1. Yanase K, Smith RM, Cizman B, et al: A subgroup of murine monoclonal anti-deoxyribonucleic acid antibodies traverse the cytoplasm and enter the nucleus in a time- and temperature-dependent manner. *Lab Invest* 71:52–60, 1994.
2. Koren E, Koscec M, Wolfson-Reichlin M, et al: Murine and human antibodies to native DNA that cross-react with the A and D SnRNP polypeptides cause direct injury of cultured kidney cells. *J Immunol* 154:4857–4864, 1995.
3. Vlahakos D, Foster MH, Ucci AA, et al: Murine monoclonal anti-DNA antibodies penetrate cells, bind to nuclei and induce glomerular proliferation and proteinuria *in vivo*. *J Am Soc Nephrol* 2:1345–1354, 1992.

Repertoire Cloning of Lupus Anti-DNA Autoantibodies

Roben P, Barbas SM, Sandoval L, et al (Univ of California, San Diego, La Jolla; Scripps Research Inst, La Jolla, Calif; Tufts Univ, Boston; et al)

J Clin Invest 98:2827–2837, 1996 3–2

Background.—High levels of circulating antibodies that react with double-stranded DNA are diagnostic markers for systemic lupus erythemato-

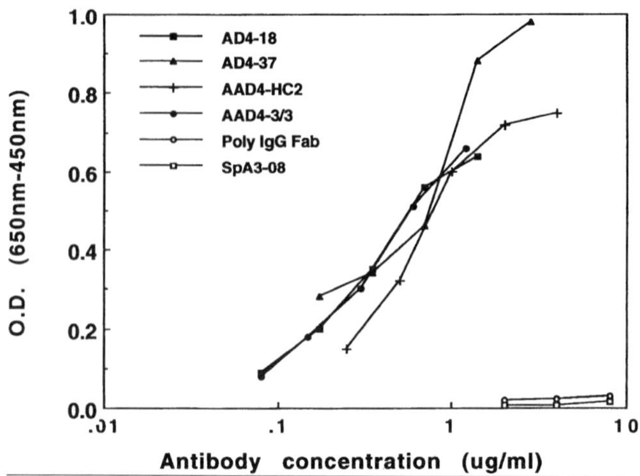

FIGURE 1.—The DNA binding activities of select autoantibodies. Binding activities of the purified monoclonal IgG Fab for double-stranded DNA precoated enzyme-linked immunosorbent assay plates are compared with adult polyclonal IgG Fab (*Poly IgG Fab*) and a control monoclonal IgG Fab (*SpA3-08*). (Reproduced from *The Journal of Clinical Investigation*, courtesy of Roben P, Barbas SM, Sandoval L, et al: Repertoire cloning of lupus anti-DNA autoantibodies. *J Clin Invest* 98:2827–2837, 1996, by copyright permission of the American Society for Clinical Investigation.)

sus (SLE) and are associated with the development of lupus nephritis. Repertoire cloning has been used to generate a library of lymphocyte-expressed heavy and light antibody chains that can be expressed in vitro and selected for binding specificity. The authors had previously described such a library from the lymphocytes of an active SLE patient, S1. This work was expanded with 2 new IgG Fab libraries constructed from the lymphocytes of a set of identical twins who are discordant for SLE. The anti-DNA autoantibodies present in these libraries were characterized and compared with those present in the circulation of the donors.

Methods.—The SLE patients S1 and AA were diagnosed according to the criteria of the American Rheumatism Association. AA had an identical twin with no symptoms of SLE. Peripheral blood samples were used as a source of messenger RNA (mRNA) to generate IgG1 libraries. Polymerase chain reaction was used to rescue the antibody genes and clone them into a phage display vector.

Results.—The selecting antigen for each IgG Fab library was human placental double-stranded DNA. This antigen selected antibodies from the library of the twin with SLE (Fig 1), but not from the library of the twin without SLE. The libraries of both twins had large numbers of fragments from the V_H5 family. Both SLE libraries had IgG anti–double stranded DNA autoantibodies (Fig 5), which are characteristic of SLE. In the twin with SLE, one of these antoantibodies contained the V_H5 fragment, with a targeted cluster of mutations that might improve binding efficiency. The recovered IgG anti–double stranded DNA autoantibodies expressed the same idiotypes as the in vivo IgG anti–double stranded DNA response in the respective donor.

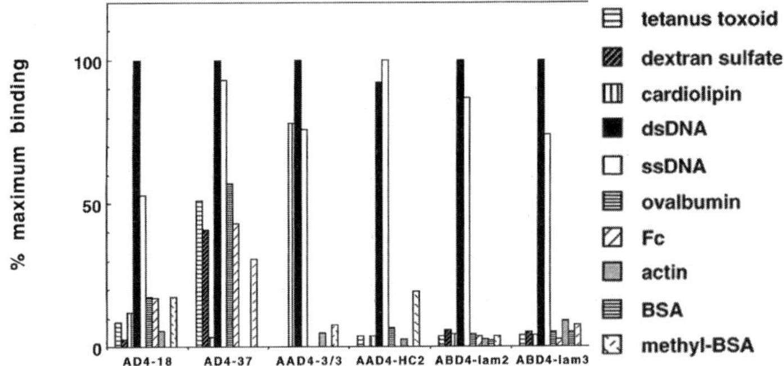

FIGURE 5.—Cross-reactivities of Fabs to a panel of solid-phase antigens tested by enzyme-linked immunosorbent assay. Reactivities are compared for each monoclonal IgG Fab at 2 µg/mL. Values are reported as a percentage of the maximum absorbance attained. (Reprinted from *The Journal of Clinical Investigation*, courtesy of Roben P, Barbas SM, Sandoval L, et al: Repertoire cloning of lupus anti-DNA autoantibodies. *J Clin Invest* 98:2827–2837, 1996, by copyright permission of the American Society for Clinical Investigation.)

Conclusion.—Repertoire cloning techniques were used to sample antibodies from the autoantibody response of patients with SLE. The phage display repertoire cloning method used in this study was an effective method for characterizing the disease-associated antibody responses of the donors. The comparison between an SLE-affected woman and her identical twin without SLE permitted analysis of the interaction between heredity and somatic processes that produce lupus-associated IgG antibodies. These methods have the ability to increase our knowledge of the pathogenesis of antibody-mediated autoimmune disease.

► It is well known that autoantibodies to double-stranded (ds)DNA are not only diagnostically specific for SLE but vary with disease activity and likely participate in disease expression, especially nephritis. Understanding the molecular and genetic bases of anti-dsDNA production is one of the keys to understanding the pathogenesis of SLE.

This paper reports findings in identical twins discordant for disease and anti-dsDNA production that shed light on 1 aspect of the molecular genetic bases for anti-dsDNA production. Certain genes for Ig heavy chains (V_H5) were easily shown to be enriched in both twins by repertoire cloning, a powerful method for isolating clonally restricted autoantibody expressing phage particles. The major findings were (1) that somatically hypermutated V_H5 occurred only in the disease-associated twin and (2) that, not surprisingly, restricted pairing of V_H5 heavy chains with certain Vλ light chains occurred only in the sibling with SLE.

Thus, it appears that the minimum requirements for production of IgG anti-dsDNA include activation or triggering of the hypermutation mechanism and the selection of certain specific Vλ genes that pair with the appropriate V_H5 genes. Clearly, these latter processes are not under genetic control as they did not occur in the unaffected identical twin. Application of these powerful molecular methods should improve understanding of the processes proximate to anti-dsDNA production.

M. Reichlin, M.D.

Hyperexpression of CD40 Ligand by B and T Cells in Human Lupus and Its Role in Pathogenic Autoantibody Production

Desai-Mehta A, Lu L, Ramsey-Goldman R, et al (Northwestern Univ, Chicago)

J Clin Invest 97:2063–2073, 1996 3–3

Background.—The pathogenic antinuclear autoantibodies in systemic lupus erythematosus (SLE) are driven by certain T helper cells transiently expressing the CD40 ligand, that are prevalent in patients who have active lupus nephritis but not in normal individuals or in patients in remission. The hyperexpression of CD40 ligand by B and T cells and its role in pathogenic autoantibody production in patients with lupus were reported.

Methods and Findings.—Eight patients who had active lupus, 7 patients in long-term remission, and 6 healthy individuals were included. Compared with healthy individuals and patients in remission, patients who had active lupus had a 21-fold increase in the frequency of CD40L-expressing CD4+ T cells in periphral blood mononuclear cells. CD40 molecules on

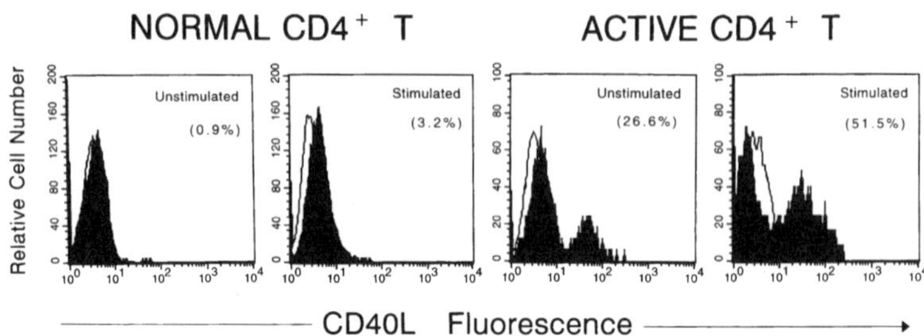

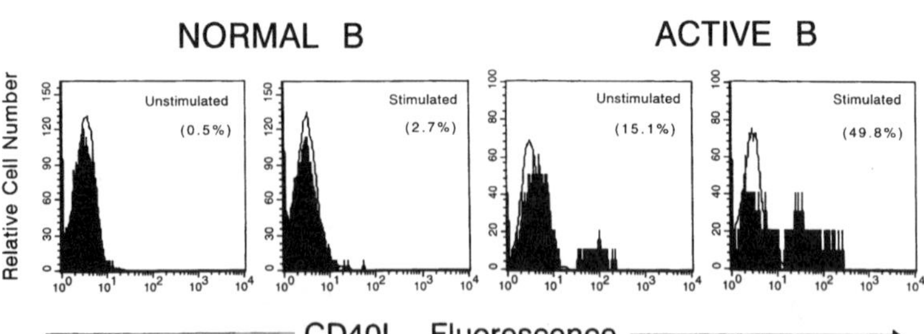

FIGURE 4.—Histograms showing the hyperexpression of CD40L (*solid black*) by gated CD4+ T cells and B cells (CD20+) of patients who have active lupus (*active*) as compared with those from normal individuals. Percentage CD40L+ cells are indicated in *parentheses*. (Reproduced from Desai-Mehta A, Lu L, Ramsey-Goldman R, et al: Hyperexpression of CD40 ligand by B and T cells in human lupus and its role in pathogenic autoantibody production. *J Clin Invest* 97:2063–2073, 1996, by copyright permission of the American Society for Clinical Investigation.)

autologous B cells downregulated the mitogenic stimulation–induced expression of CD40L in lupus and in normal T cells equally well. Patients who had active lupus had a 22-fold increase in the percentage of CD8+ T cells that expressed CD40L, which is consistent with their unusual helper activity in SLE. Unexpectedly, patients who had active disease had a 20.5-fold increase in B cells that spontaneously expressed high CD40L levels as strongly as T cells. Although the patients in remission had low levels of CD40L+ cell (within the normal range), mitogen-induced upregulation of CD40L expression in T and B cells was substantially higher than in healthy individuals, which suggests the presence of an intrinsic defect. In patients who had active, established lupus, a monoclonal antibody to CD40L significantly blocked the ability of lymphocyte to produce the pathogenic variety of antinuclear autoantibodies in vitro, which suggests the possibility of anti-CD40L immunotherapy for patients who have lupus (Fig 4).

Conclusions.—The hyperexpression of CD40L by lupus B cells was observed. Future research on this hyperexpression could define the regulatory defect in the pathogenic T and B cells of lupus. Anti-CD40L therapy in human lupus is a promising approach.

▶ This paper shows that one of the molecules that lives on the surface of lymphocytes, CD40L, is greatly hyperexpressed in the T and B cells of patients who have SLE and that this increased expression correlates with disease activity. Because this molecule is involved in the cellular interactions (with CD40) that underlie autoantibody production, these findings may have pathogenetic, and hence therapeutic, implications. As our detailed molecular knowledge of the systemic autoimmunity of diseases like SLE grows more precise, we should expect novel, specific, and effective therapies to emerge. This particular area looks promising for just such developments.

M. Reichlin, M.D.

Fas Ligand Mutation in a Patient With Systemic Lupus Erythematosus and Lymphoproliferative Disease

Wu J, Wilson J, He J, et al (Univ of Alabama at Birmingham; Jackson Veterans Affairs Med Ctr, Miss; Brigham and Women's Hosp, Boston)

J Clin Invest 98:1107–1113, 1996 3–4

Background.—Systemic lupus erythematosus (SLE) has a multifactorial and multigenetic pathogenesis; genes that are candidates for contributing to SLE in humans include the apoptosis genes *fas* and *fas* ligand (*fas*L). Mutations of these genes have resulted in autoimmunity in murine models, and *fas* gene mutations have resulted in a familial autoimmune lymphoproliferative syndrome in humans. However, no defects in the *fas*L gene in humans have yet been identified.

Methods.—Single-stranded conformational polymorphism analysis was used to screen the DNA from 75 patients with SLE in a search for potential mutations of the extracellular domain of *fas*L. Further analyses were conducted with molecular cloning and sequencing.

Results.—In 1 patient with SLE (who had lymphadenopathy), a heterozygous single-stranded conformational polymorphism for *fas*L was identified. This patient's DNA contained an 84–base-pair deletion within exon 4 of the *fas*L gene that resulted in a predicted 28–amino-acid in-frame deletion. Peripheral blood mononuclear cells were analyzed, revealing decreased *fas*L activity, decreased activation-induced cell death, and increased postactivation T-cell proliferation.

Conclusion.—This is the first reported case of a mutation of the *fas*L gene in a human with SLE that was related to defective *fas*L-mediated apoptosis. *fas*L mutations may be an uncommon cause of human SLE.

► In the 1994 YEAR BOOK OF RHEUMATOLOGY (pp 355–356) we reported on a paper that was sweeping the immunology world and was promising to reveal new and startling insights into the mechanisms of systemic autoimmunity in humans. That paper described the nature of the genetic defect in the MRL 1pr mouse, which greatly accelerated a lupus-like disease in the mouse.[1] The defect was in the *fas* gene, which mediates apoptosis, and was accompanied by massive lymphoproliferation caused by accumulation of double negative T lymphocytes. When the defect is in *fasL*, the model is the *gld* mouse, which also features lymphoproliferation and lupus.

It soon became apparent that *fas* function was basically normal in human SLE, so the excitement soon waned. A search for genetic abnormalities in the *fasL* has uncovered a single patient with SLE with a mutation in the *fasL* and defective *fasL* function with accompanying defective apoptosis. So the moral of this story is, if you look long enough you can find a human with SLE who behaves like a lupus mouse.

M. Reichlin, M.D.

Reference

1. Watanche-Fukunaga R, Brannan CI, Copeland NG, et al: Lymphoproliferation disorder in mice explained by defects in Fas antigen that mediates apoptosis. *Nature* 356:314–317, 1992.

Impaired Recovery and Cytolytic Function of CD56+T and Non-T Cells in Systemic Lupus Erythematosus Following In vitro Polyclonal T Cell Stimulation: Studies in Unselected Patients and Monozygotic Disease-discordant Twins

Stohl W, Elliott JE, Hamilton S, et al (Univ of Southern California, Los Angeles)

Arthritis Rheum 39:1840–1851, 1996 3–5

Background.—Although T cells are generally thought to play an important role in the pathogenesis of systemic lupus erythematosus (SLE), the abnormalities that have been reported were either limited to or markedly more pronounced in patients with active disease. Thus, such T-cell abnormalities may actually be consequences of the disease rather than predisposing factors. In a recent study, impaired in vitro anti-CD3-driven polyclonal generation of cytologic activity in SLE was found to be an abnormality independent of disease activity and immunosuppressive medications. Also, this abnormality does not occur in patients with a variety of systemic inflammatory rheumatologic disorders. The study determined whether the generation and cytolytic function of CD56+ T cells and non-T cells in human SLE are impaired.

Methods and Findings.—Seventy-three patients with SLE, 39 healthy controls, and 9 pairs of monozygotic (MZ) twins discordant for SLE were studied. The percentage of recovered CD56+ T cells was 1.6-fold lower and the percentage of total CD56+ cells was 1.8-fold lower in patients with SLE than in healthy individuals. Patients also had decreased cytologic activities of isolated total CD56+ cells and CD56+ T cells. These defects were independent of SLE activity and immunosuppressive drugs, which reflected impaired maturation of cytolytic effector cells rather than a deficiency in precursor cell number. In the MZ twins, 4 of 8 with SLE had very low recovered percentages of CD56+ cells, and 6 of 9 had low cytolytic responses. In cell-mixing experiments with the peripheral blood mononuclear cells of the twins, the E+ cell fractions from the co-twins with SLE had a reduced capability to generate cytolytic activity compared with those from the healthy co-twins. However, recovered percentages of CD56+ and non-T cells were depressed in 4 of 8 healthy co-twins, and cytolytic responses were depressed in 4 of 9 healthy co-twins.

Conclusions.—Impaired CD56+ T cells and non-T cell responses are features of SLE. These characteristics may occur before the onset of clinical disease.

► It has long been recognized that hyperactivity of B cells with florid autoantibody production is a characteristic feature of SLE; equally obvious for the past decade is a major deficiency in T lymphocyte–derived functional activities associated with almost universal lymphopenia that is sometimes profound. The conundrum has been understanding whether this defect in T-lymphocyte activity is primary and of pathogenic significance or secondary and of no consequence to the etiopathogenesis of the disease. This paper suggests that generation of CD56+ cells with cytolytic activity is deficient in SLE, and studies of monozygotic twins discordant for SLE suggests that, in many instances, this defect antedates disease onset. How could deficiency of cytolytic T cells be involved in pathogenesis of autoimmunity? One could think of several mechanisms, the most prominent 1 being failure to remove virus-infected cells (e.g., T or B lymphocytes) that are a constant stimulus to autoimmunity. In any case, recognition of such a defect should focus clinical investigators' interest on such potential targets for the deficient cytolytic T cells in patients with SLE.

M. Reichlin, M.D.

Transplantation With Allogenic Bone Marrow From a Donor With Systemic Lupus Erythematosus (SLE): Successful Outcome in the Recipient and Induction of an SLE Flare in the Donor

Sturfelt G, Lenhoff S, Sallerfors B, et al (Univ Hosp of Lund, Sweden)
Ann Rheum Dis 55:638–641, 1996 3–6

Background.—Recent research has shown that systemic lupus erythematosus (SLE)–related autoantibody production is determined by bone marrow-derived cells. This suggests that allogenic bone marrow transplantation (ABMT) may produce an autoimmune reaction in the recipient. The clinical and laboratory features of an ABMT recipient with acute myeloid leukemia in second remission after transplantation from a donor with stable inactive SLE were reported.

Patients and Findings.—The transplant recipient was a man, 43 years, with AML in remission, and the donor was his histocompatibility leukocyte antigen–identical brother with mild SLE. Autoantibodies were measured before and after transplantation. In the weeks after transplantation, transient mild graft-vs.-host disease (GVHD) developed in the recipient. In the donor, concentrations of anti-C1q antibodies to the collagenous region of the complement component C1q were persistently high. Anti-C1q antibodies developed in the recipient 3 months after transplantation and persisted for 2 months. There was no evidence of autoantibodies or SLE-like manifestations. Five months after transplantation, chronic GVHD developed but responded to intensified immunosuppressive therapy. The patient was in unmaintained remission 3 years after receiving the transplant. In the donor, SLE was exacerbated a few weeks after marrow was donated. Severe pulmonary alveolitis developed and was treated with cyclophosphamide.

Conclusions.—There was no evidence of transfer of SLE after bone marrow transplantation in the current patient. However, he did temporarily produce anti-C1q antibodies, a characteristic feature of the donor's SLE. Also, the donor's disease was exacerbated, possibly in association with the bone marrow tap.

▶ Two things were noted when allogenic but major histocompatibility complex–identical bone marrow was given from a donor with SLE to his brother with acute myeloid leukemia. First, the graft was successful, undoubtedly prolonging the life (if not curing) the recipient. Of great interest is that sustained autoimmunity was not transferred to the recipient, which shows that a bone marrow graft is not sufficient to transfer the serologic findings of SLE. Second, more perplexing is a major flare in disease in the donor who had previously had 6 years of quiescent disease. The authors make much of this, but, as the flare consisted primarily of alveolitis, an unusual if not rare complication of SLE, one wonders if that aspect of his disease was even related to his SLE. In any case, it is clear that it takes more than a successful bone marrow transplant to transfer either the serologic or clinical findings of SLE.

M. Reichlin, M.D.

Nucleosomes and Histones Are Present in Glomerular Deposits in Human Lupus Nephritis

van Bruggen MCJ, Kramers C, Walgreen B, et al (Univ Hosp Nijmegen, The Netherlands; Univ Hosp Groningen, The Netherlands; CNRS, Strasbourg, France; et al)

Nephrol Dial Transplant 12:57–66, 1997 3–7

Background.—Anti-double-stranded (ds)DNA antibodies are thought to play a pathogenic role in the initiation of glomerular disease in patients with systemic lupus erythematosus (SLE). In a previous study, the authors showed that certain anti-dsDNA antibodies can bind to heparan sulfate (HS), an intrinsic component of the glomerular basement membrane, in experimental animals via the histone part of the nucleosome. This study determined whether histones or nucleosomes could be identified in glomerular deposits in human lupus nephritis and whether there was a correlation between the presence of these nuclear components and the absence of HS staining.

Methods.—Renal biopsy specimens were obtained from 17 patients with SLE, 11 with diffuse proliferative glomerulonephritis (DPGN), and 6 with membranous glomerulonephritis (MGN). Renal biopsy specimens of

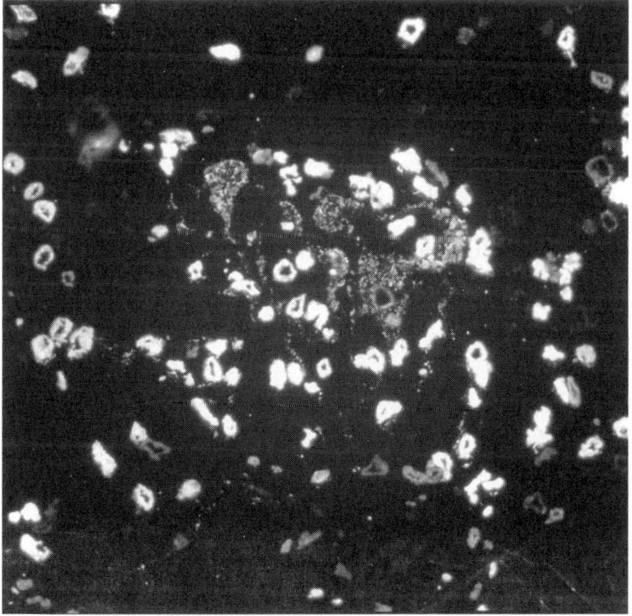

FIGURE 1.—Immunofluorescence of a kidney biopsy of patient with systemic lupus erythematoseus with diffuse proliferative glomerulonephritis stained with a mouse antinucleosome monclonal antibody (LG10–1). Besides staining of the capillary loops and the mesangium, prominent nuclear staining can be seen. Original magnification, ×300. (Courtesy of van Bruggen MCJ, Kramers C, Walgreen B, et al: Nucleosomes and histones are present in glomerular deposits in human lupus nephritis. *Nephrol Dial Transplant* 12:57–66, 1997. By permission of Oxford University Press.)

4 patients with non-SLE mesangiocapillary glomerulonephritis and 5 patients with non-SLE MGN were evaluated as controls. Biopsy sections were stained for histones, DNA, nucleosomes, IgG, and HS.

Results.—With use of a polyclonal anti-H3 1-21 antiserum, investigators detected histones in all 11 patients with DPGN and in 2 of 6 with SLE-MGN. A monoclonal antihistone antibody led to detection of histones in 3 patients with DPGN but in none of the biopsy specimens from patients with MGN. Nucleosome specific monoclonal antibodies allowed detection of nucleosomes in 5 patients with DPGN (Fig 1) and in 2 with MGN; this finding was absent in all biopsy specimens with non-SLE glomerulonephritis. Whereas HS staining was nearly absent in patients with DPGN, it was only moderately reduced in controls and those with MGN.

Conclusion.—This study presents the first demonstration that nucleosomes can be identified in immune deposits of patients with SLE nephritis, which is a finding that serves to emphasize the importance of nucleosomes for the pathogenesis of SLE. Histones were identified in all patients with DPGN, and nucleosomes were identified in 5 of 11 patients; 2 of 6 patients with MGN also exhibited nucleosomes.

► Much has been made recently of autoantibodies in patients with SLE, which react specifically with nucleosomes, small subunits of chromatin composed of histones and DNA. It appears that, in murine SLE, antibodies to nucleosomes precede the appearance of antibodies to native (or ds) DNA. Circumstantial evidence suggests that antinucleosome antibodies may be important in the human disease as well, although most SLE scholars in the past 20 years have favored the idea that anti-dsDNA antibodies are the crucial, specific autoantibodies involved in active disease, especially of the kidney. This paper shows that, in at least half the human biopsy specimens from kidneys of patients with lupus nephritis, nucleosome and histone antigens could be identified in the renal deposits. This strongly implicates antinucleosome antibodies in the pathogenesis of the nephritis.

We thus have come full circle because it is these antinucleosome antibodies that are responsible for the lupus erythematosus (LE) cell phenomenon, which was involved in the first serologic test for SLE described by Hargraves in 1948.[1] It is an interesting corollary that this LE phenomenon was signaling, from the very beginning, its involvement in the immunopathogenesis of the disease.

M. Reichlin, M.D.

Reference

1. Hargraves MM, Richmond H, Morton R. Presentation of 2 bone marrow elements; "tart" cell and "L.E." cell. *Proc Staff Meet Mayo Clin* Jan 1948, pp 25–28.

Quinolinic Acid in Patients With Systemic Lupus Erythematosus and Neuropsychiatric Manifestations

Vogelgesang SA, Heyes MP, West SG, et al (Walter Reed Army Med Ctr, Washington, DC; Fitzsimons Army Med Ctr, Aurora, Colo; Natl Insts of Mental Health, Bethesda, Md; et al)

J Rheumatol 23:850–855, 1996 3–8

Background.—Neuropsychiatric manifestations, a major feature of systemic lupus erythematosus (SLE), can result in significant morbidity and mortality. Cognitive and memory impairments, psychiatric disturbances, seizures, cerebrovascular accidents, and myelitis are among the manifestations that can occur. The diagnostic methods available for assessing the presence of neuropsychiatric involvement are not sensitive or specific. Increased CSF levels of quinolinic acid, a neuroactive metabolite of L-tryptophan, have been associated with CNS immune activation and neuropsychologic deficits. The relationship between quinolinic acid and neuropsychiatric manifestations of SLE was investigated.

Methods and Findings.—Forty CSF specimens were obtained from 39 patients with SLE who had a total of 40 episodes of neuropsychiatric dysfunction. The samples were assessed blindly. In 30 patient-episodes, neuropsychiatric dysfunction was confirmed to be SLE related. In the remaining 10 episodes, other causes were thought to explain CNS dysfunction. The median CSF levels of quinolinic acid were 232.5 nmol/L in the first group and 38.2 nmol/L in the second group, a significant difference. Although CSF and serum levels of quinolinic acid were significantly correlated, there was no association between CSF levels of quinolinic acid and CSF levels of protein or white blood cell counts.

Conclusions.—Increased CSF and serum levels of quinolinic acid may be associated with neuropsychiatric dysfunction in SLE. Quinolinic acid, a neurotoxin and convulsant in high concentrations, may play a role in the pathogenesis of such neuropsychiatric involvement.

▶ Understanding neuropsychiatric disease in SLE remains a daunting challenge. Welcome a new candidate for participation in this part of the disease in the form of quinolinic acid, a metabolite of L-Tryptophan, which is found in high concentrations in the CSF of patients with SLE who have CNS disease. Whether the quinolinic acid is made in the brain or is diffused in from the serum is not clear, but the present evidence suggests that there are contributions from both compartments. Quinolinic acid is a neurotoxin and could play a role in CNS disease. Time will tell.

M. Reichlin, M.D.

Is Immunogenetic Susceptibility to Neuropsychiatric Systemic Lupus Erythematosus (SLE) Different From Non-neuropsychiatric SLE?

Silva LM, Donadi EA (Univ of São Paulo, Brazil)
Ann Rheum Dis 55:544–547, 1996 3–9

Introduction.—More than 50% of patients with systemic lupus erythematosus (SLE) have neuropsychiatric abnormalities, whereas neuropsychiatric lupus (NPSLE) may occur in the absence of generalized disease. There is controversy as to whether the pathogenesis of SLE without neuropsychiatric involvement differs from that of NPSLE. Patients with SLE were evaluated for histocompatibility leukocyte antigen (HLA) class II antigens to determine the frequency of these antigens and lymphocytotoxic autoantibodies in those with and without neuropsychiatric involvement.

Methods.—The study participants were 93 patients with SLE; 51 (median age, 30 years) did not have neuropsychiatric features and 42 (median age, 34 years) had a variety of neuropsychiatric abnormalities. Both groups were predominantly white and female. The controls were 191 healthy blood donors of similar ethnic background who were typed for HLA class II antigens; 30 healthy individuals were also assayed for lymphocytotoxic autoantibodies.

Results.—The most common neuropsychiatric features in these patients with SLE were organic brain syndrome (33.3%), psychosis (30.9%), generalized seizures (30.9%), and cranial neuropathies (28.6%). Specificity for HLA-DR3 was significantly increased in the total group of patients. Compared with controls, those with NPSLE exhibited a significantly increased HLA-DR3 antigen; HLA-DR4 specificity was overrepresented in patients without neuropsychiatric features and underrepresented in the NPSLE subgroup. The neuropsychiatric subgroup also showed increased HLA-DR9 and HLA-DQ2 antigens, and those with HLA-DR9 specificity had an increased frequency of lymphocytotoxic autoantibodies. Whereas all controls were negative for lymphocytotoxic autoantibodies, this finding was present in 12 of 38 patients with NPSLE and CNS involvement and in only 1 of 20 randomly selected patients with nonneuropsychiatric SLE.

Conclusion.—Patients with SLE and neuropsychiatric features have specific immunogenetic markers. Histocompatibility leukocyte antigen–DR4 was associated with protection against the development of NPSLE, whereas HLA-DR3, HLA-DR9, and HLA-DQ2 were associated with susceptibility. An association was also found between HLA-DR9 antigen and the presence of lymphocytotoxic autoantibodies. Increased frequency of HLA-DR9 and HLA-DQ2 antigens has not been previously reported in NPSLE.

► This paper nicely shows, that at least in this series of patients with SLE, patients with neuropsychiatric involvement have different major histocompatibility complex (MHC) class II genes than those who don't, as well as a vastly different prevalence of lymphocytotoxic autoantibodies. The conventional interpretation of how MHC genes would affect disease expression is via their influence as immune response genes. These would determine which autoantibodies are expressed. In this case, lymphocytotoxic autoantibodies are the only such antibodies that segregate with neuropsychiatric disease, but they didn't examine antiribosomal P antibodies, which, in other studies, have been associated with neuropsychiatric disease. Notwithstanding, it is of great interest that such a strong relationship exists between neuropsychiatric disease in SLE and HLA class II antigens.

M. Reichlin, M.D.

Antinuclear Antibodies and Other Autoantibodies

Antinuclear Antibody Determination in a Routine Laboratory

Feltkamp TEW (Athron, Research Centre for Rheumatic Diseases Amsterdam, The Netherlands)

Ann Rheum Dis 55:723–727, 1996 3–10

Background.—There are several pitfalls in the use of the indirect immunofluorescence technique (IFT) for demonstrating antinuclear antibodies (ANAs). The problems associated with IFT for demonstrating ANAs in a normal routine laboratory for clinical immunology were discussed.

Pitfalls.—Determining ANAs by the IFT is associated with several variable factors: nuclear antigen substrate; ANA specificity and avidity; the specificity, avidity, fluorochrome labeling, and concentration of the conjugate; incubation conditions, washing, and mounting; and microscopy and reading. Because many serum samples contain mixtures of different ANAs, the findings of routine tests are best expressed in titers or expressions of the intensity of fluorescence. The ANA test using the IFT should be done as a screening method for other tests that allow for a more defined interpretation of the ANA (Fig).

Conclusions.—Each laboratory is a unique setting and must define its own method. Each laboratory should also determine the borderline between positive and negative findings. Regular participation in national and international quality control rounds is necessary for all laboratories.

► Although this article is directed to individuals running laboratories performing ANA determinations, appreciation of the limitations of the ANA test are even more important for the clinician than for the laboratory director. It is a myth that the ANA test is a standardized test; indeed, the pitfalls are numerous, and the variation between licensed laboratories is astounding for the same samples. The essential lesson, then, is that this is a screening test that acquires meaning only in the context of solid clinical findings, as, for example, in the diagnosis of systemic lupus erythematosus. If ever "caveat emptor" had meaning, it is in the use of the screening tests for ANA determination.

M. Reichlin, M.D.

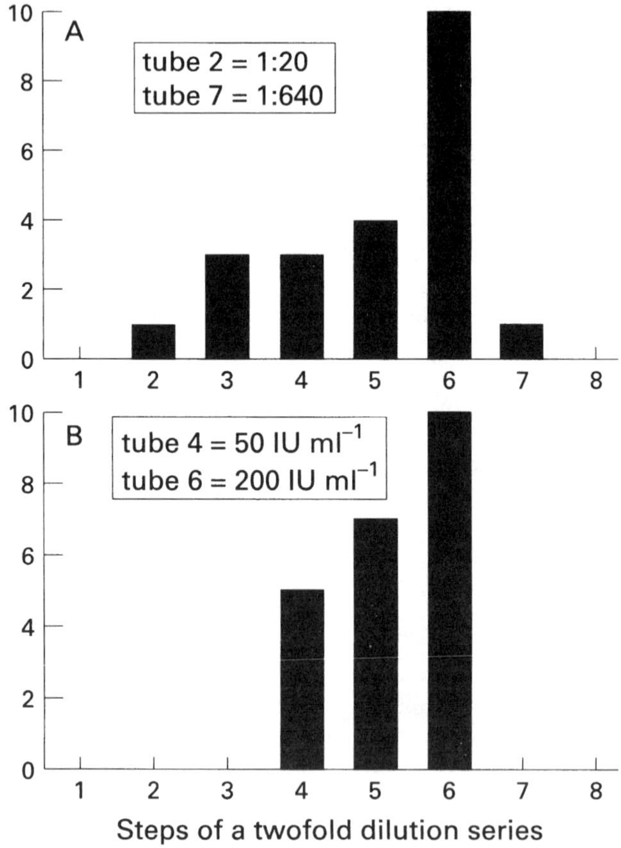

FIGURE.—Results found by 11 laboratories testing serum for antinuclear antibodies (homogenous) on human laryngeal tumor cells on 2 occasions: **A**, expressed as titres; **B**, expressed as IU/mL. (Courtesy of Feltkamp TEW: Antinuclear antibody determination in a routine laboratory. *Ann Rheum Dis* 55:723–727, 1996.)

Screening for Antinuclear Antibodies by Enzyme Immunoassay
Jaskowski TD, Schroder C, Martins TB, et al (Univ of Utah, Salt Lake City)
Am J Clin Pathol 105:468–473, 1996 3–11

Background.—Indirect fluorescent antibody (IFA) is the most commonly used method for screening for autoantibodies against a wide range of nuclear antigen in clinical laboratories. A number of antinuclear antibody (ANA) enzyme immunoassay (EIA) screens, marketed as alternatives to the IFA method for ANAs, have recently become available. A suitable EIA method for such screening would be useful in laboratories that have large sample volumes, given the subjectivity of IFA interpretation and the high number of ANA-negative samples.

Methods.—Five ANA EIA screens were compared with IFA in the human epithelial cell line HEp-2. Sera from 601 patients submitted for autoimmune testing and from 202 healthy blood donors were assessed.

Findings.—Sensitivity and specificity for each ANA EIA screens were determined by comparison with IFA. For the Elias screen, agreement was 87%; sensitivity, 69.5%; and specificity, 97.9%. For the Helix, these values were 95.6%, 90.2%, and 97.3%, respectively; for the Sanofi, 95%, 93.7%, and 95.9%; for the TheraTest, 95.3%, 97.7%, and 93.5%; and for the Zeus, 87.1%, 96.2%, and 81.4%.

Conclusions.—Antinuclear antibody screening by EIA using several commercial assays was sensitive and specific compared with IFA. When screening a large number of clinical specimens, EIA is objective and much less labor intensive. Because none of the EIAs were 100% sensitive, they may not detect a few of the nonspecific ANAs with atypical or classic IFA patterns. Confirming titers and patterns of sera that have positive EIA screens by using classic IFA methods with HEp-2 cells is still recommended.

▶ Screening for ANA has been traditionally done by using either cryostat tissue sections or tissue culture cells as substrate in indirect immunofluorescent assays. This approach has been very successful and has helped establish the autoimmune profiles that aid clinicians in the diagnosis and classification of systemic rheumatic diseases. The use of indirect immunofluorescence, however, has several limitations. Among these are the semiquantitative nature of the measurement, the need for skilled observers to read the tests, the inability to automate the test, and the subjectivity that accompanies an observer-controlled test.

One alternative is EIA with various kinds of fixed cells or cell extracts as antigen. There are several such commercial kits on the market, and they are evaluated in this paper. Most, but not all, kits have acceptable agreement, sensitivity, and specificity with IFA, and one can look for increasing utilization of such methods for ANA screening in the future. For positive samples, pattern recognition will still be required by the old IFA methods.

M. Reichlin, M.D.

Utility of Anti-Sm, Anti-RNP, Anti-Ro/SS-A, and Anti-La/SS-B (Extractable Nuclear Antigens) Detected by Enzyme-Linked Immunosorbent Assay for the Diagnosis of Systemic Lupus Erythematosus

Sánchez-Guerrero J, Lew RA, Fossel AH, et al (Brigham and Women's Hosp, Boston; Harvard Med School, Boston)

Arthritis Rheum 39:1055–1061, 1996 3–12

Background.—Antibodies to extractable nuclear antigens (ENAs) are found in patients with systemic lupus erythematosus (SLE) and may be markers of particular manifestations of that disease. Previous studies of these antibodies have used immunodiffusion methods, but enzyme-linked immunosorbent assay (ELISA) may now also be applied. The value of using ELISA to detect anti-ENA antibodies as a predictor for SLE was evaluated.

Methods.—Antinuclear antibodies (ANAs) were detected in 259 consecutive patients via testing of 2,185 serum samples; the medical records of these patients were reviewed, and the diagnoses were established with American College of Rheumatology criteria. Clinical differences between patients with SLE who did or did not show anti-ENA antibodies were examined. For analysis, 3 patient groups were defined: all patients positive for ANAs (ANA+), patients positive for ANAs and anti-double stranded DNA (ANA+/anti-dsDNA+), and patients positive for ANAs and negative for anti-dsDNA (ANA+/anti-dsDNA−).

Results.—Among ANA+/anti-dsDNA− patients, the predictive diagnostic value of anti-ENA antibodies, especially anti-Ro/SS-A, was high. Among ANA+/anti-dsDNA+ patients, however, the antibodies showed no predictive value. Only 2 clinical manifestations proved more common among patients with SLE who showed anti-ENA antibodies: pleuritis and use of hydroxychloroquine.

Conclusions.—The presence of anti-ENA antibodies may be a useful predictor of SLE, at least in patients positive for ANA and negative for anti-dsDNA. Patients with SLE who are positive for ANA did not differ significantly in clinical presentation of their disease depending on the presence or absence of anti-ENA antibodies.

► This paper defines the diagnostic utility of measuring antibodies to the small RNA proteins Ro/SS-A, La/SS-B, U_1RNP, and Sm by ELISA in the diagnosis of SLE. The bottom line is that, in referral rheumatologic centers, the measurement of anti-Ro/SS-A is a useful predictor of SLE in patients who are ANA+ but anti-dsDNA−. This is another example of how the use of defined antigen-specific immunoassays in the recognition of systemic rheumatic diseases is sharpening and will sharpen our diagnostic tools.

M. Reichlin, M.D.

Some Autoantibodies to Ro/SS-A and La/SS-B Are Antiidiotypes to Anti–double-stranded DNA

Zhang W, Reichlin M (Univ of Oklahoma, Oklahoma City)

Arthritis Rheum 39:522–531, 1996 3–13

Background.—Antibodies to native, or double-stranded, DNA (dsDNA) play an important role in systemic lupus erythematosus (SLE). Research suggests that the low prevalence of an overt anti-dsDNA response in many patients who have SLE and produce anti–Ro/SS-A and/or anti–La/SS-B indicates that these antibodies may behave as anti-idiotypes to anti-dsDNA and downregulate the production of anti-dsDNA. The relationship between anti–Ro/SS-A and anti–La/SS-B antibodies to anti-dsDNA in sera from patients who had SLE was studied.

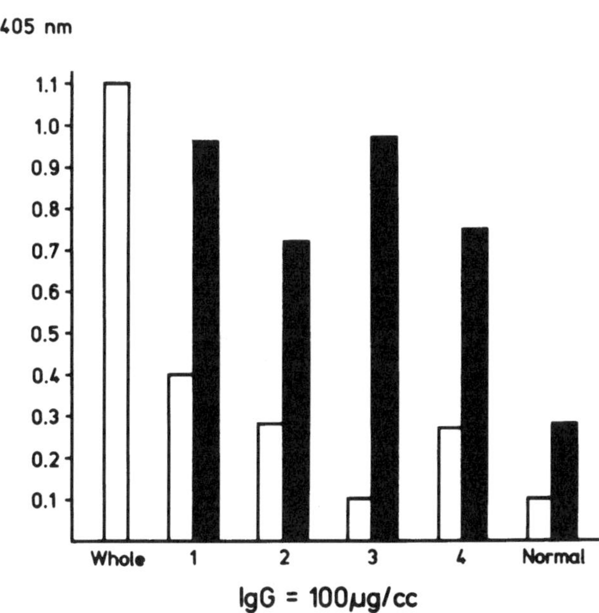

FIGURE 4.—Results of studies in which serum 1 (with anti–Ro/SS-A), sera 2–4 (with anti–La/SS-B), and a normal control serum were separately isolated on a double-stranded DNA (dsDNA) affinity column. The same concentration of serum IgG (100 µg/mL) was compared with IgG isolated from a dsDNA cellulose column. *White bars* represent whole sera; *black bars* represent the affinity-purified IgG from the DNA cellulose column. The *first white bar* is from a serum containing high levels of anti-dsDNA, as a positive control. Values are the absorbance at 405 nm ($A_{405\ nm}$). (Courtesy of Zhang W, Reichlin M: Some autoantibodies to Ro/SS-A and La/SS-B are antiidiotypes to anti–double-stranded DNA. *Arthritis Rheum* 39:522–531, 1996, copyright American College of Rheumatology.)

Methods.—Sera from 5 patients who had anti–Ro/SS-A alone and from 7 who had anti–Ro/SS-A and anti–La/SS-B were absorbed with purified Ro/SS-A and La/SS-B, respectively. The absorbed sera were then assessed for reactivity with MOLT-4 extract by Western blot and dsDNA by enzyme-linked immunosorbent assay (ELISA). In selected samples, anti-dsDNA was isolated on DNA cellulose columns, and anti–Ro/SS-A and anti–La/SS-B were isolated on antigen-affinity columns.

Findings.—All sera showed reactivity with small nuclear ribonucleoprotein A and D bands in Western blots after absorption. In addition, some showed reactivity with dsDNA by ELISA. Anti-dsDNA populations were purified on dsDNA cellulose columns, and anti–Ro/SS-A and anti–La/SS-B were affinity purified from the same sera as the anti-dsDNA. In all cases, anti-dsDNA bound autologous anti-Ro/SS-A and anti-La/SS-B much more strongly than normal pooled IgG. These interactions were blocked by dsDNA but not RNA. In the same interactions, Ro/SS-A blocked anti–Ro/SS-A and La/SS-B blocked anti–La/SS-B (Fig 4).

Conclusions.—Subpopulations of anti–Ro/SS-A and anti–La/SS-B that bind and mask anti-dsDNA exist in sera with these antibodies. These antibodies may be anti-idiotypes to idiotypes on anti-dsDNA and may mask and downregulate these anti-dsDNA antibodies.

► One of the most interesting aspects of the clinical and serologic characteristics of patients who have SLE is why subsets with certain precipitin profiles have a low prevalence of antibodies to dsDNA. Not surprisingly, these same patients have a low prevalence of glomerulonephritis, as dsDNA–anti-dsDNA immune complexes are thought to be an important proximate cause of this manifestation of in SLE. This paper shows that some fraction of anti–Ro/SS-A and anti–La/SS-B from patients who had SLE without anti-dsDNA are in fact antibodies (or anti-idiotypes) to anti-dsDNA. The implications of this are twofold. First, these anti–Ro/SS-A and anti–La/SS-B antibodies with this activity mask and/or downregulate anti-dsDNA antibodies. Second, such antibodies could be used therapeutically as immunologically specific therapy for high levels of anti-dsDNA antibody in patients who have SLE.

M. Reichlin, M.D.

Coexistence of Serum Anti-DNA Topoisomerase I and Anti-Sm Antibodies: Report of 3 Cases

Kameda H, Kuwana M, Hama N, et al (Keio Univ, Tokyo)

J Rheumatol 24:400–403, 1997 3–14

Background.—Because serum antinuclear antibodies (ANAs) are closely associated with clinical features in patients with rheumatic diseases, they are useful indicators of diagnosis and classification of disease subsets. Three Japanese patients whose sera were found to contain anti-topoisomerase I and anti-Sm antibodies at the same time were reported.

> *Case Reports.*—The patients were a 14-year-old girl and 2 women, aged 24 and 39 years. The typical characteristics of systemic lupus erythematosus (SLE), such as glomerulonephritis, were present in all 3 patients. In addition, the patients had skin thickening and systemic sclerosis–related organ involvement, including pulmonary interstitial fibrosis and renal crisis. Of note, when the symptoms of SLE developed in the third patient, her serum contained anti-Sm antibody that had not been detected many years previously, when she had only the features of systemic sclerosis (Fig 2).

Conclusion.—The coexistence of these 2 disease-specific antibodies has not been reported previously. The clinical presentations of these 3 patients support the notion that ANA-clinical associations are strong.

► In the United States, patients with an overlap of scleroderma and SLE are well known and have a variety of autoantibodies corresponding to the 2

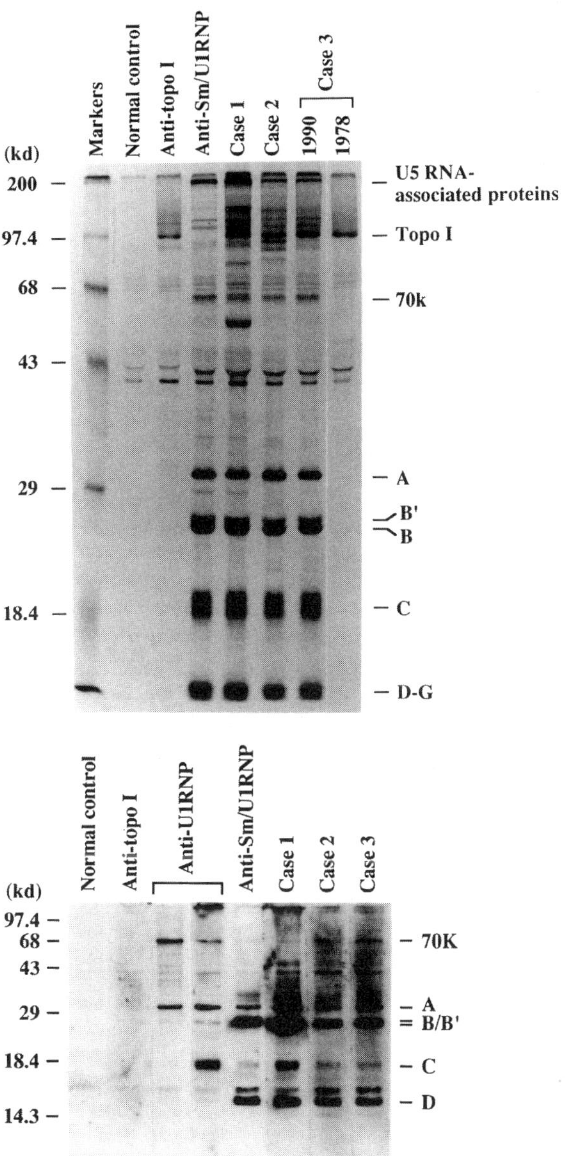

FIGURE 2.—Analysis of sera from cases 1–3 by immunoprecipitation assay using ^{35}S-labeled HeLa cell extracts (A) and by immunoblots using purified Sm antigen (B). (Courtesy of Kameda H, Kuwana M, Hama N, et al: Coexistence of serum anti-DNA topoisomerase I and anti-Sm antibodies: Report of 3 cases. *J Rheumatol* 24:400–403, 1997.)

diseases. No North American case, however, has ever been recognized in which autoantibodies to Sm, which are SLE-specific, and autoantibodies to DNA topoisomerase I (Scl-70), which are specific for scleroderma, coexist.

In this report from Japan, 3 cases of scleroderma-SLE overlaps are described in which all three patients had both anti-Sm and antitopoisomerase

I. This difference bespeaks the probable existence of racially determined genetic factors that control autoantibody production, and clinical expression in the 2 populations.

M. Reichlin, M.D.

Cross-Reactivity of Human IgG Anti-F(ab')$_2$ Antibody With DNA and Other Nuclear Antigens

Williams RC Jr, Malone CC, Cimbalnik K, et al (Univ of Florida, Gainesville; Florida State Univ, Tallahassee; Univ of Bari, Italy)
Arthritis Rheum 40:109–123, 1997 3–15

Background.—Human antibodies to determinants on the F(ab')$_2$ portion of IgG or anti-F(ab')$_2$ have been seen as examples of natural antiidiotypes. This anti-F(ab')$_2$ antibody response has been considered to be completely different from anti-DNA specificity in patients with systemic lupus erythematosus (SLE), because during active disease serum anti-DNA levels are high and anti-F(ab')$_2$ levels are depressed, while during remission, serum anti-F(ab')$_2$ levels increase and anti-DNA levels decrease. The immunologic specificity and antiidiotype activity of IgG and anti-F(ab')$_2$ were characterized from normal individuals and from SLE patients with active and inactive disease. The results presented demonstrate that anti-F(ab')$_2$ antibodies have anti-DNA and anti-nuclear ribonucleoproteins (Sm/RNP) specificities.

Methods.—Anti-F(ab')$_{2a}$ IgG and anti–double-stranded DNA (anti-dsDNA) were affinity purified using immunoadsorption columns. This affinity-purified IgG anti-F(ab')$_2$ (APAF) and affinity-isolated IgG anti-dsDNA (APAD) were tested by enzyme-linked immunosorbent assay (ELISA) for cross-reacting specificities, including anti-Sm, anti-Sm/RNP, and anti-*Crithidia*. Anti-DNA specificity was examined by S1 nuclease treatment of heat-denatured DNA. Rabbit antiidiotype antisera were prepared by immunization with APAF and APAD from both normal and SLE volunteers. The APAF and APAD were examined by high-resolution electron microscopy for ring forms indicating antiidiotypic V-region interactions.

Results.—The APAF derived from normal individuals had significant concentrations of both anti-F(ab')$_2$ and anti-DNA, as well as anti-Sm, and anti-Sm/RNP reactivity. The anti-DNA reactivity of APAF and APAD from normal volunteers was much more sensitive to S1 nuclease treatment than anti-DNA reactivity from SLE patients. Control APAF and APAD did not produce positive antinuclear immunofluorescence or positive *Crithidia* staining, whereas SLE APAF and APAD were strongly positive for both. Absorbed rabbit anitsera to normal or SLE APAF and APAD had strong ELISA reactivity to both APAF and APAD, but no activity with normal Cohn fraction II. Sequencing of monoclonal human IgM antibodies with anti-F(ab')$_2$ and anti-DNA reactivity demonstrated that they were relatively V_H3 and/or V_κ restricted. High-resolution electron microscopy did not reveal any forms indicative of antiidiotypic V-region interactions from either normal or SLE APAD or APAF.

Conclusions.—Anti-F(ab')$_2$ from both healthy controls and patients with SLE consists of a polyreactive Ig subfraction that contains anti-DNA, anti-Sm, and anti-Sm/RNP reactivities. Anti-DNA and anti-F(ab')$_2$ antibodies appear to share cross-reactivity and V-region antigens. The anti-DNA reactivity from healthy controls is much more sensitive to S-nuclease digestion of denatured dsDNA than the anti-DNA reactivity of SLE patients. These surprising results suggest that healthy individuals are more similar immunologically to patients with SLE than has been previously supposed.

▶ Dr. Williams and his colleagues have been teaching us for the past 15 years that antibody activity against normal pepsin-digested IgG (or F(ab')$_2$) is high in normals and low in active SLE, implying that in some way these anti-F(ab')$_2$ antibodies are part of normal immunoregulation. In SLE, this "control" mechanism is disturbed or deficient, and indeed in remission, anti-F(ab')$_2$ antibodies rise in titer as patients improve. This paper comes up with some surprising and paradoxical findings: analysis of affinity purified anti-F(ab')$_2$ from normals shows antibody activity against the autoantigens DNA and Sm/nRNP not exhibited by unfractionated IgG from the same normal individuals. These results are very surprising and bring normal individuals immunologically close to SLE patients.

The authors offer no simple explanation for these surprising and complex findings; but one has the feeling that when these phenomena are understood, some of the threshold events in the induction of the autoimmunity of SLE will be revealed.

M. Reichlin, M.D.

Antiphospholipid Syndrome and Antibodies

Long-Term Outcome of Mothers of Children With Complete Congenital Heart Block

Press J, Uziel Y, Laxer RM, et al (Univ of Toronto)
Am J Med 100:328–332, 1996 3–16

Purpose.—Complete congenital heart block (CHB) occurs as an intrauterine complication of neonatal lupus erythematosus syndrome. It is probably caused by transplacental passage of maternal antibodies to Ro/SSA and La/SSB ribonucleoproteins. Some reports have suggested that the mothers of children with CHB are at risk of connective tissue diseases, especially systemic lupus erythematosus (SLE) or Sjögren's syndrome (SS). However, these studies have been small or had problems with referral bias. The short- and long-term health outcomes of mothers of infants born with CHB were analyzed.

Methods.—The study included 64 mothers of 64 infants born with CHB. Information for the analysis was collected by questionnaire, telephone interview, and/or from the attending physicians. The mothers were

TABLE 2.—Health Status of 64 Mothers of Children With Congenital Heart Block

Maternal Health Status at Delivery	Maternal Health Status at Follow-Up
Mothers with a defined disease	
2 patients had SLE	2 patients continued to have SLE
2 patients had linear scleroderma	2 patients continued to have linear scleroderma
2 patients had RA	1 patient developed SLE
	1 patient continued to have RA
3 patients were clinically well with a history of rheumatic fever	2 patients remained clinically well
	1 patient developed SS
1 patient had SS	1 patient continued to have SS
Mothers with undifferentiated autoimmune disease (UAS)	
12 patients had UAS	6 patients continued to have UAS
	3 patients developed SLE
	2 patients developed SS
	1 patient became clinically well
Healthy mothers	
42 mothers were healthy	3 developed UAS
	1 developed ankylosing spondylitis
	1 developed hyperthyroidism
	1 developed SLE

Abbreviations: SLE, systemic lupus erythematosus; *SS*, Sjögren's syndrome; *UAS*, undifferentiated autoimmune syndrome.

(Reprinted by permission of the publisher, courtesy of Press J, Uziel Y, Laxer RM, et al: Long-term outcome of mothers of children with complete congenital heart block. *Am J Med* 100:328–332, copyright 1996 by Excerpta Medica, Inc.)

classified as having a definite rheumatic disease, as having an undifferentiated autoimmune syndrome (UAS), or as being healthy currently and at the time they delivered the infant with CHB. Serum samples from 53 mothers were analyzed by enzyme-linked immunosorbent assay for anti-Ro and anti-La antibodies.

Results.—The mothers' mean age at delivery was 28 years, at which time 66% were healthy. Two (3%) had SLE, 2 (3%) had linear scleroderma, 2 (3%) had RA, 3 (5%) had a history of rheumatic fever but were currently well, and 1 (2%) had SS. Nineteen percent of the mothers had a UAS at the time of delivery, with symptoms including arthralgias, myalgia, photosensitivity, skin vasculitis, and Raynaud's phenomenon. The mean age at the time of the study was 38 years. Of the 12 mothers who had a UAS at delivery, 3 had progressed to SLE, 2 had SS, and 1 had gone into remission. Of the 42 mothers who had been healthy at delivery, 1 had SLE, 1 had hyperthyroidism, 1 had ankylosing spondylitis, and 3 had UAS (Table 2). The mean follow-up was 123 months for the mothers who remained healthy and 121 months for those in whom autoimmune diseases developed.

Sixty percent of the women tested positive for anti-Ro and/or anti-La antibodies. At the time of the study, 26% were symptomatic. Serum samples obtained at delivery were positive for anti-Ro and/or anti-La antibodies in 12 of 13 patients.

Conclusion.—Most mothers of children with CHB who are healthy at delivery remain healthy over the long term. Systemic lupus erythematosus may develop in approximately one fourth of mothers who have UAS at the time of delivery, compared with a very small proportion of initially healthy mothers. The rate at which autoimmune disease developed in asymptomatic mothers after the birth of a child with CHB was lower in this study than in previous reports. However, mothers who have a UAS need close follow-up.

▶ From one half to two thirds of women who give birth to children with complete CHB are healthy despite the very common presence of high titers of antibodies to the Ro/SSA antigen. This informs us that these antibodies are not, by themselves, sufficient to cause disease expression and provides a potential cohort of patients with which to unravel the possible additional factors that are critical for disease expression. This study tells us that even in a 10-year follow-up period (on average), in only 6 of 42 asymptomatic women did clinical disease develop. This not only gives us something to tell these people about their prognosis, it also shows that the recruitment of the additional factors that mediate disease expression is quite uncommon.

M. Reichlin, M.D.

Antiphosphatidylethanolamine Antibodies as the Only Antiphospholipid Antibodies. I: Association With Thrombosis and Vascular Cutaneous Diseases

Berard M, Chantome R, Marcelli A, et al (Hôpital St Louis, Paris)
J Rheumatol 23:1369–1374, 1996 3–17

Background.—Antiphospholipid antibodies (aPLs) occur in various conditions. Few laboratories screen for antibodies against phosphatidylethanolamine (PE), a zwitterionic phospholipid (PL) occurring in both layers of cell membranes. In a large number of serum samples sent to 1 laboratory for aPL detection, the frequency of anti-PE antibodies (aPEs) as the sole aPL was determined, and the presence of these antibodies correlated with clinical manifestations.

Methods.—Serum was obtained from 41 patients with autoimmune diseases, 34 with thromboembolic episodes (TEEs), 31 with livedo reticularis with or without thrombosis or recurrent fetal loss (RFL), 10 with systemic vasculitides, and 6 with miscellaneous disorders. Samples were tested for antibodies against 4 anionic PLs (cardiolipin, phosphatidylserine, inositol, and phosphatidic acid) and lupus anticoagulant in addition to aPEs.

Findings.—Fifteen patients had aPEs but not antibodies to anionic PL, including lupus anticoagulant. Seven patients had IgM, 4 had IgG plus IgM, and 4 had IgG. The aPEs were associated with TEE alone, TEE and livedo reticularis, or livedo reticularis alone significantly more often than with autoimmune disorders (Table 4).

Conclusion.—The detection of aPEs alone in a patient with mesenteric infarcts and RFL made possible the diagnosis of primary antiphospholipid syndrome. The follow-up of 3 patients showed that aPEs are not transient. Thus, patients with clinical symptoms suggesting antiphospholipid syn-

TABLE 4.—Antiphospholipid Antibody Distribution According to Disease Category and the Type of Phospholipid Recognized

Group	Disease Category (n)	Patients with a-Anionic aPL† or LAC, n=49	aPE* Alone, n=15
I	Autoimmune disorders (28)	26	2
II	Thromboembolic episodes (15)	9	6
III	LR (without thrombosis or RFL) (7)	4	3
IV	LR + thrombosis or RFL (8)	4	4
V	Systemic vasculitides (5)	5	0
VI	Miscellaneous disorders (1)	1	0

Note: Statistical analysis (Yates' corrected chi-squared): Group I/group II: $P = 0.025$; III: ns; /IV: $P = 0.02$; /II+III+IV: $P = 0.004$.

*Antiphosphatidylethanolamine antibodies (*aPEs*) without antianionic antiphospholipid antibodies (*aPLs*) (a-anionic aPLs) and lupus anticoagulant (*LAC*).

†a-anionic aPLs were screened by enzyme-linked immunosorbent assay using cardiolipin and/or phosphatidylinositol, phosphatidylserine, phosphatidic acid as antigens. Patients with a-anionic aPLs may also have aPEs, as they were not screened for aPEs.

Other abbreviations: LR, livedo reticularis; *RFL*, recurrent fetal loss.

(Courtesy of Berard M, Chantome R, Marcelli A, et al: Antiphosphatidylethanolamine antibodies as the only antiphospholipid antibodies: I. Association with thrombosis and vascular cutaneous diseases. *J Rheumatol* 23:1369–1374, 1996.)

drome but with sera negative for antibodies to cardiolipin or another anionic PL should be screened for aPEs, especially patients with thrombosis, RFL, and/or livedo reticularis.

▶ This paper tells us that if all the available tests for anticardiolipin antibodies and the lupus anticoagulant are performed, we may still not detect some aPLs which are clinically associated with thrombosis. A few such patients with recurrent thrombosis and a moderate level of aPEs were identified in this study. Thus, the absence of antibodies to anionic phospholipids and/or lupus anticoagulant does not detect all the patients with aPLs related to thromboses.

M. Reichlin, M.D.

Anti-Phospholipid Autoantibodies Bind to Apoptotic, But Not Viable, Thymocytes in a β_2-Glycoprotein I-Dependent Manner

Price BE, Rauch J, Shia MA, et al (Boston Univ; McGill Univ, Montreal)
J Immunol 157:2201–2208, 1996 3–18

Background.—Antiphospholipid autoantibodies (aPLs) have been associated with a wide range of infectious and autoimmune diseases, including a clinical syndrome of hypercoagulability, thrombocytopenia, and fetal loss. Many aPLs do not have a pure phospholipid target in vitro, but instead target either a complex between anionic phospholipids and the plasma protein β-2-glycoprotein I (β-2-GPI) or β-2-GPI alone. Anionic proteins are not normally found on the extracellular cell membrane surface, but during apoptosis they are redistributed from the inner to the outer leaflet. The binding characteristics of aPLs were further examined.

Methods.—The aPLs were obtained from the serum of a patient with primary aPL syndrome; apoptosis was induced in freshly isolated murine thymocytes. Immunofluorescent staining and fluorescence-activated cell sorter analysis were performed.

Results.—The aPLs bound specifically to apoptotic thymocytes and not to viable thymocytes. This binding was dependent on the presence of β-2-GPI. The β-2-GPI bound selectively to the surface of the apoptotic thymocytes, generating an epitope for antiphospholipid autoantibodies.

Conclusion.—The data suggest that the natural immunogen and/or target for aPLs may be apoptotic cells. Interaction between redistributed anionic phospholipids and circulating β-2-GPI may generate a novel ligand by which apoptotic cells are recognized directly for phagocytic clearance. By interfering with the normal clearance of apoptotic cells and the autoantigens they contain, aPLs may contribute to the development of autoimmunity.

Antiphospholipid Antibodies Are Directed Against Epitopes of Oxidized Phospholipids: Recognition of Cardiolipin by Monoclonal Antibodies to Epitopes of Oxidized Low Density Lipoprotein

Hörkkö S, Miller E, Dudl E, et al (Univ of California, San Diego; Scripps Research Inst, La Jolla, Calif; Univ of Louisville, Ky; et al)

J Clin Invest 98:815–825, 1996 3–19

Background.—Management of antiphospholipid antibody syndrome (APS) is hampered by lack of understanding of the mechanism behind it. Why antiphospholipid antibodies (aPLs) form against such ubiquitous compounds as phospholipids has not been explained. The hypothesis that most aPLs do not bind to "native," unmodified phospholipids was explored.

Findings.—Many, if not most, aPLs appear to be directed toward either neoepitopes of oxidized phospholipids or neoepitopes produced by adduct formation between breakdown products of oxidized phospholipids and associated proteins. Rapid oxidation occurs when cardiolipin molecules are plated and exposed to air. As cardiolipin is exposed to air for increasing periods, a striking time-dependent increase occurs in its binding to sera from apo E–deficient mice (which have high autoantibody titers to oxidized low-density lipoprotein). The oxidized cardiolipins also bound to monoclonal antibodies to oxidized low-density lipoprotein (cloned from apo E–deficient mice) and to sera and affinity-purified aCL-IgG from patients with APS. A reduced cardiolipin analogue that was unable to undergo peroxidation, in contrast, did not bind to any of these substances.

Conclusion.—Oxidative events may be important in the pathophysiology of APS, as evidenced by these data, which show that many aPLs are directed at neoepitopes of oxidized phospholipids. The possibility of new therapeutic strategies, such as intensive antioxidant therapy, is suggested.

▶ These 2 papers (Abstracts 3–18 and 3–19) provide information about the immunologic specificity of aPLs, as well as the physiologic state of cells that can bind these antibodies. The paper on specificity shows that at least some antibodies are directed at new epitopes related to oxidized phospholipids. This links in an interesting way with past work that suggests that oxidized phospholipids are involved in atherosclerosis. It could be more than coincidence that this biochemical state of lipids that affect atherosclerosis and the molecular target of antiphospholipids are on a continuum with biological events resulting in thrombosis.

The second aspect of these reports relates to antiphospholipids binding cells that are apoptotic. This is not surprising because the redistributed phospholipids characteristic of apoptotic cells might be ideal for reactivity with aPLs. This reaction may also play a positive role in marking cells for phagocytosis, perhaps enhanced by the binding of aPLs.

M. Reichlin, M.D.

Similarities of Specificity and Cofactor Dependence in Serum Antiphospholipid Antibodies From Patients With Human Parvovirus B19 Infection and From Those With Systemic Lupus Erythematosus

Loizou S, Cazabon JK, Walport MJ, et al (Royal Postgraduate Med School, London; Centre Hospitalier Universitaire Vadois, Lausanne, Switzerland)
Arthritis Rheum 40:103–108, 1997 3–20

Background.—Parvovirus B19 is a small, single-stranded DNA virus associated with a variety of clinical manifestations in humans. The phospholipid specificity and immunoglobulin isotype of antiphospholipid antibodies (aPLs) in affected patients were reported.

Methods.—Serum samples were obtained from 12 patients with acute parvovirus B19 infections, 10 with other acute viral infections, and 15 with syphilis. Enzyme-linked immunosorbent assays were used to measure the specificity of aPL and isotype distribution in the negatively charged

TABLE 2.—Effects of β_2-Glycoprotein I on IgG Anticardiolipin Antibody–Binding in Patients With Parvovirus B19, Other Viral Infections, Syphilis, or Systemic Lupus Erythematosus

Patient group	Total no.	No. (%) of β_2-GPI-dependent sera	No. of β_2-GPI-independent sera
Parvovirus B19	12	8 (66.7)*	4
SLE	11	6 (54.5)†	5
Other viruses	10	2 (20)	8
Syphilis	11	1 (9.1)	10

Note: β_2-glycoprotein I (β_2-GPI)–dependent binding was expressed as a > 10% increase in the optical absorbence readings in the presence of β_2-GPI above those for the same serum samples in the absence of β_2-GPI. Independent binding of β_2-GPI was expressed as reductions in optical absorbence ≤ 10%.

*$P < 0.034$ vs. other viruses; $P < 0.007$ vs. syphilis, by Fisher's exact test.

†$P < 0.03$ vs. syphilis, by Fisher's exact test.

(Courtesy of Loizou S, Cazabon JK, Walport MJ, et al: Similarities of specificity and cofactor dependence in serum antiphospholipid antibodies from patients with human parvovirus B19 infection and from those with systemic lupus erythematosus. *Arthritis Rheum* 40:103–108, 1997, copyright American College of Rheumatology.)

phospholipids, cardiolipin and phosphatidylserine, and the neutral phosphopholipid, phosphatidylethanolamine. The dependence of anticardiolipin (aCL) binding on the presence of β_2-glycoprotein I (β_2-GPI) as a binding cofactor was also determined and compared with sera from 11 patients with systemic lupus erythematosus (SLE) with increased aCL antibody reactivity.

Findings.—Sera from all 3 groups of infected patients showed antibodies against any of the 3 phospholipids. The sera from patients with B19 infections contained mostly IgG antibodies against the negatively charged phospholipids, cardiolipin, and phosphatidylserine. The specificity and isotype distribution differed from those in the other 2 patient groups. B19-related aCL increased binding to antigen in the presence of β_2-GPI as a binding cofactor. This was similar to aCL in patients with SLE but unlike the antibodies from patients with other viral infections or with syphilis (Table 2).

Conclusion.—The specificity of aPLs in B19-infected patients is remarkably similar to that in patients with SLE. This raises the question as to whether parvovirus infection may trigger the development of aPLs in autoimmune diseases.

▶ This paper reports another finding that draws the wake of parvovirus infection into convergence with systemic rheumatic disease. The finding reported is the similarity of specificity and cofactor dependence of aPLs after parvovirus infection with these properties in the aPLs of patients with SLE. In contrast, patients with several other viral infections and syphilis have aPLs that do not depend on β_2-glycoprotein I and are either largely IgM (viral infections) or directed frequently against phosphatidylethanolamine (syphilis).

These findings suggest a possible role for parvovirus in the induction of aPLs. Long-term follow-up of these patients should tell us whether parvovirus is a possible trigger for the antiphospholipid syndrome or whether the results seen here represent an interesting but trivial coincidence.

M. Reichlin, M.D.

A Monoclonal IgG Anticardiolipin Antibody From a Patient With the Antiphospholipid Syndrome Is Thrombogenic in Mice

Olee T, Pierangeli SS, Handley HH, et al (Sam and Rose Stein Inst for Research on Aging, La Jolla, Calif; Univ of California, San Diego, La Jolla; Univ of Louisville, Ky; et al)

Proc Natl Acad Sci USA 93:8606–8611, 1996 3–21

Background.—Antiphospholipid syndrome (APS) is characterized by recurrent episodes of thrombosis and pregnancy loss in patients with systemic lupus erythematosus and serum antiphospholipid antibodies (APAs). Recurrent thrombosis in patients with APS is strongly associated with APAs, including anticardiolipin antibodies (ACAs). The binding specificity and role of ACAs in thrombosis have not been clearly determined. In vivo assays have been developed that allow assessment of the pathogenic procoagulant activity of a patient's autoantibodies, but the particular species responsible for in vivo thrombosis have not been identified. The involvement of ACAs in recurrent thrombosis in patients with APS was evaluated.

Methods.—Two human monoclonal IgG ACAs were generated by cultivating peripheral blood mononuclear cells from a patient with primary APS, high titers of serum ACAs, and recurrent thrombosis. The thrombotic events in the patient were determined to not be caused by abnormal levels of protein C, protein S, or factor V.

Findings.—These antibodies bound to cardiolipin in the presence, but not in the absence, of 10% bovine serum. They were reactive against phosphatidic acid but not against purified human β-2 glycoprotein 1, DNA, heparan sulfate, or 4 other test antigens. The monoclonal antibodies did not inhibit prothrombinase activity and lacked lupus anticoagulant activity. When tested with an in vivo mouse model, 1 of the monoclonal antibodies had thrombogenic properties.

Conclusions.—This is the first evidence demonstrating that monoclonal ACAs derived from a patient with APS can have thrombogenic properties. These data support, but do not establish, the belief that this type of ACA can be thrombogenic in patients with APS.

► One of the clinical autoimmune syndromes that has captured the attention and interest of clinicians is APS. Part of the excitement originates from the hope and expectation that the antiphospholipids themselves are the proximate cause of the clinical event, the thrombosis. This lends optimism to the proposition that effective interventions can be found once the target of therapy is identified. This paper elegantly shows that an IgG monoclonal APA prepared from a patient with recurrent thrombosis can promote thrombosis in an in vivo mouse model. This finding not only supports the idea that it is true that APAs directly promote thrombosis but also provides the experimental milieu in which to find potentially useful interventions.

M. Reichlin, M.D.

Anticardiolipin Antibodies: Clinical Consequences of "Low Titers"

Silver RM, Porter TF, van Leeuween I, et al (Univ of Utah, Salt Lake City; Univ of Iowa, Iowa City)

Obstet Gynecol 87:494–500, 1996 3–22

Background.—The clinical consequences of IgM anticardiolipin antibodies or low levels of IgG anticardiolipin antibodies are unclear. However, most patients with positive tests for antiphospholipid antibodies either have isolated IgM or low-positive IgG anticardiolipin antibodies. The implications of low levels of IgG or IgM anticardiolipin antibodies were investigated.

Methods.—Four groups of women who underwent clinically indicated testing for antiphospholipid antibodies were assessed. The high-positive group, included 131 women who had lupus anticoagulant or more than 19 IgG binding units of anticardiolipin antibodies. The low-positive IgG group included 93 who had fewer than 20 IgG binding units. Ninety-seven women comprised a group with IgM only; these women had more than 9 IgM binding units. The last group included 153 women who had negative findings.

Findings.—The women with high-positive findings were more likely to have at least 1 new medical complication during the median study period of 4 years or more compared with the other groups. By contrast, the other 3 groups showed a similar low risk for the development of new disorders. On retesting, 9.3% of women in the low-positive IgG, IgM only, or negative groups had lupus anticoagulant or more than 19 IgG binding units. At least 1 new disorder developed in half these patients.

Conclusions.—Women who have IgM or low levels of IgG anticardiolipin antibodies are distinct from women who have lupus anticoagulant or moderate to high concentrations of igG anticardiolipin antibodies. The former are not at risk for disorders related to antiphospholipid antibody beyond the risk associated with their medical histories. New or recurrent clinical symptoms in such women, however, merit repeat testing.

Natural History and Risk Factors for Thrombosis in 360 Patients With Antiphospholipid Antibodies: A Four-year Prospective Study From the Italian Registry

Finazzi G, Brancaccio V, Moia M, et al (Ospedali Riuniti, Bergamo, Italy; Ospedale Cardarelli, Naples, Italy; IRCCS Ospedale Maggiore Univ, Milan, Italy; et al)

Am J Med 100:530–536, 1996 3–23

Background.—The presence of antiphospholipid antibodies (APA) has been associated with the clinical features of antiphospholipid syndrome, including arterial and venous thrombosis, recurrent fetal loss, and thrombocytopenia. The risk for thrombosis in patients who have APAs, however, has been difficult to determine. The natural history and risk factors for thrombosis in a large cohort with APAs were reported.

Methods.—Three hundred sixty consecutive, unselected patients, from 16 Italian centers, who met the criteria for the diagnosis of lupus anticoagulant and/or increased IgG anticardiolipin antibodies (IgG ACA) were studied. The group included 242 female and 118 male patients, aged from 2–78 years.

Findings.—During a median observation of 3.9 years, thrombotic complications developed in 34 patients. The total incidence was 2.5% patient-years. In a multivariate logistic regression analysis, previous thrombosis and IgG ACA titer exceeding 40 units were independent risk factors for thrombotic events. Twenty-five women had a total of 28 pregnancies, 39%

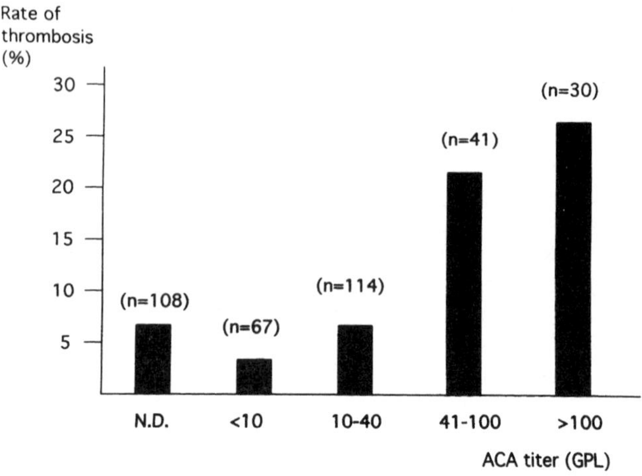

FIGURE 1.—Rate of thrombosis during the follow-up of 360 patients who had antiphospholipid antibodies according to the titer of anticardiolipin (*ACA*) IgG, expressed in GPL units. In *parentheses*, the number of patients in each group. *Abbreviation: ND*, not determined. (Reprinted by permission of the publisher from Finazzi G, Brancaccio V, Moia M, et al: Natural history and risk factors for thrombosis in 360 patients with antiphospholipid antibodies: A four-year prospective study from the Italian Registry. *Am J Med* 100:530–536, copyright 1996 by Excerpta Medica, Inc.)

of which were unsuccessful. Adverse pregnancy outcomes were significantly more common among women who had a history of miscarriage or vascular occlusion than in those who had no symptoms. Non-Hodgkin's lymphoma developed in 4 patients. Eighteen patients died during follow-up, most commonly of vascular events and hematologic malignancies (Fig 1).

Conclusions.—Previous thrombosis and ACA titers of more than 40 units independently predict thrombosis. These findings also show that history of miscarriage is significantly associated with adverse outcomes in pregnant women. In addition, hematologic malignancies can develop in patients who have APAs.

▶ These 2 papers (Abstracts 3–22 and 3–23) bear the same message and do so with large numbers of patients from both sides of the Atlantic. Patients who have low titers of IgG APAs or IgM APAs alone have no more risk of anticardiolipin-related problems than do individuals who have negative tests for APA. Correspondingly, IgG APA of high titer or previous thrombotic episodes are the key risk factors for thrombosis. These data should help in clinical decision making regarding therapy and follow-up.

M. Reichlin, M.D.

Randomised Controlled Trial of Aspirin and Aspirin Plus Heparin in Pregnant Women With Recurrent Miscarriage Associated With Phospholipid Antibodies (or Antiphospholipid Antibodies)
Rai R, Cohen H, Dave M, et al (Imperial College, London)
BMJ 314:253–257, 1997 3–24

Introduction.—Women with persistently positive results for phospholipid antibodies have a 90% rate of fetal loss when they receive no specific treatment during pregnancy. The favored treatments in such cases are low-dose aspirin or heparin. A randomized controlled trial compared the rate of live births among women given low-dose aspirin alone and those treated with low-dose aspirin plus low-dose heparin.

Methods.—Ninety patients were recruited from a recurrent miscarriage clinic between April 1993 and July 1995. The women had a median age of 33 years and a median of 4 miscarriages. All had persistently positive results for phospholipid antibodies. Low-dose aspirin (75 mg daily) was administered as soon as the women had a positive pregnancy test. When fetal heart activity was seen on US, 45 patients were allocated to continuing low-dose aspirin and 45 received the addition of self-administered subcutaneous calcium heparin (5,000 U every 12 hours). Treatment was continued until miscarriage or 34 weeks of gestation.

Results.—The 2 treatment groups were similar in age and in the number and gestation of previous miscarriages. More live births were achieved in the aspirin plus heparin group (32 [71%]) than in the aspirin only group (19 [42%]), a significant difference (Table 2). In both groups, most miscarriages occurred in the first trimester. Once a pregnancy had progressed beyond 13 weeks of gestation, the outcome did not differ according to treatment arm. Overall, 24% of successful pregnancies were delivered before 37 weeks of gestation. None of the infants had congenital abnormalities. Both low-dose aspirin and heparin were well tolerated, but women in the aspirin plus heparin group had a decrease (median, 5.4%) in lumbar spine bone density.

Conclusion.—Compared with aspirin alone, the combination of low-dose aspirin and low-dose heparin led to a significantly higher rate of live births in pregnant women with phospholipid antibodies and a history of

TABLE 2.—Details of Pregnancies of Patients in Trial

	Aspirin (n=45)	Aspirin and heparin (n=45)	P value
Median gestation (range) at randomisation (weeks)	6.6 (5.1–8.3)	6.7 (5.0–8.0)	0.32*
No of live births	19	32	0.01†
No of miscarriages	26	13	

*Mann-Whitney U test.
†Fisher's Exact Test.
(Courtesy of Rai R, Cohen H, Dave M, et al: Randomised controlled trial of aspirin and aspirin plus heparin in pregnant women with recurrent miscarriage associated with phospholipid antibodies [or antiphospholipid antibodies]. *BMJ* 314:253–257, 1997.)

recurrent miscarriages. The combination of aspirin and heparin may promote successful embryonic implantation and protect against thrombosis of the uteroplacental vasculature.

▶ The appropriate therapy for pregnant women with recurrent miscarriages and antiphospholipid antibodies has not been determined. Steroids are controversial in this setting and are not routinely recommended. This study shows that the administration of aspirin plus heparin produces more live births than the administration of aspirin alone. This study seems to be a step in the right direction and perhaps sets the stage for further interventions in the future.

M. Reichlin, M.D.

Clinical Aspects

Age-Specific Incidence Rates of Myocardial Infarction and Angina in Women With Systemic Lupus Erythematosus: Comparison With the Framingham Study

Manzi S, Meilahn EN, Rairie JE, et al (Univ of Pittsburgh, Pa; Boston Univ)
Am J Epidemiol 145:408–415, 1997 3–25

Background.—Several conditions appear to increase the risk of cardiovascular events in premenopausal women. The age-specific incidence rates of myocardial infarction and angina pectoris in a large number of women with systemic lupus erythematosus (SLE) were reported.

Methods.—Four hundred ninety-eight women with SLE seen at 1 center between 1980 and 1993 were included in the study. Cardiovascular event

TABLE 2.—Incidence Rates of Cardiovascular Events per 1,000 Person-Years in Women With Systemic Lupus Erythematosus Vs. Women Without the Disease

Age	SLE*		Framingham		Rate	
(years)	Rate	95% CI*	Rate	95% CI	ratio	95% CI
			Myocardial infarction			
15–24	6.33	0.2–35.3	0.00	0.0–11.8	∞	
25–34	3.66	0.8–10.7	0.00	0.0–1.2	∞	
35–44	8.39	4.2–15.0	0.16	0.0–0.9	52.43	21.6–98.5
45–54	4.82	1.0–14.1	1.95	0.9–3.6	2.47	0.8–6.0
55–64	8.38	1.7–24.5	1.99	0.6–4.6	4.21	1.7–7.9
65–74	7.94	1.0–28.7	0.00	0.0–17.1	∞	
			Angina			
15–24	0.00	0.0–23.4	0.00	0.0–11.8	∞	
25–34	1.22	0.0–6.8	0.62	0.1–2.3	1.96	0.0–9.0
35–44	1.53	0.2–5.5	0.65	0.2–1.7	2.35	0.4–11.1
45–54	1.61	0.0–8.9	1.56	0.7–3.1	1.03	0.2–4.6
55–64	5.59	0.7–20.2	2.39	0.9–5.2	2.33	0.9–5.5
65–74	15.87	4.3–40.6	0.00	0.0–17.1	∞	

Abbreviations: SLE, systemic lupus erythematosus; *CI,* confidence interval.

(Courtesy of Manzi S, Meilahn EN, Rairie JE, et al: Age-specific incidence rates of myocardial infarction and angina in women with systemic lupus erythematosus: Comparison with the Framingham Study. *Am J Epidemiol* 145:408–415, 1997.)

rates in this group were compared with those occurring among 2,208 women without SLE of similar age during the same period.

Findings.—Thirty-three first events occurred among the women with SLE after the diagnosis of lupus. There were 11 cases of myocardial infarction, 10 of angina pectoris, and 12 of both. Two thirds of the women were younger than 55 years at the time of these events. Women with SLE, aged 35 to 44 years, were more than 50 times more likely to have a myocardial infarction as women in that age group but without SLE. Compared with women with SLE who did not have an event, those with SLE who did have such an event were older at the time of their lupus diagnosis, had a longer duration of disease and of corticosteroid use, and were more likely to have hypercholesterolemia and to be postmenopausal (Table 2).

Conclusion.—Premature cardiovascular disease is much more common in premenopausal women with SLE than in unaffected women of similar age. Because improved treatment has increased the life expectancy of patients with SLE, cardiovascular disease has become a significant threat to the health of these patients.

▶ This large study dramatically and numerically illustrates two things regarding coronary artery disease (CAD) in patients with SLE which signal a call for action. Premature CAD, be it manifest as myocardial infarction or angina pectoris, is a serious problem in women of all ages with SLE. No one has previously reported the age-specific incidence of CAD in SLE, and it is this figure that most dramatically describes the increased risk of premature CAD in SLE. This is underappreciated, and an aggressive approach to modifiable risk factors needs to be set in motion among physicians caring for these patients. Aggressive therapy of hypercholesterolemia, stringent blood pressure control, thoughtful reduction of steroids (and elimination where possible), and aggressive antismoking measures are some of the major actions that can be instituted to reduce the risk of premature CAD in SLE.

M. Reichlin, M.D.

Subacute Cutaneous Lupus Erythematosus Arising in the Setting of Calcium Channel Blocker Therapy

Crowson AN, Magro CM (Misericordia Gen Hosp, Winnipeg, Man; Harvard Med School, Boston; Pathology Services Inc, Cambridge, Mass)

Hum Pathol 28:67–73, 1997 3–26

Background.—One percent to 14% of patients treated with calcium channel blockers (CCBs) for various disorders ultimately have skin eruptions. However, the development of lupus erythematosus in association with CCB treatment has not been thoroughly studied. The development of subacute cutaneous lupus erythematosus (SCLE) in 9 patients taking CCBs was described.

Methods and Findings.—Photoinduced annular or papulosquamous eruptions clinically consistent with SCLE developed after 6 months to 5 years of CCB therapy for arterial hypertension in the 9 patients. Four patients were taking diltiazem; 4, verapamil; and 1, nifedipine. Serologic assessment showed antinuclear antibodies in 7 patients, anti-Ro antibodies in 5, and anti-La antibodies in 5. Three patients had anti-La antibodies only. All patients underwent skin biopsy. The specimens were found to be characteristic of SCLE based on light microscopy and direct and indirect immunofluorescence. Treatment with CCB was stopped in all patients, and the eruptions resolved in 8 patients.

Conclusion.—The CCBs may induce Ro and La antigen displacement by changing cytosolic calcium levels and provoking immune perturbation. This would allow the emergence of autoantibodies that may bind to Ro or La, initiating complement-mediated lysis and antibody-dependent cytoxicity against keratinocytes in the manner postulated for idiopathic SCLE.

▶ Add CCBs to the list of drugs that can induce a form of lupus erythematosus. In this case, and in distinction to the systemic disease induced by Pronestyl and hydralazine, CCBs induce SCLE accompanied by the characteristic autoantibodies of that syndrome, anti Ro and anti La. The case for the drugs being implicated is good but not perfect because, although the clinical disease faded quickly after cessation of drug therapy, no patients were challenged with the drug after remission of clinical skin disease to see whether clinical disease could be exacerbated. Why and how CCBs induce SCLE and anti Ro and anti La are most interesting questions; the answers should elucidate important aspects of the pathogenesis of SCLE and the regulation of autoantibody production.

M. Reichlin, M.D.

Association of Anti-Ribosomal P Protein Antibodies With Neuropsychiatric Systemic Lupus Erythematosus

Isshi K, Hirohata S (Teikyo Univ, Tokyo)

Arthritis Rheum 39:1483–1490, 1996 3–27

Background.—The clinical correlation between antiribosomal P protein antibodies (anti-Ps) and systemic lupus erythematosus (SLE) has not been clearly defined, although anti-Ps are reportedly highly specific for lupus psychosis. The association between anti-P and neuropsychiatric SLE was re-evaluated.

Methods.—With the use of glutaraldehyde, human serum albumin (HSA) was conjugated with highly purified synthetic ribosomal P peptides of the carboxyterminal 22–amino-acid sequence. An enzyme-linked immunosorbent assay (ELISA) using HSA-ribosomal P peptide conjugates as antigens was used to analyze anti-P in the sera of 26 patients with SLE and no CNS disease, 28 patients with SLE and lupus psychosis, and 21 patients with SLE and nonpsychotic CNS involvement. Nonspecific binding activities to HSA were subtracted to quantitate anti-P levels.

TABLE 3.—Frequency of Anti-Ribosomal P Protein Antibodies in Different Groups of Systemic Lupus Erythematosus Patients

Patient group	n	Anti-ribosomal P Positive	Anti-ribosomal P Negative	% positive
SLE without CNS manifestation	26	2	24	7.7
Lupus psychosis*	28	14	14	50.0†
Nonpsychotic CNS lupus	21	5	16	23.8

Note: Values are the number of patients, except where indicated. Positive is defined as ≥ 3 SD above the mean serum anti-P values for normal healthy individuals.

*These patients have organic brain syndrome ($n = 9$) or nonorganic psychosis ($n = 19$).

†Significant at $P < 0.005$ compared with the other 2 patient groups, as determined by χ^2 test.

Abbreviation: SLE, systemic lupus erythematosus.

(Courtesy of Isshi K, Hirohata S: Association of anti-ribosomal P protein antibodies with neuropsychiatric systemic lupus erythematosus. *Arthritis Rheum* 39:1483–1490, 1996, copyright American College of Rheumatology.)

Results.—As compared with Western blotting, the ELISA proved specific for anti-P. Patients with lupus psychosis (either organic or nonorganic) had significantly higher levels of anti-P in serum than did patients with non-CNS SLE or nonpyschotic CNS lupus (Table 3). Serum anti-P levels did not differ with regard to organic brain syndrome vs. nonorganic psychosis. Serum anti-P levels significantly decreased in 6 patients with lupus psychosis after they were treated (Fig 3). Neither patients with lupus psychosis or with nonpsychotic CNS lupus had anti-P antibodies in CSF.

Conclusion.—These data confirm the correlation between serum anti-P and lupus psychosis. The conflicting results reported in the literature for this association may have been affected by differences in the purity of the ribosomal P peptides used. Anti-P in serum, but not in CSF, could play a nonspecific role in the development of diffuse cerebral damage.

► Since Bonfa and colleagues demonstrated an association between lupus psychosis and anti-P in 1987,[1] there has been controversy regarding this association.[2] This study from Japan finds a clear-cut association between lupus psychosis as well as nonpsychotic CNS disease and anti-P. One of the suggestions from this paper is that the synthetic 22–amino-acid carbonyl terminus—which is the immunodominant epitope when bound to human serum albumin—is a particularly suitable antigen for quantitative ELISA. Furthermore, in 6 patients followed serially, improvement in the psychosis was associated with a decline in serum anti-P titers. This paper provides powerful evidence of the reality of this association and may offer useful insights as to appropriate forms of the antigen.

M. Reichlin, M.D.

References

1. Bonfa E, Golombek S, Kaufman L, et al: Association between lupus psychosis and anti-ribosomal P protein antibodies. *N Engl J Med* 317:265–271, 1987.
2. Teh L-S, Isenberg DA: Anti-ribosomal P protein antibodies in systemic lupus erythematosus: A reappraisal. *Arthritis Rheum* 378:307–315, 1994.

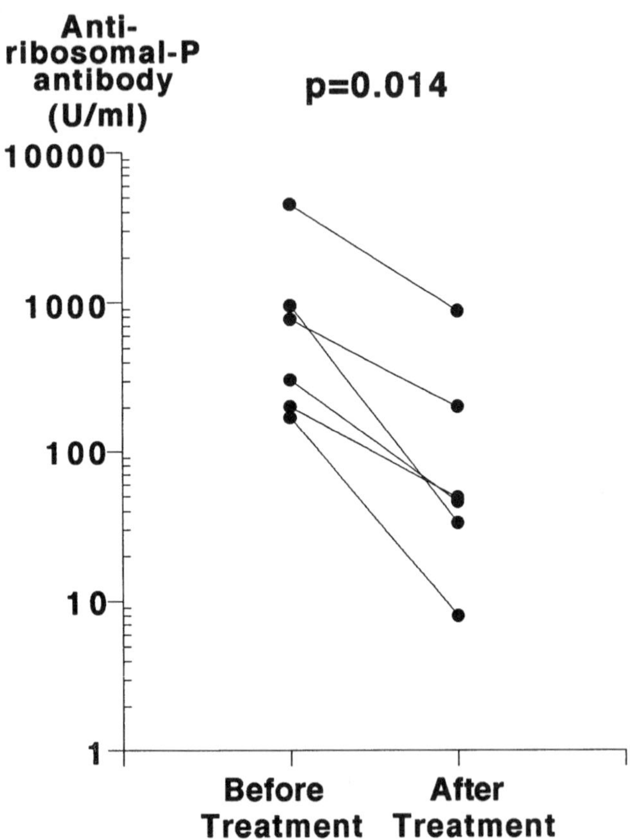

FIGURE 3.—Changes in serum anti-ribosomal P antibody levels (units per milliliter) after treatment in 6 patients with lupus psychosis. Statistical analysis was performed with Wilcoxon signed rank test. (Courtesy of Isshi K, Hirohata S: Association of anti-ribosomal P protein antibodies with neuropsychiatric systemic lupus erythematosus. *Arthritis Rheum* 39:1483–1490, 1996, copyright American College of Rheumatology.)

Therapy

Serum Complement Determinations in Patients With Quiescent Systemic Lupus Erythematosus

Sullivan KE, Wisnieski JJ, Winkelstein JA, et al (Children's Hosp of Philadelphia; Cleveland Veterans Affairs Med Ctr, Ohio; Johns Hopkins Univ, Baltimore, Md)

J Rheumatol 23:2063–2067, 1996 3–28

Background.—Systemic lupus erythematosus (SLE) is a multisystem inflammatory syndrome characterized by flares and remissions. Hypocomplementemia is believed to be a characteristic of patients with SLE at risk for organ damage. This hypocomplementemia is the result of the

TABLE 3.—New Onset of Clinical Features of the Complement Consumption Group Compared With the Control Population

	Consumption Group, %	Control Group, %	P
Anti-dsDNA*	8	2	0.19
False positive RPR	0	1	1.00
Arthritis	8	2	0.13
Malar rash	3	1	0.07
Livedo reticularis	0	2	1.00
Proteinuria	4	1	0.31
Hematuria	8	3	0.26
Renal insufficiency	20	0	<0.0001†
Renal failure	0	1	1.00
Hemolytic anemia	8	1	0.07
Leukopenia	4	1	0.31
Thrombocytopenia	4	1	0.31
Pericarditis	0	1	1.00
Pleuritis	4	1	0.31
Vasculitis	4	0	0.17
Stroke	4	0	0.17
Seizures	4	0	0.17

*ANA, anti-Sm, anti-Ro, anti-RNP, and anti-La titers were not serially recorded.
†Significance remains if adjusted for multiple comparisons.
Abbreviation: RPR, rapid plasma reagin.
(Courtesy of Sullivan KE, Wisnieski JJ, Winkelstein JA, et al: Serum complement determinations in patients with quiescent systemic lupus erythematosus. *J Rheumatol* 23:2063–2067, 1996.)

consumption of early complement components in the activation of the classical complement pathway. During inactive disease periods, complement levels might define an at-risk SLE subpopulation. To examine whether complement component determinations during a period of inactive disease could be used to define clinically important subgroups or predict morbidity, patients from the Johns Hopkins Lupus Cohort were evaluated when their disease was inactive.

Methods.—The Johns Hopkins Lupus Cohort has enrolled patients with SLE since 1987. Patients are seen at least 4 times each year, when laboratory studies and clinical activity are monitored. Sera were obtained during a period of disease inactivity in 277 patients with SLE who were followed for an average of 4 years. These sera were analyzed for levels of Clq, Clr, Cls, C3, C4, and CH100.

Results.—Of the 277 SLE patients in the study group, 25 had hypocomplementemia and another 24 had a very low level of a single complement component. The group with hypocomplementemia was significantly more likely to progress over time to renal insufficiency than those in the study group with normal complement levels (Table 3), but there were no other clinical associations with low levels of complement factors.

Conclusion.—In a group of patients with inactive SLE studied to examine the relationship between complement levels and prognosis, the only association detected was between hypocomplementemia and eventual renal insufficiency. Complement component evaluation during periods of inactive disease is not useful in predicting long-term outcome but may identify those at increased risk of long-term renal insufficiency.

▶ It has long been suspected that persistent hypocomplementemia in the face of clinical quiescence may not mean all is well, especially in the kidneys of patients with SLE. That is the message of this paper. Inactive SLE with multiple low complement determinations is associated with increased risk of renal insufficiency. The question then becomes Does the risk of complement normalization with steroids and/or immunosuppressives exceed the risk of doing nothing and observing patients as they slip into renal insufficiency? This was a point not addressed by the authors, but it is surely one faced by clinicians in day-to-day practice. At the moment, treatment decisions in this setting have to be made without benefit of controlled trials.

M. Reichlin, M.D.

Hydroxychloroquine in Pregnant Patients With Systemic Lupus Erythematosus

Parke A, West B (Univ of Connecticut, Farmington)

J Rheumatol 23:1715–1718, 1996 3–29

Background.—Antimalarial drugs containing the 4-aminoquinoline radical are useful for controlling the manifestations of systemic lupus erythematosus (SLE) and discoid lupus. Discontinuing these agents may result in disease flare ups. In pregnant women, the discontinuation of antimalarial drugs not only puts the mother's health at risk but also compromises pregnancy outcomes. The safety of continuing antimalarial drugs during pregnancy was investigated.

Methods and Findings.—Nine pregnancies in 8 patients with SLE were documented. All the women took hydroxychloroquine throughout their pregnancies. All 9 babies were born alive; 5 were preterm and 4 were at term. None of the infants had congenital abnormalities. At a mean follow-up of 33 months, no other abnormalities were found in the children. In 1 woman, a 1-month discontinuation of hydroxychloroquine precipitated a disease flare up, which was documented clinically and serologically.

Conclusions.—These findings show that continuing hydroxychloroquine during pregnancy is safer than discontinuing it. The authors are not aware of any reports of fetal toxicity associated with hydroxychloroquine exposure at the dosages recommended for women with connective tissue disorders.

▶ A common practice among rheumatologists and obstetricians is to discontinue hydroxychloroquine in patients with SLE when they become pregnant. Two major reasons have formed the basis for this practice: the 4-aminoquinoline drugs cross the placenta, and hydroxychloroquine is related to the more toxic and now infrequently used drug, chloroquine. In fact, because it has been shown that discontinuing hydroxychloroquine increases the risk of flare ups, there is good reason to continue it during pregnancy. Moreover, accumulating evidence suggests a low if unmeasurable level of toxicity of hydroxychloroquine for the fetus.

Such is the message of this paper. The risk of not using hydroxychloroquine in pregnancy exceeds the risk of continuing the drug, especially with regard to successful completion of pregnancy.

M. Reichlin, M.D.

Methotrexate in Nonrenal Lupus and Undifferentiated Connective Tissue Disease: A Review of 36 Patients

Wise CM, Vuyyuru S, Roberts WN (Med College of Virginia, Richmond)
J Rheumatol 23:1005–1010, 1996 3–30

Introduction.—Methotrexate (MTX) has become an increasingly popular therapy for patients with RA and may be of value in the treatment of other inflammatory diseases. Medical records were reviewed for 21 patients with systemic lupus erythematosus (SLE) and 15 with undifferentiated connective tissue disease to determine the efficacy, toxicity, and steroid-sparing effect of MTX in these conditions.

Methods.—Patients were identified from a database of 467 patients seen for connective tissue diseases. Charts were reviewed for duration of illness, disease activity, other disease manifestations, previous and concurrent drug therapy, toxicity, and steroid reduction during MTX treatment.

Results.—Patients with SLE ranged in age from 50 to 62 years; 18 were women, 11 were white, and 10 were black. Common clinical manifestations of disease were arthritis and rashes, each reported in 18 patients. Nine patients had hematologic disorders. In 11 cases, MTX was given in an effort to reduce steroid requirements. During the course of MTX, 16 patients received corticosteroids for SLE manifestations, 13 were given hydroxychloroquine, and 2 were treated with azathioprine. Most patients began receiving MTX with a dose of 7.5 mg weekly. Mean doses increased in those continuing to receive the drug to 17.9 mg/week at 18 months (36% of those starting treatment). Response to MTX was sustained in 6 patients and partial in 6. The drug was more effective in patients treated for arthritis and cutaneous disease than in those given MTX for CNS dysfunction or serositis. Toxicities were reported in 62% of the patients, and one third had to discontinue treatment. The most common adverse effects were stomatitis and infections. Prednisone dosage was able to be reduced substantially in 9 patients and discontinued in 3. Patients with undifferentiated connective tissue disease showed a similar pattern of response and toxicity to MTX. Half of the evaluable patients had discontinued MTX by 12 months.

Discussion.—Methotrexate was of modest efficacy in SLE. Most responses were in patients with arthritis and cutaneous disease. Although steroid requirements were usually reduced, few patients could discontinue these agents. Compared with patients with RA who received MTX, these patients with SLE had a higher rate of toxicity and a lower rate of response.

▶ The irreversible toxicities of steroids—osteopenia and accelerated atherosclerosis—are sufficiently disabling and lethal that any steroid-sparing approach is welcome. Perhaps, as the authors suggest, cyclophosphamide can be used for renal and CNS lupus involvement and MTX for skin, serosal, and synovial involvement. Even here, toxicities are substantial (62% of patients, 33% sufficient to discontinue) but perhaps more manageable.

E.C. LeRoy, M.D.

Dosing Implications of a Clinical Interaction Between Grapefruit Juice and Cyclosporine and Metabolite Concentrations in Patients With Autoimmune Diseases

Ioannides-Demos LL, Christophidis N, Ryan P, et al (Monash Univ, Victoria, Australia)

J Rheumatol 24:49–54, 1997 3–31

Background.—Cyclosporine is frequently used to treat patients with various autoimmune conditions, including RA. In inflammatory diseases such as RA, cyclosporine exerts effects on T cells and on bone, cartilage, and synovial cells. Cyclosporine concentrations in blood can be influenced by various medications and food constituents. The effect of long-term grapefruit juice administration on blood concentrations of cyclosporine was examined in a group of 9 patients.

Methods.—The randomized crossover study included adult patients with autoimmune diseases. All had been stabilized with administration of cyclosporine oral capsules. The morning and evening cyclosporine doses were taken with either 150 mL grapefruit juice or water. Whole blood samples were collected before the morning dose and during the 12-hour interdose interval. A relatively specific homogeneous enzyme immunoassay was used to measure whole blood cyclosporine; total metabolite concentrations were estimated with a nonspecific assay.

Results.—The 9 patients had a mean age of 36.1 years and a mean daily dose of cyclosporine of 3.4 mg/kg. One patient experienced significant side effects when taking grapefruit juice. Administration of the juice was associated with an increase of 68.9% in her cyclosporine trough concentrations and 214% in total metabolite levels. For the group as a whole, the mean steady-state cyclosporine trough concentrations were 128 µg/L with water and 182 µg/L with grapefruit juice. The mean steady-state metabolite trough concentrations were 203 µg/L with water and 295 µg/L with grapefruit juice (Fig 1). Exposure to grapefruit juice also produced significant increases in the area under the cyclosporine and metabolite blood concentration–time curves.

Conclusion.—Ingestion of grapefruit juice by patients receiving cyclosporine for various autoimmune diseases led to variable but significant

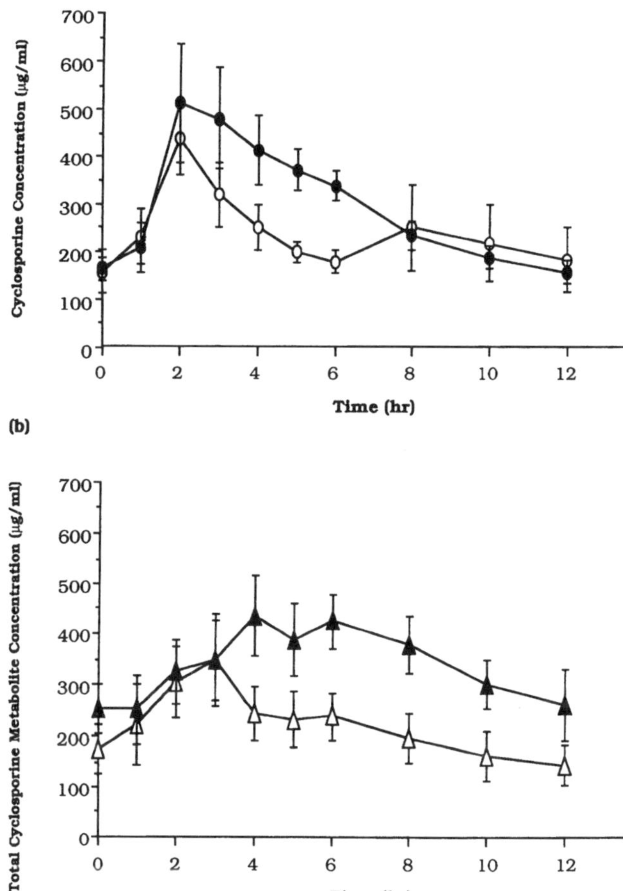

FIGURE 1.—Cyclosporine data normalized for a 3-mg/kg dose and presented as mean plus or minus standard error of the mean ($n = 9$). **A**, steady-state cyclosporine concentrations with water (*open circle*) or grapefruit juice (*closed circle*), and **B**, total steady-state cyclosporine metabolites after water (*open triangle*) or grapefruit juice (*closed triangle*). (Courtesy of Ioannides-Demos LL, Christophidis N, Ryan P, et al: Dosing implications of a clinical interaction between grapefruit juice and cyclosporine and metabolite concentrations in patients with autoimmune diseases. *J Rheumatol* 24:49–54, 1997.)

changes in the kinetics of cyclosporine and metabolites. In 1 patient, these pharmacokinetic changes were associated with an adverse neurologic episode. Cyclosporine dosing needs to be individualized in all patients because of the possibility of metabolic interactions.

► Rheumatologists who treat patients with cyclosporine are in ever-increasing numbers as the number of patients with rheumatic diseases treated with this agent grows. As with all drugs, interactions with other pharmaceuticals can increase or decrease levels of this agent by interfering with or enhancing its metabolism, its binding to serum proteins, etc. It now appears that grapefruit juice profoundly affects cyclosporine levels, probably by interfering with cytochrome p450 activity, the metabolic pathway for cyclosporine. Having struggled with erratic cyclosporine levels in a patient recently treated, I am now alerted to a common food that can greatly elevate cyclosporine levels.

M. Reichlin, M.D.

Reduction in Circulating dsDNA Antibody Titer After Administration of LJP 394

Weisman MH, Bluestein HG, Berner CM, et al (Univ of California, San Diego)
J Rheumatol 24:314–318, 1997 3–32

Background.—LJP 394 is a novel immunomodulant designed to reduce double-stranded DNA antibodies (anti-dsDNA) by inducing highly selective B-lymphocyte tolerance. This agent has been shown to delay the progression of renal disease and to extend survival in the BXBS experimental murine lupus nephritis model. The safety and immunologic effects of this novel toleragen agent in patients with systemic lupus erythematosus (SLE) were investigated.

Methods.—Four women with stable SLE received a 100-mg infusion of LJP 394. Follow-up was 4 weeks. Measures of safety variables and anti-dsDNA, circulating immune complexes, complement, and complement split products were obtained.

Findings.—Double-stranded DNA antibody titers declined promptly with treatment. Four weeks after the infusion, titers in 2 patients were still less than baseline values. In the remaining 2, titers returned to pretreatment levels. Although transient increases occurred in some complement split products, there were no adverse clinical events during or immediately after infusion.

Conclusion.—In these 4 patients with SLE, LJP 394 infusion safely and effectively reduced anti-dsDNA. The most likely explanation for this finding is immune complex formation and rapid elimination.

► Antibodies to dsDNA are highly specific for SLE, their titer fluctuates with disease activity, and they are likely involved in tissue damage. Treatment with steroids and/or immunosuppressive drugs is usually required for a decrease in titer of these antibodies and for clinical improvement. Therapy with a dsDNA analogue described in this paper has several attractive features. First, it is immunologically specific and, second, its administration did not provoke any adverse effects. Conceivably, such therapies could eventually induce tolerance and provide an aspect of treatment much safer than that presently used by rheumatologists, as described above. If this therapy works, it will eventually find its place in the armamentarium used in the treatment of SLE.

M. Reichlin, M.D.

Ongoing Immunologic Activity After Short Courses of Pulse Cyclophosphamide in the NZB/W Murine Model of Systemic Lupus Erythematosus

Austin HA III, Patel AD, Cadena CA, et al (Natl Inst of Diabetes and Digestive and Kidney Diseases, Bethesda, Md)

J Rheumatol 24:61–68, 1997 3–33

Background.—Systemic lupus erythematosus (SLE) is characterized by hyperactive B cells that secrete immunoglobulins reactive to a range of self and nonself antigens. Cytotoxic drug therapy can be an effective treatment for this disorder, but it has serious side effects. To overcome some of these side effects, pulse cyclophosphamide (CY) has been used as a treatment for SLE, but relapses are not uncommon. To determine the efficacy of short-term pulsatile CY therapy on SLE, a mouse model of SLE, the female NZB/NZW (B/W) mouse, was used.

Methods.—Five-month-old female B/W mice were randomly assigned to treatment with either a single or 4 monthly intraperitoneal injections of CY or served as controls (no treatment). At intervals, control and treatment animals were sacrificed and the phenotypic and functional characteristics of their spleen lymphocytes were compared.

Results.—After one dose of CY, spleen lymphocyte subpopulations decreased rapidly, but recovered within 4 weeks. After 4 monthly doses of CY, there was a sustained reduction in spleen lymphocyte subpopulations

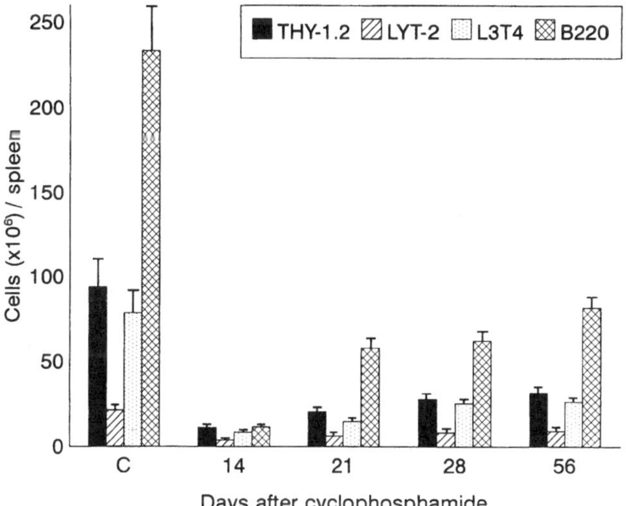

FIGURE 2.—Spleen lymphocyte populations in 8.5- to 10-month-old NZB/NZW (B/W) mice 14–56 days after 4 monthly intraperitoneal cyclophosphamide injections (250 mg/kg; initiated at 5 months of age) and in 8.5-month-old untreated control B/W mice (C). Results represent the mean +/− standard error of the mean of 5 control mice and 4 treated mice at each time point. Key refers to cell subsets. (Courtesy of Austin HA III, Patel AD, Cadena CA, et al: Ongoing immunologic activity after short courses of pulse cyclophosphamide in the NZB/W murine model of systemic lupus erythematosus. *J Rheumatol* 24:61–68, 1997.)

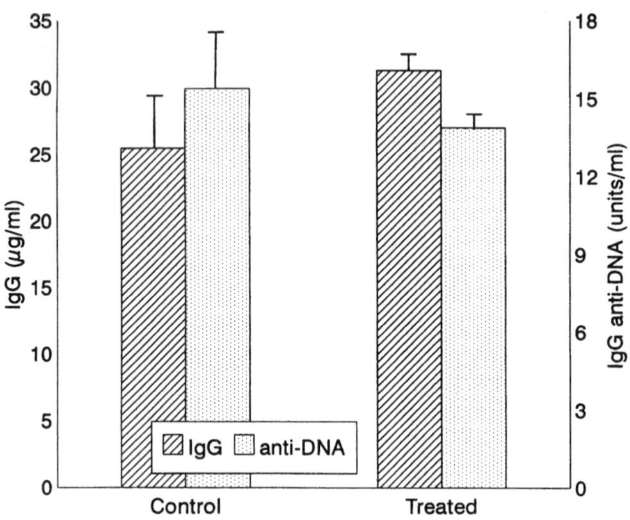

FIGURE 6.—Supernatant concentrations of IgG (**left axis**) and IgG anti-ssDNA antibody (**right axis**) after spleen cell suspensions were cultured for 5 days with 50 μg/mL of lipopolysaccharide. Spleen cells were obtained from 9-month-old NZB/NZW (B/W) mice 28 days after 4 monthly injections of intraperitoneal cyclophosphamide (treated) and from 9-month-old untreated (control) B/W mice. Results represent the mean +/− standard error of the mean of 6 mice in each group. (Courtesy of Austin HA III, Patel AD, Cadena CA, et al: Ongoing immunologic activity after short courses of pulse cyclophosphamide in the NZB/W murine model of systemic lupus erythematosus. *J Rheumatol* 24:61–68, 1997.)

and a decrease in the number of spleen cells that spontaneously secreted immunoglobulin and anti-DNA antibody to approximately 30% of the number in control mice (Fig 2). Lipopolysaccharide-induced secretion of total IgG and anti-DNA IgG by cultured spleen cells was not decreased 1 month after completion of the 4-month CY treatment cycle (Fig 6).

Conclusion.—When female B/W mice were treated with a 4-month course of intraperitoneal CY, there was a significant reduction in the number of activated B cells that produced autoantibody, but immunomodulation was not sustained. This suggests that there will be a continued susceptibility to flare-ups of SLE after brief, intense courses of cytotoxic drug therapy. Further studies are needed to define the optimal approach to treatment of SLE.

► The use of immunosuppressive therapy, especially with cytoxan, is of continuing concern in patients with SLE. Continuous oral therapy is probably most effective but has considerable toxicity. Intravenous pulse therapy seems safer but may be less immunosuppressive. This paper shows that 4 months of intraperitoneal pulse therapy in B/W mice reduces, but does not eliminate, autoreactive B cells. Clearly, short term intraperitoneal cytoxan therapy prolongs life from a median survival of about 300–485 days but does not eliminate the autoreactivity that eventually kills the mouse. Longer-term intermittent therapies are more effective in B/W mice, but for humans, it would appear that strategies other than simply intermittent cytoxan are needed to completely control this disease.

M. Reichlin, M.D.

Sjögren's Syndrome

Sudden Onset Unilateral Renomegaly as an Initial Manifestation of Primary Sjögren's Syndrome in a Teenage Girl

Manthorpe R (Malmö Univ, Sweden)

Scand J Rheumatol 25:186–188, 1996 3–34

Introduction.—Primary Sjögren's syndrome usually appears between the ages of 30 and 50 years, and diagnosis is often delayed because disease symptoms are complex. The case reported is unusual in the age of the patient (18 years) and initial manifestation (sudden onset of unilateral renomegaly).

Case Report.—Woman, 18, reported left-sided abdominal pain. She had no genetic history of connective tissue or kidney disease and her routine clinical examination was normal. Abdominal studies with CT and ultrasound showed the left kidney to be clearly enlarged, with perirenal fluid spreading to the pelvic region and left pleural cavity (Fig 1). The patient's pain decreased during the following days, and the kidney had returned to normal at 2 months. Biopsy specimens from perirenal fluid showed a very high ANA titer, normal anti-DNA, and positive anti-SS-A and anti-SS-B antibodies. A lower lip biopsy was then done, revealing autoimmune sialadenitis with a focus score of 2 (Fig 2, B). Tests subse-

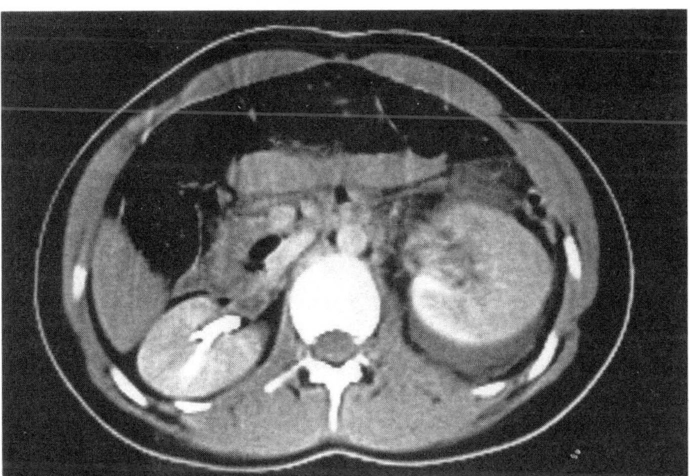

FIGURE 1.—Computed tomography of the abdomen in woman, 18 years, with sudden onset of left-sided abdominal pain. The left kidney—at the right side of the picture—measures 60 × 62 mm (transverse × anterior/posterior diameter) at the hilum of the kidney. The right kidney measures 40 × 51 mm at the hilum. Both kidneys are 10 cm in length—not shown. The unilateral renomegaly is surrounded by fluid. The renomegaly started to diminish after 10 days and both kidneys had equal size at 2 months. (Courtesy of Manthorpe R: Sudden onset unilateral renomegaly as an initial manifestation of primary Sjögren's syndrome in a teenage girl. *Scand J Rheumatol* 25:186–188, 1996.)

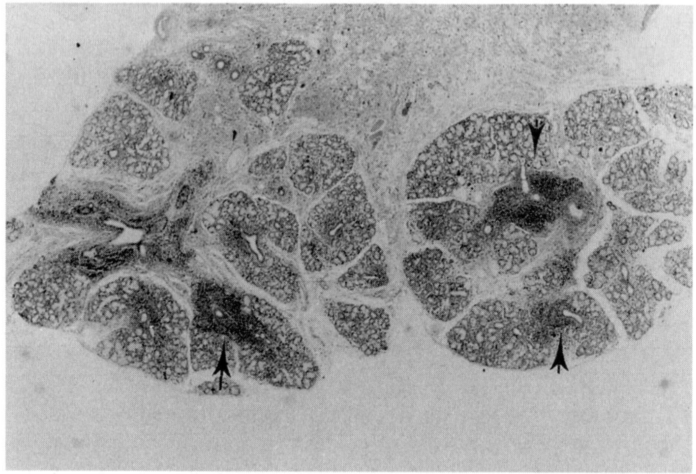

FIGURE 2, B.—Biopsy specimen from lower lip (hematoxylin-eosin; original magnification, ×35) showing larger *(arrows)* and smaller lymphoid aggregates (autoimmune sialadenitis) with focus score of 2. (Courtesy of Manthorpe R: Sudden onset unilateral renomegaly as an initial manifestation of primary Sjögren's syndrome in a teenage girl. *Scand J Rheumatol* 25:186–188, 1996.)

quently performed at a Sjögren's syndrome research center confirmed that the patient fulfilled classification criteria for primary Sjögren's syndrome. Although she was not experiencing persistent dry eyes and dry mouth, all objective tests for keratoconjunctivitis sicca and xerostomia were abnormal.

Discussion.—The most common cause of left-sided abdominal pain in a teenager or young adult is urolithiasis. In this case, however, there was no history of stone attacks or groin pain. Histologic examinations of perirenal fluid and the renal biopsy seemed to favor a nonurologic explanation. Because there are morphologic and functional similarities among kidney and salivary/lacrimal glands, the case suggests that sudden-onset 1-sided renomegaly may be related to the more common sudden-onset unilateral swelling of the salivary and lacrimal glands occurring in patients with primary Sjögren's syndrome.

▶ The kidney is not usually considered a part of Sjögren's syndrome, although interstitial nephritis is recognized by authorities such as Jacob Churg. In this case, the nephritis was essentially unilateral, as is often the case with the parotitis, which may wax and wane for years before becoming a more generalized sialadenitis. This is a worthy topic for a search for cross-reactive epitopes in renal tubules and salivary ductular epithelium or basal lamina. Could laminin or nidogen be involved? With precise epitope information, could a blocking immune response be devised?

E.C. LeRoy, M.D.

Identification of α-Fodrin as a Candidate Autoantigen in Primary Sjögren's Syndrome

Haneji N, Nakamura T, Takio K, et al (Tokushimia Univ, Japan; Inst of Physical and Chemical Research, Wako, Japan)

Science 276:604–607, 1997 3–35

Background.—The pathogenesis of Sjögren's syndrome (SS) is still unknown. The role of organ-specific autoantigens is not clear. Protein immunoblot analysis was done to detect a salivary gland autoantigen reactive with affinity-purified IgG from the sera of a mouse model of human SS.

Methods and Findings.—A 120-kd organ-specific autoantigen was purified from the salivary gland tissues of 3-d-Tx NFS/*sld* mice. The amino-terminal residues were identical to α-Fodrin, a human cytoskeletal protein. The purified antigen induced proliferative T-cell responses. In addition, it induced the production of interleukin-2 and interferon-τ in vitro. Neonatal immunization with the 120-kd antigen prevented SS in this mouse model. Sera obtained from patients with SS reacted positively with purified antigen and recombinant human α-fodrin protein. Sera from patients with systemic lupus erythematosus and rheumatoid arthritis did not (Fig 4).

Conclusion.—The identification of the salivary gland 120-kd α-fodrin will help to elucidate the crucial role of this autoantigen in the development of primary SS. If the 120-kd α-fodrin plays a critical role in initiating exocrinopathy, preventing or reversing the autoimmune response to it in the salivary and lacrimal glands may constitute a therapeutic approach.

▶ There are several outstanding questions regarding the etiology and pathogenesis of primary SS. Among the most important questions is why the salivary and lacrimal glands are targeted for destruction. An immunologic answer would involve the identification of an organ-specific immune response, which until now has been lacking. These workers in Japan claim to have found the responsible antigen in 2 systems: (1) a mouse model with the cryptic designation 3-d-Tx NFS/*sld,* which translates into 3-day-old NFS/*sld* mice that have been thymectomized, and (2) humans with primary SS.

The culprit antigen is α-fodrin, a 120-kd protein which is a proteolytic product of 240-kd α-protein which forms a heterodimer with a 235-kd β-protein. This is a cytoskeletal protein which dramatically rearranges when the parotid gland does the business of secretion. Moreover, the 120-kd α-protein is cleaved from the larger α-protein during apoptosis. The data are impressive in the mouse model where this disease can be prevented by neonatal injection of purified recombinant protein, and antibodies to the purified or recombinant protein are specifically found in humans with primary SS.

We now await confirmation of these findings by others, as well as an explanation of the mechanics underlying the selection of this antigen as the inciting event in the exocrinopathy of primary SS. Time will tell whether this work is as important as it appears to be.

M. Reichlin, M.D.

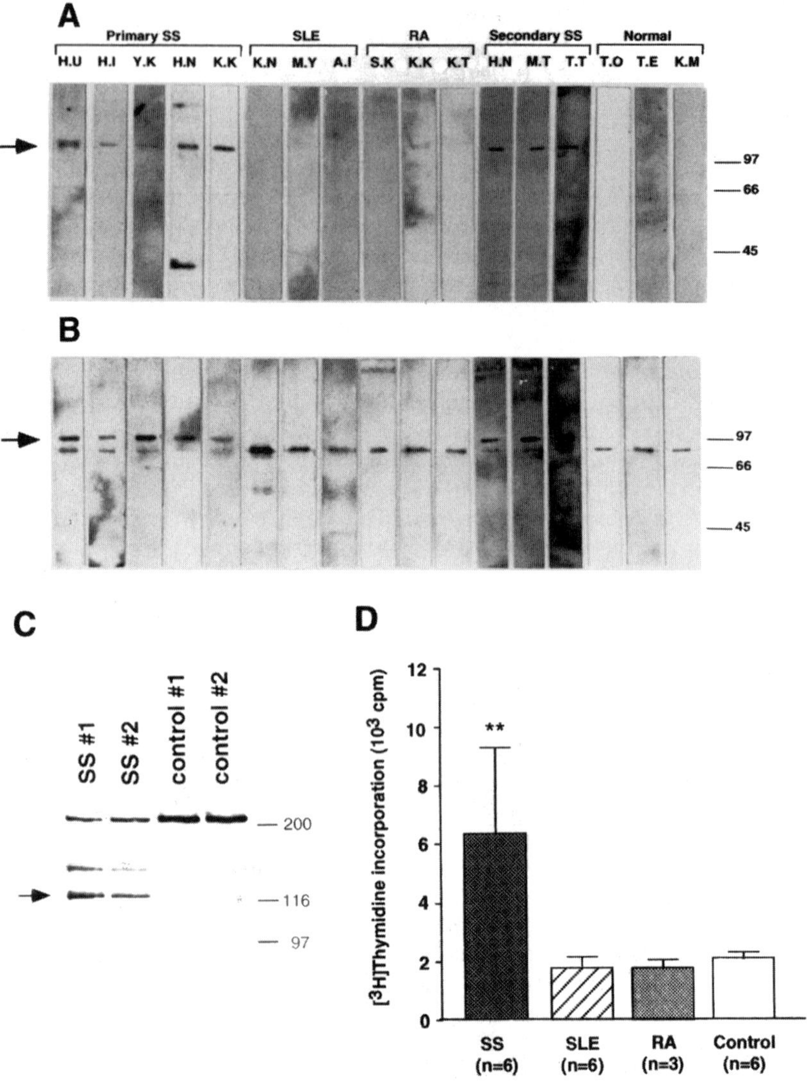

FIGURE 4.—Protein immunoblot analysis of the 120-kd α-fodrin and recombinant fusion protein JS-1 with sera from patients with various autoimmune diseases. Serum samples were tested in duplicate at a 1:250 dilution. Representative immunoblotting profiles were selected from each group. **A**, protein immunoblots of the purified 120-kd α-fodrin. **B**, protein immunoblots of JS-1 (70-kd protein is an artifact band of *Escherichia coli* degradation). **C**, protein immunoblot analysis of mouse monoclonal antibody to α-fodrin (AFFINITI, Exeter, England) with labial gland homogenates from patients with primary Sjögren's syndrome (*SS*) (N = 2), and control individuals with labial gland mucous cyst (N = 2). D, Proliferative response of peripheral blood mononuclear cells (PBMCs) to the purified 120-kd antigen. A significant response was detected in PBMCs from patients with primary SS (N = 6) but not with systemic lupus erythematosus (*SLE*) (N = 6), rheumatoid arthritis (*RA*) (N = 3), or healthy controls (N = 6). Data are mean counts per minute per culture ± standard deviation of triplicate samples (*double asterisks, P* < 0.001). (Reprinted with full permission from *Science,* courtesy of Haneji N, Nakamura T, Takio K, et al: Identification of α-fodrin as a candidate autoantigen in primary Sjögren's syndrome. *Science* 276:604–607. Copyright 1997, American Association for the Advancement of Science.)

***FAS* and *FAS* Ligand Expression in the Salivary Glands of Patients With Primary Sjögren's Syndrome**

Kong L, Ogawa N, Nakabayashi T, et al (Univ of Texas, San Antonio)
Arthritis Rheum 40:87–97, 1997 3–36

Background.—The mechanism of glandular parenchyma destruction in primary Sjögren's syndrome (SS) remains obscure. The role of the *Fas*-mediated apoptosis in the salivary glands of patients with this syndrome was investigated.

Methods.—Biopsy specimens of 20 labial salivary glands and 2 parotid glands were obtained from 21 women and 1 man meeting criteria for primary SS. Immunohistochemical staining and reverse transcriptase–polymerase chain reaction were performed to detect expression of *Fas*, *Fas* ligand (*Fas*L), and *bcl*-2. The enzymatic incorporation of labeled nucleotides was performed to assess DNA fragmentation in apoptotic cells.

Findings.—The acinar epihhelial cells were positive for *Fas* and *Fas*L. These cells died by apoptosis. Most infiltrating lymphocytes in SS were positive for *Fas* and *bcl*-2, whereas few lymphocytes expressed *Fas*L. Cell death of lymphocytes was minimal, especially in dense periductal foci, in the in situ detection of apoptosis. Compared with that in the interstitium, lymphocytic cell death was significantly decreased in these foci.

Conclusion.—In patients with SS, infiltrating lymphocytes in the focal lesions of the salivary glands are blocked in their ability to commit to apoptosis, although they may express *Fas*. This inability to undergo apoptosis may be explained by the presence of *bcl*-2. By contrast, the acinar epithelial cells may undergo *Fas*-mediated apoptosis. Thus, the *Fas* death pathway may be an important mechanism in the glandular destruction associated with SS.

► We know that the glandular epithelium in SS is destroyed either by, or in association with, the invasion of the gland and its replacement by dense collections of lymphocytes, most of them carrying the CD4 marker. It now appears that the glandular cells may be dying from programmed cell death (apoptosis) mediated by *Fas* (the molecule mediating the signals of apoptosis), and the lymphocytes infiltrating the gland may be egged on and sustained by increased levels of the factor *bcl*-2, which inhibits apoptosis. Knowledge of these perverse pathologic events may sharpen our focus on methods for better understanding the stimuli that lead to these pathophysiologic phenomena and help us devise better strategies for saving these glands.

M. Reichlin, M.D.

Common T Cell Receptor Clonotype in Lacrimal Glands and Labial Salivary Glands From Patients With Sjögren's Syndrome

Matsumoto I, Tsubota K, Satake Y, et al (Chiba Univ, Japan; Tokyo Dental College, Chiba; Toho Univ, Chiba, Japan; et al)
J Clin Invest 97:1969–1977, 1996 3–37

Background.—Sjögren's syndrome (SS), an autoimmune disease, involves lymphocytic infiltration into lacrimal and salivary glands that results in dry eyes and mouth. Immunohistologic studies have shown that most infiltrating lymphocytes around the lacrimal and labial salivary glands are CD4 positive αβ T cells. The pathogenesis of T cells infiltrating into lacrimal and labial salivary glands was investigated.

Methods and Findings.—Four patients were studied. The T-cell clonotype of the cells infiltrating into both glands was examined with the use of polymerase chain reaction–single-strand conformation polymorphism (SSCP) and sequencing. Some infiltrating T cells in both glands expanded clonally, suggesting that the cells proliferate by antigen-driven stimulation. Commonly, 6–16 identical T-cell receptor (TCR) Vβ genes were detected in lacrimal and labial salivary glands from individual patients, indicating that some T cells infiltrating into both glands recognize the shared epitopes on autoantigens. Also, highly conserved amino acid sequence motifs occurred in the TCR CDR3 region with the same TCR Vβ family gene from the patients, suggesting that the shared epitopes on antigens are limited.

Conclusions.—In patients with SS, some T cells recognize shared epitopes on autoantigens from labial salivary and lacrimal glands. The targets recognized by autoreactive T cells should become clearer with the establishment of T-cell transfectants or T-cell lines from infiltrating T cells in several organs. Identifying the autoantigens at the amino acid level may enable the development of a new specific treatment approach to SS through the selective inactivation of autoreactive T cells by vaccination with analogue peptides.

► The central and characteristic pathologic feature of SS is the lymphocytic infiltration and destruction of the lacrimal and salivary glands. These lymphocytes have long been recognized to be CD4 positive, and there have been hints that they are restricted to a few Vβ gene families, which suggests a restricted response to a specific autoantigen. This paper emphasizes resoundingly that the lymphocytes in the gland are very restricted with 6–16 identical T-cell receptor Vβ genes, and that in an individual patient there are identical clonotypes in the 2 types of glands. It is then fairly certain that there is a shared epitope on a common autoepitope that drives this response. The question now: What is this antigenic target that drives this T-cell response and leads to the glandular destruction? Knowledge of this target should lead us to a clearer understanding of the immunopathogenesis of SS.

M. Reichlin, M.D.

Hepatitis C Virus Infection in 'Primary' Sjögren's Syndrome: Prevalence and Clinical Significance in a Series of 90 Patients

Garcia-Carrasco M, Ramos M, Cervera R, et al (Hosp Clinic, Barcelona)

Ann Rheum Dis 56:173–175, 1997 3–38

Background.—Patients with Sjögren's syndrome (SS) in the absence of an associated systemic autoimmune disease are classified as having "primary" SS. Although an association between hepatitis C virus (HCV) and SS has been postulated, little is known about the prevalence of HCV infection in primary SS.

Methods.—Eighty-three women and 7 men with SS were followed up prospectively. Patient age ranged from 31 to 80 years. Complete histories were obtained, together with physical examination and biochemical and immunologic assessment for liver disease. Serum was tested for antibodies to HCV by third generation enzyme-linked immunosorbent assay. Positive findings were confirmed by polymerase chain reaction.

Findings.—Fourteen percent of the patients with primary SS had antibodies to HCV. Compared with those without HCV infection, those with such infection had a greater prevalence of hepatic involvement. Transcutaneous liver biopsy, performed in 5 patients with HCV infection, showed chronic active hepatitis in all patients, with varying degrees of portal inflammation.

Conclusion.—Patients with primary SS commonly have HCV infection. All such patients have liver involvement. The possible pathogenic role of HCV infection in primary SS is not yet clear.

▶ A Spanish group has studied 90 consecutive patients with primary SS and found that 13 of these patients (14%) were infected with HCV and had active liver disease. The prevalence of HCV infection in the general population in that part of Spain is 1.2%, far less than in this group of patients with primary SS. This observation raises more questions than it answers. Are patients with primary SS more susceptible to HCV infection than persons without primary SS? Alternatively, is HCV infection the cause in a subset of patients with primary SS? How will α-interferon therapy for HCV infection affect the sicca components in such patients? It is of interest that α-interferon therapy for chronic myelocytic leukemia has been associated with the development of lupus-like syndromes, so untoward outcomes may follow appropriate therapy for the viral infection.

However, it will be of interest to see whether these observations are replicated in other parts of the world. If so, the answers to the kinds of questions raised above should improve our understanding of both primary SS and HCV infection.

M. Reichlin, M.D.

Mixed Monoclonal Cryoglobulinemia and Monoclonal Rheumatoid Factor Cross-Reactive Idiotypes as Predictive Factors for the Development of Lymphoma in Primary Sjögren's Syndrome

Tzioufas AG, Boumba DS, Skopouli FN, et al (Natl Univ of Athens, Greece; Univ of Ioannina, Greece)

Arthritis Rheum 39:767–772, 1996 3–39

Background.—Primary Sjögren's syndrome is a common chronic autoimmune disease involving lymphocytic infiltration of exocrine glands. In some affected patients, B-cell lymphoma develops. Whether mixed monoclonal cryoglobulinemia (MMC) and monoclonal rheumatoid factor (mRF)–associated cross-reactive idiotypes (CRIs) are predictive factors of B-cell lymphoma in these patients was prospectively assessed.

Methods.—From 1986 to 1991, 103 consecutive patients with primary Sjögren's syndrome were evaluated. The cryoglobulin content was measured with ultraviolet absorption at 280 nm and 260 nm, and the cryoglobulinemia type was determined with agarose gel electrophoresis and immunofixation. Enzyme-linked immunosorbent assay of sera was used to determine the presence of 3 immunoglobulin idiotypes.

Results.—During the first evaluation, MMC was found in 17.4% of patients with primary Sjögren's syndrome. The presence of MMC correlated significantly with a higher prevalence of autoantibodies to Ro/SS-A and La/SS-B and to extraglandular manifestations. Lymphomas developed in 7 patients during 5 years. Six of these patients (86%) had previous MMC, whereas only 12 of the 96 other patients (12.4%) had MMC. Cryoglobulin levels were higher in patients in whom lymphomas developed. Two of the 3 CRIs (17109 and G-6) occurred with the development of lymphomas, but this was dependent on the presence of MMC.

Conclusions.—Lymphoma development in patients with primary Sjögren's syndrome may be predicted by determination of MMC. It may also be predicted by the CRIs 17109 and G-6, particularly when the monoclonal component is absent. Prospective studies determining the sensitivity and specificity of these methods are needed.

► One of the serious complications of primary Sjögren's syndrome is the development of lymphomas. This paper teaches us that the presence of MMC is a predictive factor for the development of lymphomas. Of 7 patients with primary Sjögren's syndrome in whom lymphomas developed in a 5-year follow-up, 6 had MMC (86%), whereas of 96 patients in whom lymphomas did not develop 12 had MMC (12.4%). Two other serologic markers for CRIs were also predictive for lymphoma development but added nothing to the determination of MMC. The determination of the monoclonality of the cryoglobulin requires only agarose electrophoresis with immunofixation, a technique available in clinical laboratories all over the world. Thus, a simple method is at hand to predict the development of lymphomas when patients are first seen with primary Sjögren's syndrome.

M. Reichlin, M.D.

Decreased Reflex Tearing Is Associated With Lymphocytic Infiltration in Lacrimal Glands

Tsubota K, Xu K-P, Fujihara T, et al (Tokyo Dental College, Chiba; Keio Univ, Tokyo; Saitama Med Ctr, Japan)

J Rheumatol 23:313–320, 1996 3–40

Background.—The finding of dry eye is necessary but not sufficient by itself to diagnose Sjögren's syndrome. Results of the Schirmer test, used to assess lacrimal function, may be affected by causes other than lymphocytic infiltration of the lacrimal gland. The Schirmer test with nasal stimulation has been proposed to evaluate reflex tearing.

Methods.—Two hundred seventy-two patients with dry eye and regular Schirmer test results of less than 10 mm underwent the test again with nasal stimulation. The patients were then divided into 2 groups depending on those results. Twenty-four age- and sex-matched patients from each group underwent lacrimal gland biopsy. Ten patients from each group underwent salivary gland biopsy (Fig 1).

Findings.—Sixty-nine percent of the whole group showed good reflex tearing, and 31% had poor reflex tearing. The 2 groups were comparable in age and sex distribution. Seven of the 24 patients with good reflex tearing and 22 of the 24 with poor reflex tearing had lymphocytic infiltration of the lacrimal gland. In addition, lymphocytic infiltration of the salivary gland was noted in 6 of the 10 patients with poor reflex tearing compared with only 2 of the 10 with good reflex tearing.

Conclusions.—Assessing reflex tearing using the Schirmer test with nasal stimulation enables clinicians to identify 2 groups of patients with dry eye. Patients with poor reflex tearing are more likely to have autoantibodies and lymphocytic infiltration of the exocrine glands, consistent with the diagnosis of Sjögren's syndrome.

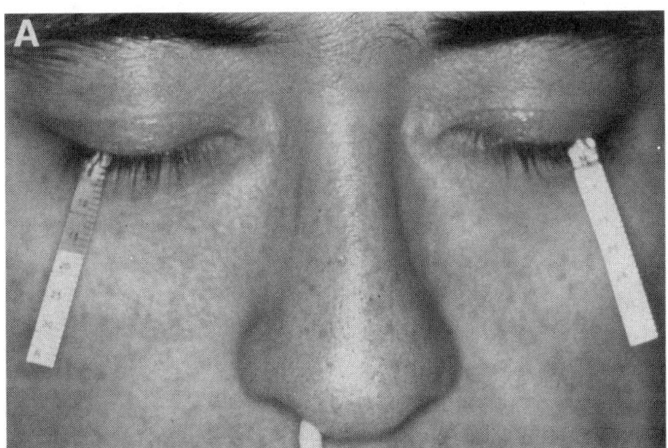

(*Continued*)

FIGURE 1 (cont.)

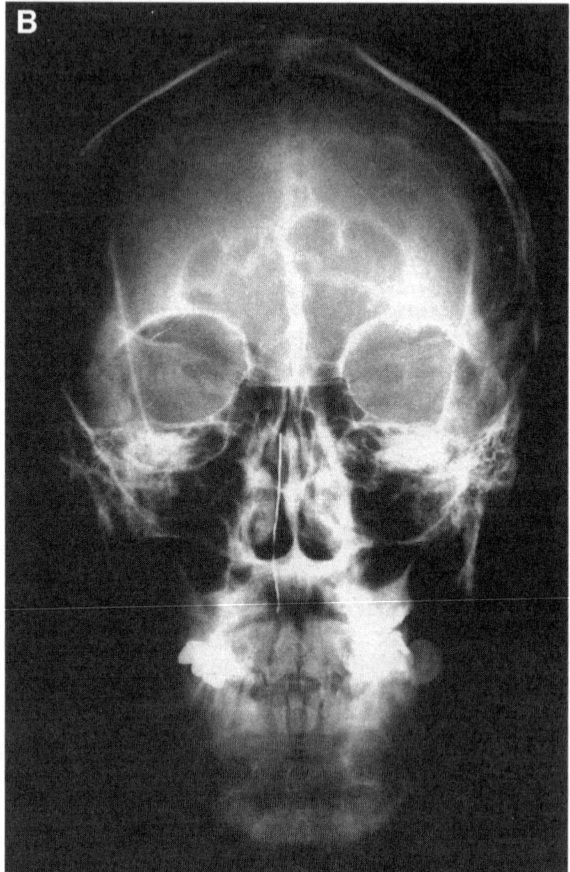

FIGURE 1.—**A,** the cotton swab is inserted almost to the top of the nasal cavity. The ordinary Schirmer test was performed for 5 minutes. Note that only the stimulated side showed wetting of the Schirmer test strip. **B,** radiograph of the inserted cotton swab. Wire was placed inside the swab before insertion into the nasal cavity. Note the swab is parallel to the median line of the nasal cavity. (Courtesy of Tsubota K, Xu K-P, Fujihara T, et al: Decreased reflex tearing is associated with lymphocytic infiltration in lacrimal glands. *J Rheumatol* 23:313–320, 1996.)

▶ Those of us who screen patients suspected of having Sjögren's syndrome with Schirmer tests now need to put a cotton swab into the nasal cavity in addition to the filter papers into the conjunctival spaces. Our patients will love us even more than before for tormenting them in this way, but they should be informed before the experience that such a maneuver greatly enhances the value of the exercise because *reflex*, not *spontaneous*, tearing is what correlates best with lymphocytic infiltration of the lacrimal glands, one of the pathologic hallmarks of the keratoconjunctivitis sicca of Sjögren's syndrome. The illustrations seen here beautifully show the power of this maneuver.

M. Reichlin, M.D.

Development of Complete Heart Block in an Adult Patient With Sjögren's Syndrome and Anti–Ro/SS-A Autoantibodies

Lee LA, Pickrell MB, Reichlin M (Univ of Oklahoma, Oklahoma City; Austin Diagnostic Clinic, Tex)

Arthritis Rheum 39:1427–1429, 1996 3–41

Background.—The occurrence of complete heart block in an adult with systemic lupus erythematosus and anti-Ro autoantibodies has been reported only 3 times. Complete heart block has not been previously reported in an adult with Sjögren's syndrome and anti-Ro autoantibodies.

Case Report.—Woman, 39, had a history of parotid gland swelling, progressive polyarticular pain, and synovitis. Rheumatoid factor was present in her serum (1:20), as were antinuclear antibodies (1:1,280) with a nuclear speckled pattern. She was treated with methotrexate (discontinued because of headache and nausea), then low-dose prednisone, then hydroxychloroquine. The patient was clinically stable for 2 years, then showed recurrent episodes of near syncope. Telemetry revealed intermittent complete heart block (pauses of 3–4 seconds). Echocardiography revealed no evidence of cardiomyopathy or infiltration of the cardiac tissue. Antibodies to both the 60-kd and 52-kd Ro proteins were found in the patient's serum. The patient had no family history of heart disease, including her 2 children. A permanent pacemaker was implanted, and the patient remains stable.

Discussion.—This is the first report of complete heart block occurring in an adult with Sjögren's syndrome and anti-Ro autoantibodies. Although the presence of anti-Ro autoantibodies in this patient's serum does not prove a causal relationship to heart block, the patient had no other known risk factors for this condition. Hence, although the adult atrioventricular node appears relatively resistant to heart block associated with anti-Ro antibodies, the potential for such an interaction should be considered.

▶ It is well known that the most common cause of complete congenital heart block is neonatal lupus erythematosus in which mothers with anti–Ro/SS-A antibodies bear children with complete congenital heart block. That this can happen in adults is illustrated by this case report in which complete heart block developed in a 39-year-old woman with Sjögren's syndrome and anti–Ro/SS-A antibodies. Identification and study of such patients might provide clues as to why this does not happen more often in adults and, conversely, why it happens so frequently in children.

M. Reichlin, M.D.

4 Systemic Sclerosis and Related Disorders

Introduction

Thirty excellent publications relevant to the understanding and management of patients with systemic sclerosis (SSc) were selected; their uniform high quality made choosing a "Pick of the Year" selection particularly difficult. Consideration was given to all publications reviewed. Several merit special mention: the report of three-fold elevation of urinary isoprostanes in SSc patients, which supports a free radical hypothesis of pathogenesis (Abstract 4–14); color Doppler ultrasound to pre-select SSc patients at risk for scleroderma renal crisis (Abstract 4–24); cardiac stress thallium scans as an independent predictor of death in diffuse SSc patients (Abstract 4–22); the elegant demonstration of endothelial apoptosis in SSc lesions and in the chicken model of scleroderma (Abstract 4–13); and the distinct physiologic delineation of digital vascular response to cold between subjects with Raynaud's phenomenon only, systemic sclerosis, and controls (Abstract 4–28). My "Pick of the Year" demonstrated the capacity of relaxin to block bleomycin associated pulmonary fibrosis (Abstract 4–1).

E. Carwile LeRoy, M.D.

I was struck by the explosion of insightful observations pertaining to the pathogenesis of systemic sclerosis—good studies in immunogenetics, genes, gene products, adhesion molecules, fibroblasts, collagen, interleukins and other biologically active mediators, proteoglycans, antibodies, apoptosis, endothelium, free radicals, and even chickens. I don't pretend to understand it as well as Carwile, nor is it yet clear to me what picture is being formed by all these pieces. We used to think of systemic sclerosis as a dismal disease, with a dismal prognosis, and we were clueless about pathophysiology or management. Both Carwile's selections suggest that systemic sclerosis now seems closer to where RA was some years ago, with bright prospects for understanding and perhaps even some breakthroughs.

Richard S. Panush, M.D.

Lead Article

Relaxin Induces an Extracellular Matrix-degrading Phenotype in Human Lung Fibroblasts In Vitro and Inhibits Lung Fibrosis in a Murine Model In Vivo

Unemori EN, Pickford LB, Salles AL, et al (Connective Therapeutics Inc, Palo Alto, Calif)

J Clin Invest 98:2739–2745, 1996 4–1

Introduction.—Fibrosis is a common outcome of interstitial lung disease, characterized by enhanced collagen deposition and an increase in fibroblast number. In the connective tissue phenotype of human dermal fibroblasts, the polypeptide cytokine-growth factor, relaxin, has been found to decrease the synthesis and secretion of interstitial collagens, to decrease the production of tissue inhibitor of metalloproteinases by these cells, and to increase the expression of the matrix of metalloproteinase, procollagenase. The ability of recombinant human relaxin to alter the connective tissue phenotype of human lung fibroblasts in vivo and in vitro was examined.

Methods.—Cell cultures were taken from young adult donors. Collagen was labeled biosynthetically. Western immunoblotting, detection of matrix metalloproteinases by zymography, induction of lung fibrosis with bleomycin, histology, hydroxyproline assay, and quantitation of serum levels of relaxin by enzyme-linked immunosorbent assay were performed.

Results.—Transforming growth factor-β–induced overexpression of procollagen types I and II was decreased by 80% by relaxin (100 ng/mL) by normal human lung fibroblasts in vitro. The synthesis and secretion of procollagenase was increased by up to 45% in a dose-dependent manner. Basal levels of collagen expression were not affected by relaxin in the absence of added transforming growth factor-β. Bleomycin-induced pulmonary fibrosis in mice was blocked by relaxin in vivo, as assessed biochemically and histologically. The relaxin was given at a steady state circulating concentration of ~50 ng/mL. As measured by lung hydroxyproline content, relaxin treated bleomycin-induced collagen accumulation was similar to normal levels.

Conclusion.—Excessive collagen deposition in disease states characterized by pulmonary fibrosis can be modulated by relaxin. A matrix degradative phenotype in human lung fibroblasts was induced by relaxin in vitro. In a murine model, relaxin inhibited bleomycin-induced fibrosis in vivo.

► Unemori, Amento, and colleagues have studied the birth canal hormone relaxin both in vitro and in vivo in an established model of pulmonary fibrosis. Relaxin antagonized (at the 50% level) the profibrogenic influence of TGBFβ1 but did not affect basal fibroblast collagen synthesis. Even more impressive was the capacity of relaxin to strongly inhibit the induction of pulmonary fibrosis by the anti-cancer drug bleomycin. While blocking extracellular matrix synthesis, relaxin promotes the induction of procollagenase synthesis, leading to a matrix-degrading atmosphere that, at least in the bleomycin model, serves an antifibrotic function.

A truly antifibrotic agent that is safe would be a major therapeutic advance. One must remain cautious regarding relaxin because so many putative anti-fibrotic drugs have not proved clinically effective. For example, prednisone inhibits collagen synthesis in the test tube but only complicates life for scleroderma patients. Potaba, vitamin E, and others have not really helped; D-pencillamine is presently under intense, multicenter restudy, so the jury is out. Immunosuppression may be antifibrotic but, over the long haul, has the risks of causing marrow suppression and neoplasia. And that's about it. Thus, a new addition to the antifibrotic armamentarium would be welcome.

In vivo, relaxin must be given by continuous IV pump infusion. Extrapolating this proposed therapy to humans with systemic sclerosis at risk for interstitial lung disease 4 to 6 years with continuous pump infusion therapy at costs exceeding $50,000 per year can be anticipated. At this level of cost and inconvenience, including the risks of indwelling central venous catheters, relaxin will be required to be substantially superior to all other antifibrotic therapies. The authors of the present report are principals in a corporation which expects to market relaxin. Nonetheless, this is a promising new drug in a fairly weak antifibrotic therapeutic armamentarium.

E.C. LeRoy, M.D.

Immunogenetics and Pathophysiology

Up-Regulation of Class II Major Histocompatibility Complex and Intercellular Adhesion Molecule 1 Expression on Scleroderma Fibroblasts and Endothelial Cells by Interferon-γ and Tumor Necrosis Factor α in the Early Disease Stage

Gruschwitz MS, Vieth G (Univ of Erlangen-Nürnberg, Erlangen, Germany)

Arthritis Rheum 40:540–550, 1997 4–2

Objective.—Patients with systemic sclerosis (SSc) have enhanced expression of class II major histocompatibility complex (MHC) and intercellular adhesion molecule 1 (ICAM-1). The cytokines responsible for this enhanced expression are unknown. Patients at varying stages of SSc were studied to determine their patterns of interferon (IFN)-γ and tumor necrosis factor (TNF)-α in the circulation and the codistribution of these cytokines with HLA-DR and ICAM-1 in skin lesions.

Methods.—Skin lesions, cultured fibroblasts, and peripheral blood mononuclear cells (PBMCs) of 15 patients with acute or chonic SSc were studied. Laboratory methods used included immunohistochemistry, reverse transcriptase–polymerase chain reaction, dot-blot hybridization, and cytomeric analysis. Enzyme-linked immunosorbent assay was performed to measure the patients' serum TNF-α levels.

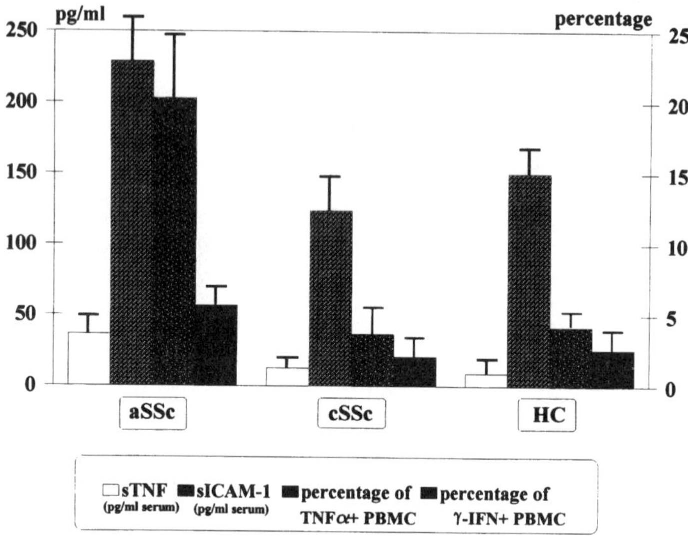

FIGURE 4.—Serum levels of soluble tumor necrosis factor α (*sTNF*) and soluble intercellular adhesion molecule 1 (*sICAM-1*), as well as the percentage of *TNFα*+ and interferon-γ (*γ-IFN*)+ peripheral blood mononuclear cells (*PBMC*), in patients with acute-phase systemic sclerosis (*aSSc*) in contrast to patients with chronic-phase (*cSSc*) and healthy controls (*HC*). $P < 0.01$, aSSc vs. both cSSc and HC. *Bars* show the mean and standard deviation values for each group. (Courtesy of Gruschwitz MS, Vieth G: Up-regulation of class II major histocompatibility complex and intercellular adhesion molecule 1 expression on scleroderma fibroblasts and endothelial cells by interferon-γ and tumor necrosis factor α in the early disease stage. *Arthritis Rheum* 40:540–550, 1997, copyright American College of Rheumatology.)

Results.—Patients in the early inflammatory stage of SSc had detectable class II MHC and ICAM-1 expression on endothelial cells and fibroblasts. This expression was noted particularly on cells in perivascular areas surrounded by infiltrating lymphocytes, which are T–helper 1 cells that express IFN-γ and TNF-α. Cultured dermal fibroblasts and PBMCs showed enhanced TNF-α expression. In addition, the patients had elevated serum levels of soluble TNF-α (Fig 4). For patients with SSc in the chronic fibrotic stage, class II MHC and ICAM-1 expression were comparable to the findings in healthy controls.

Conclusion.—Fibroblast and endothelial expression of class II MHC antigens and ICAM-1 may trigger an autoimmune response in the early stages of SSc. This pattern of cytokine expression appears to result from lymphoid infiltration with local release of TNF-α and IFN-γ. Altered class II MHC and ICAM-1 expression during the acute inflammatory phase of SSc may play an important role in the persistent fibrosis of this disease.

▶ The Erlangen dermatology group has evaluated skin biopsy specimens from acute and stable patients with SSc and noted perivascular accumulation of lymphocytes associated with endothelial cells and fibroblasts that demonstrate class II MHC and ICAM-1 expression. The lymphocytes appear to be of the T–helper 1 persuasion expressing IFN-γ and TNF-α. This is the microenvironment in which perivascular fibrosis occurs, and these cytokine cascades may be relevant to the vasculopathy and, possibly indirectly, the fibrosis. It was also shown in vitro that TNF-α induces the expression of ICAM-1, confirming earlier studies by others. Bring on the monoclonal anti–TNF-α trials.

E.C. LeRoy, M.D.

Inhibition of Synoviocyte Collagenase Gene Expression by Adenosine Receptor Stimulation

Boyle DL, Sajjadi FG, Firestein GS (Gensia Inc, San Diego, Calif)
Arthritis Rheum 39:923–930, 1996 4–3

Background.—In chronic RA, the main effector molecules involved in the degradation of the articular extracellular matrix may be the neutral matrix metalloproteinases (MMPs). Studies using methotrexate to inhibit MMP production suggest that the drug's anti-inflammatory actions may be at least partly mediated by endogenous adenosine production. An in vitro study of the regulation of MMP regulation by adenosine was performed.

Methods.—Cultures of fibroblast-like synoviocytes were prepared and stimulated with interleukin-1 in the presence or absence of adenosine receptor agonists, such as the nonselective adenosine receptor agonist 5'-*N*-ethylcarboxamidoadenosine (NECA). Enzyme-linked immunosorbent assays were used to determine the levels of immunoreactive MMPs. Northern blot analysis was performed to assess gene expression.

Results.—The presence of NECA reduced mean collagenase expression in culture from 196 to 66 ng/mL. This agonist had little effect on stromelysin production. Studies using selective adenosine receptor agonists suggested that the A2b adenosine receptor was involved, and reverse transcriptase–polymerase chain reaction confirmed that this receptor was expressed by the cultured cells. The presence of NECA reduced levels of collagenase messenger RNA (mRNA), but not of stromelysin or tissue inhibitor of metalloproteinases 1 (TIMP-1) mRNA. This suggested a pretranslational mechanism of action. The presence of NECA also decreased collagenase gene expression in fibroblast-like synoviocytes that had been stimulated with tumor necrosis factor α, not interleukin-1 (Fig 4). The nonselective NECA increased cyclic adenosine monophosphate (cAMP) levels, whereas the direct adenylate cyclase activator forskolin suppressed collagenase gene expression. Thus, the ability of NECA to inhibit collagenase production appeared to be mediated by cAMP.

Conclusion.—In cultured fibroblast-like synoviocytes, stimulation of the A2b receptor decreases collagenase gene expression but has minimal effects of stromelysin or TIMP-1. The ability to affect collagenase expression by methotrexate, adenosine-regulating agents, or adenosine provides the opportunity to regulate a key MMP while exerting a potent anti-inflam-

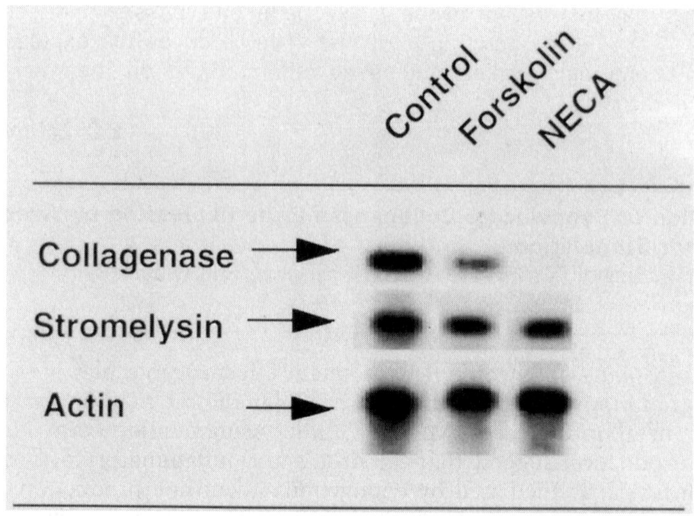

FIGURE 4.—Effect of 5'-*N*-ethylcarboxamidoadenosine (*NECA*) on tumor necrosis factor–α (TNF-α)–stimulated fibroblast-like synoviocytes (FLS). The FLS were stimulated with TNF-α in the presence or absence of forskolin (10 μM) for 24 hours. Messenger RNA was isolated, and Northern blot analysis was performed with probes specific for actin, collagenase, or stomelysin. (Courtesy of Boyle DL, Sajjadi FG, Firestein GS: Inhibition of synoviocyte collagenase gene expression by adenosine receptor stimulation. *Arthritis Rheum* 39:923–930, 1996, copyright American College of Rheumatology.)

matory action. Further research into the regulation of MMP expression by adenosine could offer new strategies for the treatment of RA.

► An adenosine agonist can selectively inhibit collagenase (MMP-1) at the transcriptional level. This in vitro observation fits well into the observations of Cronstein et al.[1] that methotrexate may exert its anti-inflammatory effects by means of increased adenosine release. Adenosine kinase inhibitors and adenosine agonists may have a future role in the management of RA. At present, the inhibition of collagenase may be an added reason for methotrexate's beneficial effects in our patients with RA.

E.C. LeRoy, M.D.

Reference

1. Cronstein BN, Naime D, Ostad E: The anti-inflammatory mechanism of low-dose methotrexate: Increased adenosine release at inflamed sites diminishes leukocyte accumulation in an in vivo model of inflammation. *J Clin Invest* 92:2675–2682, 1993.

Stimulation of α1 (I) Procollagen Gene Expression in NIH-3T3 Cells by the Human T Cell Leukemia Virus Type 1 (HTLV-1) Tax Gene

Muñoz E, Suri D, Amini S, et al (Thomas Jefferson Univ, Philadelphia)

J Clin Invest 96:2413–2420, 1995 4–4

Introduction.—Systemic sclerosis and idiopathic pulmonary fibrosis are prototypes of various diseases that are characterized by overproduction of connective tissue macromolecules, including the collagens, in tissue. The mechanisms responsible for the expression of genes that encode extracellular matrix proteins in fibroblasts and other mesenchymal cells are unknown. Various studies have shown that Tax enhances viral gene expression and triggers the expression of other cellular genes. Whether expression of collagen genes is modulated by Tax, the transregulatory protein from the human T cell leukemia virus type I, was investigated.

Methods.—NIH-3T3 cells were transfected with a Tax expressor plasmid and a chimeric construct of regulatory sequences (−804 to +42 base pain) of the α 1 (I) procollagen gene (COL1A1) promoter.

Results.—The promoter activity of the −804 to +42 base pain COL1A1 fragment increased 12-fold in cells that expressed Tax. It was revealed through deletion analysis that the region of COL1A1 from nucleotides −174 to −84 contained the Tax-responsive elements. A gene segment from nucleotides −187 to −67, which contains this region, was sufficient for Tax-inducible chloramphenicol acetyltransferase expression of a herpes simplex virus thymidine kinase promoter. Increased levels of α1 (I)

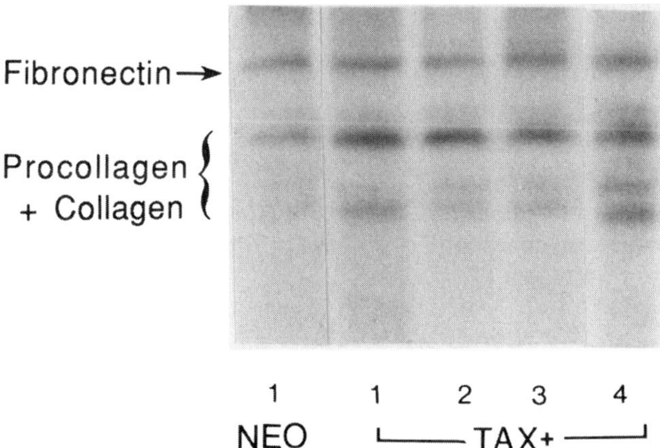

FIGURE 9.—SDS-PAGE of [^{14}C]proline extracellular matrix proteins synthesized in stable clones. NIH-3T3 cells were transfected with either pNeo alone or the pNeo plus long-terminal repeat Tax plasmid, and stably transfected clones were established. Cells from the stably transfected clones were cultured to confluency and then incubated for 24 hours with [^{14}C]proline. After dialysis, 50-µL aliquots of pooled medium and cell extract from each clone were used for the analysis. The figure represents fluorographs of SDS-PAGE of the radiolabeled media plus cell-associated proteins. *Abbreviations: NEO*, Neomycin-resistant control clone; *TAX+*, Tax + clones. (Reproduced from Muñoz E, Suri D, Amini S, et al: Stimulation of α1 [I] procollagen gene expression in NIH-3T3 cells by the human T cell leukemia virus type 1 [HTLV-1] Tax gene. *J Clin Invest* 96:2413–2420, 1995, by copyright permission of the American Society for Clinical Investigation.)

procollagen and fibronectin transcripts, and increased production and accelerated processing of type I procollagen were found in stably transfected NIH-3T3 cell clones that produce Tax (Fig 9).

Conclusion.—Retroviral proteins may have a part in the pathogenesis of systemic sclerosis and idiopathic pulmonary fibrosis characterized by collagen overproduction.

► A general observation during the past 2 decades has been that the viral transformation of mesenchymal cells is associated with downregulation of extracellular matrix genes. Now exceptions to that rule are accumulating, leading to the novel suggestion that retroviruses may be triggers of human fibrotic conditions such as scleroderma.

First, renal glomerulosclerosis was observed in mice transgenic for noninfectious human immunodeficiency virus type 1 (HIV-1) genes.[1] Next, the authors of the present report transfected glioblastoma cells with HIV-1 Tat, a transactivator of viral and host cell genes, and noted upregulation of collagen and fibronectin genes.[2] In the present report, another viral transregulatory protein, Tax, from an ancestor of HIV-1, the human T-cell leukemia virus type 1, results in upregulation of the α1(I) collagen gene. Furthermore, the promoter region involved in this upregulation is the same as that which certain cytokines use to promote collagen expression, supporting the notion that viral genes upregulate cytokine genes that promote fibrosis.

E.C. LeRoy, M.D.

References

1. Dickie P, Felser J, Eckhaus M, et al: HIV-associated neuropathy in transgenic mice expressing HIV-1 genes. *Virology* 185:109–119, 1991.
2. Taylor JP, Cupp C, Diaz A, et al: Activation of expression of genes coding for extracellular matrix proteins in Tat-producing glioblastoma cells. *Proc Natl Acad Sci USA*. 89:9617–9621, 1992.

Heterogeneity of Collagen Synthesis in Normal and Systemic Sclerosis Skin Fibroblasts: Increased Proportion of High Collagen-producing Cells in Systemic Sclerosis Fibroblasts

Jelaska A, Arakawa M, Broketa G, et al (Boston Univ)
Arthritis Rheum 39:1338–1346, 1996 4–5

Background.—Systemic sclerosis is marked by excessive accumulation of extracellular matrix in skin and internal organs. In systemic sclerosis, skin fibroblasts produce excessive amounts of several collagens, which leads to fibrosis and increased skin thickness. The presence of cellular infiltrates in vivo and fibroblast activation by immune-cell products in vitro indicates that the immune system may be involved in the pathogenesis of systemic sclerosis. Systemic sclerosis fibroblasts persistently produce excessive collagen in culture in the absence of immune stimulation, which suggests that alterations within the fibroblast itself may occur. There are

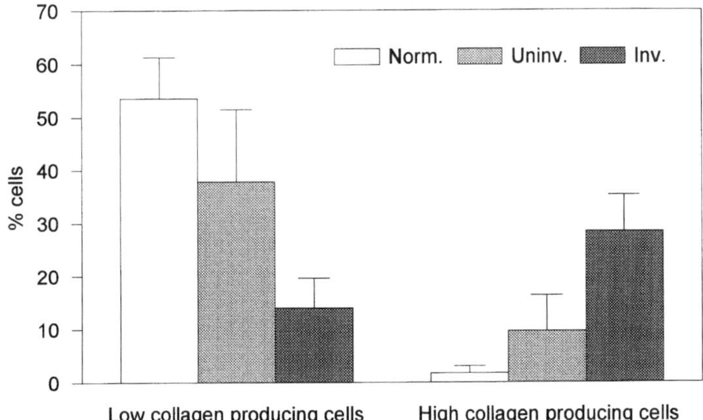

FIGURE 5.—Percentage of cells in low and high collagen-producing subpopulations. *Bars* show the mean and standard error of the mean percentage of cells in each subpopulation, which were calculated from in situ hybridization. $^*P < 0.01$ vs. normal fibroblasts. $^\dagger P < 0.05$ vs. uninvolved systemic sclerosis fibroblasts. $^\ddagger P < 0.01$ vs. uninvolved systemic sclerosis fibroblasts. *Abbreviations*: *Inv.*, involved; *Norm.*, normal; *Uninv.*, uninvolved. (Courtesy of Jelaska A, Arakawa M, Broketa G, et al: Heterogeneity of collagen synthesis in normal and systemic sclerosis skin fibroblasts: Increased proportion of high collagen-producing cells in systemic sclerosis fibroblasts. *Arthritis Rheum* 39:1338–1346, 1996, copyright American College of Rheumatology.)

various hypotheses to explain this abnormal collagen synthesis in systemic sclerosis fibroblasts. The distribution of collagen synthesis in normal and systemic sclerosis fibroblast populations was examined to learn the extent of activation in systemic sclerosis populations.

Methods.—Fibroblast cultures were obtained from involved and uninvolved skin of patients with systemic sclerosis and from healthy controls. Quantitative in situ hybridization was performed to analyze the population distribution of type I collagen synthesis. Fibroblast cultures were analyzed for levels of α1 (I) procollagen mRNA.

Results.—In situ hybridization showed that dermal fibroblasts from patients with systemic sclerosis and control subjects were heterogeneous for distribution of α1 (I) procollagen mRNA; there was a wide range of grains per cell. A somewhat homogeneous distribution of grain counts was seen in clones of neonatal fibroblasts. A larger proportion of cells in the high–collagen-producing mRNA subpopulation was seen in involved systemic sclerosis skin fibroblasts compared to normal and uninvolved fibroblasts (Fig 5). In the low–collagen-producing mRNA subpopulation, involved fibroblasts had a smaller proportion of cells than uninvolved fibroblasts. Normal fibroblasts had a majority of the cells in this subpopulation.

Discussion.—These findings show that in systemic sclerosis, only a subset of fibroblasts is activated. This was indicated by the high proportion of cells with high levels of α1 (I) procollagen mRNA. The differences between systemic sclerosis and normal fibroblasts were quantitative rather than qualitative. This may result from clonal selection or selective activation in the pathogenesis of systemic sclerosis.

▶ Virtually all biological systems studied in detail are in balance between high and low expression of the characteristic being considered. The fibrosis of systemic sclerosis and other human fibrotic disorders are examples of out-of-balance or unregulated expression and excessive deposition of extracellular matrix (ECM) material, especially types I and III collagen, in contrast to a regulated system such as wound healing. How does this happen? Sorting out the answer could open new vistas to the treatment of human fibrosis.

The thinking revolves between microenvironmental influences (cytokines from leukocytes in the perivascular lesions) that activate adjacent mesenchymal cells (fibroblasts, endothelial cells, pericytes) to express ECM genes, mRNA, and glycoproteins with the deposition of fibrosis *or* inherent, germline influences that predispose mesenchymal cells to express high levels of ECM genes, mRNA, and ECM glycoproteins. Korn & coworkers et al. have been serious students of fibroblast heterogeneity for 2 decades now. In this study, they show that up to 52% of fibroblasts within systemic sclerosis lesions are high collagen-producing ones contrasted with 0% to 6% of healthy control fibroblasts; they use an in situ hybridization technique and thus eliminate possible in vitro cell culture artifacts or total RNA isolation averaging that might obscure the presence of a minority of highly activated cells.

These are impressive differences, but they still do not answer the question "how come?" Lesional fibroblasts could be activated by the disease process, or they could be preprogrammed to respond to mitogenic stimuli [systemic sclerosis fibroblasts are selectively responsive to the mitogen tissue inhibitor of metalloproteinase (TIMP-2)] or to ECM gene regulatory factors (transforming growth factor β1 or connective tissue growth factor). If prior viral infection is involved in the pre-activation state, distinctions between exogenous and endogenous triggers become even more blurred. Whatever the basic mechanism, systemic sclerosis fibroblasts are impressively and persistently activated to deposit ECM, and there seems to be little in the way of balance to downregulate these activated cells or to resorb the fibrosis deposited.

E.C. LeRoy, M.D.

Soluble Serum Interleukin 2 Receptors in Patients With Systemic Sclerosis

Steen VD, Engel EE, Charley MR, et al (Univ of Pittsburgh, Pa)
J Rheumatol 23:646–649, 1996 4–6

Introduction.—There is considerable evidence of cellular immune abnormalities in systemic sclerosis (SSc), a connective tissue disease of unknown etiology. Findings have included reduction of T-suppressor lymphocytes and increased interleukin-2 (IL-2) activity. To determine whether soluble IL-2 receptor (sIL-2R) levels change during the course of illness and might be used to measure disease activity, patients with SSc were studied.

Methods.—Serum samples from 3 patient groups were examined: 81 consecutive new patients with SSc (group I); 21 patients with diffuse cutaneous (dc) SSc whose peripheral blood and affected skin had been analyzed for T-lymphocyte subsets (group II); and 38 patients with diffuse cutaneous SSc who had serial sIL-2R levels measured during the course of disease. A commercial double monoclonal antibody enzyme-linked immunosorbent assay technique was used in the serum sIL-2R assays.

Results.—Among group I patients, there was a significant association between sIL-2R levels and total skin thickness score. Thirty-five were classified as having diffuse cutaneous SSc and 29 as having limited cutaneous SSc; 7 cases were unclassified and 10 had overlap syndrome. All subgroups differed significantly from controls (Table 1) in mean sIL-2R levels. No other clinical features in group I patients could be correlated with levels of sIL-2R. In group II patients, there was a correlation between sIL-2R and total lymphocyte count, T lymphocytes, CD4 and CD8 cell numbers, and the peripheral blood T-helper lymphocyte: T-suppressor lymphocyte ratio. Group III patients showed a tendency, also noted in group I, for higher levels of sIL-2R during the first year of disease than later in the disease course. There was a correlation between sIL-2R level and total skin score determined at the same time the serum sample was obtained, and a significant correlation between changes in sIL-2R levels and in skin score over time (Fig 1).

Discussion.—T-cell activation appears to play a role in the pathogenesis of SSc. All patients with the disease have significantly elevated sIL-2R levels, particularly those with the diffuse cutaneous variant early in their disease course. In the first report of serial sIL-2R levels in SSc, results show

TABLE 1.—Soluble Interleukin-2 Receptor Levels in 81 Patients With Systemic Sclerosis and 35 Controls

Patient Classification	Number Studied	Mean sIL-2R Level (units ± SE)	p vs Controls
SSc	81*	821 ± 40	< 0.001
dcSSc	35	830 ± 52†	< 0.001
lcSSc	29	678 ± 52†	< 0.001
Overlap	10	1044 ± 148	< 0.001
Controls	35	389 ± 19	

*Seven unclassified patients not included.

†dcSSc vs. lcSSc, $p < 0.05$.

Abbreviations: sIL-2R, soluble interleukin-2 receptor; *SSc*, systemic sclerosis; *dcSSc*, diffuse cutaneous SSc; *lcSSc*, limited cutaneous SSc; *SE*, standard error.

(Courtesy of Steen VD, Engel EE, Charley MR, et al: Soluble serum interleukin 2 receptors in patients with systemic sclerosis. *J Rheumatol* 23:646–649, 1996.)

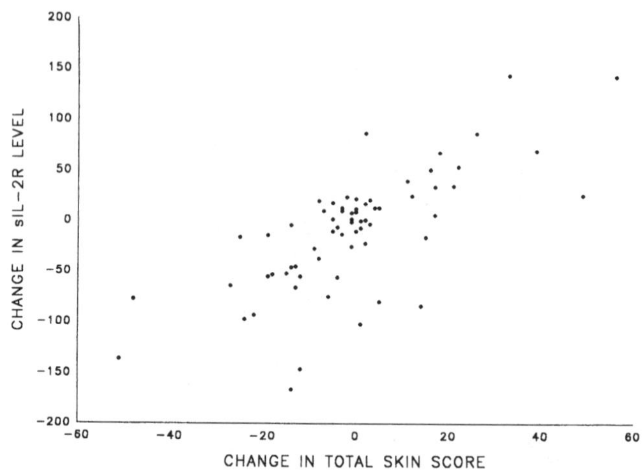

FIGURE 1.—Correlation of changes in serum soluble interleukin-2 receptor (*sIL-2R*) levels with changes in skin score in 38 patients with systemic sclerosis (*SSc*) with serial samples. (Courtesy of Steen VD, Engel EE, Charley MR, et al: Soluble serum interleukin 2 receptors in patients with systemic sclerosis. *J Rheumatol* 23:646–649, 1996.)

that measurement of sIL-2R may be useful in confirming current disease activity and monitoring progression.

▶ Physicians managing patients with SSc could be assisted by a measurement reflecting "immunologic" activity of the disease process. Steen et al. propose an enzyme-linked immunosorbent assay test for soluble IL-2 receptors shed from activated T cells (possibly also monocyte-macrophages as well) to monitor immune activity. Cautious attempts to correlate disease "activity" were positive and promising. It is reasonable to propose a prospective analysis of connective tissue (serum N-terminal type I collagen propeptide levels), vascular (plasma von Willebrand factor levels and possibly serum endothelium 1 levels), autoimmune (type and titer of serum autoantibody levels), and immune activation (serum IL-2R levels) parameters, each against the charge in total skin thickness scores and new organ-specific disease events.

E.C. LeRoy, M.D.

Expression of Interleukin-4 in Scleroderma Skin Specimens and Scleroderma Fibroblast Cultures: Potential Role in Fibrosis

Salmon-Ehr V, Serpier H, Nawrocki B, et al (Univ of Reims Champagne Ardenne, France)

Arch Dermatol 132:802–806, 1996 4–7

Background.—Scleroderma is a fibrotic disease marked by uncontrolled accumulation of collagen in tissues, mainly as a result of increased collagen synthesis by fibroblasts. At least 5 cytokines could be involved in fibroblast activation leading to fibrosis. Interleukin 4 (IL-4) activates the synthesis of extracellular matrix macromolecules by fibroblasts. Interleukin-4 stimulates collagen synthesis, as well as fibronectin and proteoglycan synthesis. Because the early stages of fibrosis are marked by infiltration of connective tissue by inflammatory cells, it was speculated that these cells might produce IL-4 in situ, which is possibly a factor in the development of the fibrotic process. The expression of IL-4 was examined with immunocytochemical analysis and in situ hybridization in normal and scleroderma skin and in fibroblast cultures.

Methods.—Biopsy specimens from 9 patients with normal skin and 11 subjects with scleroderma were obtained. Fibroblasts were obtained from skin biopsy specimens by explantation and were grown in culture flasks. Immunocytochemical studies with anti-IL-4 antibody were performed. The labeling intensity was assessed independently by 2 pathologists unaware of the diagnosis and was graded from 0 to 3.

Results.—In 8 of the 11 scleroderma skin specimens, the label was intense or strong. In 8 of the 9 normal skin specimens, the label was negative or faint. In situ hybridization showed a significant increase in the number of IL-4 messenger RNA grains in scleroderma skin specimens compared with normal skin specimens. In the 4 scleroderma fibroblast cultures, strong positive labeling with the anti–IL-4 antibody was seen. Labeling was negative in the 5 fibroblast control cultures.

Discussion.—Interleukin-4 was strongly expressed in most of the scleroderma skin specimens examined. Although a significant correlation between the expression of IL-4 and severity of disease was not found, such a correlation could be missed in a study of this size. In scleroderma, IL-4 expression by fibroblasts may be triggered by an unknown factor. Interleukin-4 may be involved in an autocrine stimulation of extracellular matrix production that may occur in fibrotic tissue. Fibrosis in scleroderma may result from a large number of cytokines, including IL-4.

▶ Interleukin-4 is a cytokine that has been prominently associated with activation of the immune system along the pathway designated T-helper 2 (TH 2), which leads to mast cell activation and is likely to be more fibrogenic than other immune activation pathways. Salmon-Ehr et al. have identified IL-4 in the lesions of localized scleroderma and have shown anti IL-4 antibody labeling of scleroderma fibroblasts in culture, which suggests that 1 of the activation characteristics of these lesional cells is a profibrogenic autocrine loop involving the production of IL-4. Further study of IL-4 gene expression may lead to a way to selectively shut off this pathway to fibrosis.

E.C. LeRoy, M.D.

Elevated Serum Levels of Interleukin 4 (IL-4), IL-10, and IL-13 in Patients With Systemic Sclerosis

Hasegawa M, Fujimoto M, Kikuchi K, et al (Kanazawa Univ, Japan; Univ of Tokyo)

J Rheumatol 24:328–332, 1997 4–8

Introduction.—Characterized by vascular alterations and fibrosis, systemic sclerosis is a disease of connective tissue. The skin, esophagus, and lungs are frequently involved sites. The pathogenesis of the disease may be affected by immunologic abnormalities. Activated T cells constitute the majority of the infiltrating cells in the skin of patients with systemic sclerosis. Many cytokines, including interleukin 2, interleukin 4, interleukin 6, interleukin 10, and interleukin 13, are released after activation. The roles of these cytokines in systemic sclerosis are poorly understood. Whether serum interleukin 4, interleukin 10, and interleukin 13, levels were elevated in patients with systemic sclerosis and whether the levels were correlated with the serologic or clinical features of this disease were investigated.

Methods.—Enzyme-linked immunosorbent assay was used to examine serum samples from 45 patients with limited cutaneous disease, from 28 patients with diffuse cutaneous disease, and from 30 controls.

Results.—In patients with limited cutaneous systemic sclerosis and diffuse cutaneous systemic sclerosis, serum interleukin 4 and interleukin 13 levels were significantly higher than in controls. Compared with controls, serum interleukin 10 levels were significantly higher in patients with diffuse cutaneous systemic sclerosis. In patients with arthralgia, elevated interleukin 10 levels were detected frequently. Erythrocyte sedimentation rates and C-reactive protein levels in patients were correlated positively with serum interleukin 13 levels.

Conclusion.—Systemic sclerosis may be affected by interleukin 4, interleukin 10, and interleukin 13. A potentially clinically useful serologic indicator of systemic inflammation in patients with systemic sclerosis may be interleukin 13.

▶ Someday, someone will measure serum cytokines in an autoimmune disease and know what it all means. At present we can only guess. Nonetheless, Professor Kazuhiko Takehara and his colleagues have demonstrated a pattern of increased cytokine levels in patients with systemic sclerosis (SSc), which is interesting. Interleukin-4, IL-10, and IL-13 are increased. In concert, these cytokines could explain both the autoantibody and profibrogenic tendencies of SSc. Interleukin 4 is certainly profibrogenic and IL-10 and IL-13, though more recently discovered, seem to be immune stimulatory. This profile may also mean that patients with SSc lean toward the T-helper 2 immune-activated profile. How to exploit these cytokine secretion patterns and immune pathway profiles for the benefit of the patient remains the future challenge.

E.C. LeRoy, M.D.

Early Expression of E-selectin, Tumor Necrosis Factor α, and Mast Cell Infiltration in the Salivary Glands of Patients With Systemic Sclerosis

Hebbar M, Gillot J-M, Hachulla E, et al (Hôpital Calmette, Lille, France)

Arthritis Rheum 39:1161–1165, 1996 4–9

Introduction.—In secondary Raynaud's phenomenon, the underlying disorder is primarily systemic sclerosis (SSc). Raynaud's phenomenon can sometimes precede the development of SSc by months or years. In such patients, abnormalities on nailfold capillaroscopy are predictive of SSc. Systemic sclerosis lesions can occur in minor salivary glands. Endothelial lesions are consistently detected in patients with SSc and indicate vascular injury. Endothelial cell activation in the skin of patients with SSc is indicated by increased expression of E-selectin, which also has a role in migration of endothelial cells into perivascular areas. Expression of E-selectin in salivary endothelial cells could result from mast cell–derived tumor necrosis factor-α. The expression of E-selectin, tumor necrosis factor-α, and mast cell infiltration in minor salivary glands were studied in patients with Raynaud's phenomenon and abnormal findings on capillaroscopy.

Methods.—Twenty-two patients (21 women) with Raynaud's phenomenon and abnormal findings on capillaroscopy had a median age of 43 years. At baseline, none of the patients met the criteria of the American College of Rheumatology for SSc. Lip biopsy specimens were obtained and immunostaining was done.

Results.—Follow-up was 1–7 years. Of 11 patients whose disease progressed to SSc, E-selectin was detected in 9, tumor necrosis factor-α was detected in 10, and mast cell infiltration was detected in 8. Of 11 patients whose disease did not progress to SSc, E-selectin was detected in 0, tumor necrosis factor-α was detected in 2, and mast cell infiltration was detected in 1 (Table 3).

Conclusions.—In patients with Raynaud's phenomenon and abnormal findings on capillaroscopy, E-selectin, tumor necrosis factor-α, and mast

TABLE 3.—Correlations Between Initial Features and Progression Systemic Sclerosis

Feature	Progression to SSc (n = 11)	No progression to SSc (n = 11)	*P**
E-selectin expression	9	0	<0.001
TNFα expression	10	2	<0.01
Mast cell infiltration	8	1	<0.01
Antinuclear antibodies	8	1	<0.01
Sclerosis	9	2	0.01
Chisholm score ≥ 3	6	2	Not significant

*Chi-square test with Yates' correction.

Abbreviations: SSc, systemic sclerosis; *TNF-α,* tumor necrosis factor-α.

(Courtesy of Hebbar M, Gillot J-M, Hachulla E, et al: Early expression of E-selectin, tumor necrosis factor-α, and mast cell infiltration in the salivary glands of patients with systemic sclerosis. *Arthritis Rheum* 39:1161–1165, 1996, copyright American College of Rheumatology.)

cell infiltration can be detected in minor salivary glands, indicating very early stages of SSc. Because of the small number of patients studied and the long follow-up period, it cannot be absolutely concluded that these 3 factors have independent predictive value.

► Patients with Raynaud's phenomenon in whom widefield low-power microscopy shows the nailfold capillary abnormalities of dilatation, loss, and distortion and hemorrhage characteristic of SSc are suspect to have SSc develop in the future. Many do not fulfill American College of Rheumatology Preliminary Classification Criteria, which were intentionally designed for specificity and not sensitivity and are thus insensitive, especially in patients with limited cutaneous SSc. Of 22 patients who had Raynaud's phenomenon and capillary abnormalities whose selection was not prospectively determined, 13 had evidence of inflammatory or sclerotic histology on lip or salivary gland biopsy specimen (E-selectin, tumor necrosis factor-α, and mast cells). Ten of the 13 patients positive for inflammation/sclerosis were among the 11 judged clinically to progress to definite SSc (all limited), whereas only 2 of the 11 judged not to progress to definite SSc were positive for inflammation/sclerosis.

The report of this promising and potentially prognostic finding is incomplete in its clinical documentation. Whereas no patients of 22 were positive for American College of Rheumatology Preliminary Classification Criteria on entry to the study, in fact only 3 of the 22 patients fulfilled these criteria on study completion. The other 8 of the 22 patients who "progressed" were characterized as having limited SSc largely on the basis of sclerodactyly, and we are not told explicitly that they were free of sclerodactyly at study entry (follow-up was for a median of 5 years). This study (among others) points up the need for a consensus set of early diagnostic criteria for limited cutaneous SSc. I propose that Raynaud's phenomenon positivity by digital cuff cold-induced vasospasm (Nielsen test) and characteristic SSc nailfold capillaroscopic findings are sufficient criteria for limited cutaneous SSc, because these findings are found in few if any other diseases (dermatomyositis may be an exception). Putting aside criteria problems, if lip biopsy specimen findings can be shown to be of prognostic significance in a prospective, blinded study by independent observers, it will be a welcome addition to the prognostic armamentarium.

E.C. LeRoy, M.D.

Elevated Serum Tumor Necrosis Factor-α Levels in Patients With Systemic Sclerosis: Association With Pulmonary Fibrosis

Hasegawa M, Fujimoto M, Kikuchi K, et al (Kanazawa Univ, Japan; Univ of Tokyo)

J Rheumatol 24:663–665, 1997 4–10

Introduction.—Findings vary regarding the relation between serum tumor necrosis factor-α (TNF-α) levels and systemic sclerosis (SSc). To

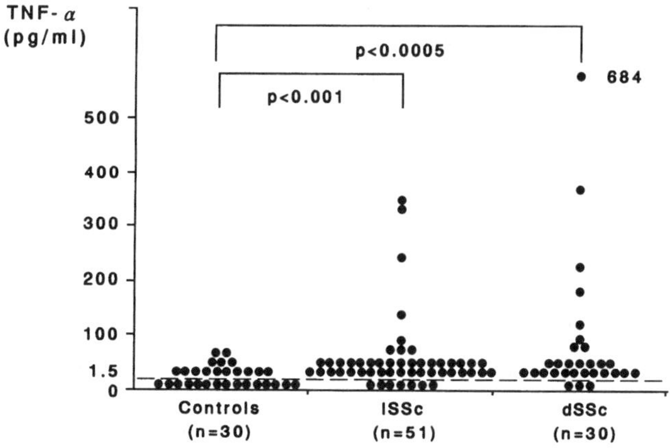

FIGURE 1.—Serum tumor necrosis factor (TNF)-α levels in patients with lSSc and dSSc. The *broken line* indicates the detection limit. *Abbreviations: lSSc*, limited cutaneous systemic sclerosis; *dSSc*, diffuse cutaneous systemic sclerosis. (Courtesy of Hasegawa M, Fujimioto M, Kikuchi K, et al: Elevated serum tumor necrosis factor-α levels in patients with systemic sclerosis: Association with pulmonary fibrosis. *J Rheumatol* 24:663–665, 1997.)

determine whether the TNF-α levels in patients with SSc were elevated and whether they correlated with clinical or serologic manifestations of the disease, these levels were measured.

Methods.—Serum TNF-α levels were measured by enzyme-linked immunosorbent assay in 51 patients with limited cutaneous SSc (lSSc), 30 patients with diffuse cutaneous SSc (dSSc), and 30 controls. Organ system involvement and pulmonary function studies were recorded.

Results.—Serum TNF-α levels were detectable more frequently in patients with lSSc (44/51) and dSSc (27/30) than in controls (15/30). Significantly higher median levels of serum TNF-α were detected in lSSc and dSSc than in controls (7.0, 7.5, and 1.5, respectively) (Fig 1). Serum TNF-α levels were not significantly different in patients treated with or without prednisolone (32% vs. 68%). There was a significant correlation between elevated TNF-α levels and presence of pulmonary fibrosis and decreased vital capacity. Serum TNF-α levels were negatively correlated with vital capacity in patients with SSc.

Conclusion.—Tumor necrosis factor-α may contribute to pulmonary fibrosis in patients with SSc.

▶ Takehara, Kikuchi, and colleagues from Kanazawa and Tokyo have found a statistically inverse correlation between serum TNF-α levels and pulmonary vital capacity in patients with SSc. Most patients with SSc have normal or only slightly elevated TNF-α levels; most of these have normal or near normal vital capacities. In contrast, the few patients with SSc with distinctly elevated serum TNF-α levels had severe pulmonary fibrosis, which may have pathogenic implications for SSc lung disease. Curiously missing from this study, which includes patients with both lSSc and dSSc, is whether TNF-α levels correlate with skin score. Tumor necrosis factor-α is an effective experimental tool for inducing interstitial lung disease in the laboratory animal, and may well be important in human SSc. Is it time for a blinded, controlled trial of monoclonal antibody to TNF-α in early alveolitis in patients with diffuse SSc?

E.C. LeRoy, M.D.

Altered Dermatan Sulfate Proteoglycan Synthesis in Fibroblast Cultures Established From Skin of Patients With Systemic Sclerosis

Westergren-Thorsson G, Cöster L, Åkesson A, et al (Lund Univ, Sweden)

J Rheumatol 23:1398–1406, 1996 4–11

Background.—Systemic sclerosis (SSc) almost always involves the skin. Research of SSc fibroblasts has shown increased expression of messenger RNA (mRNA) for collagen types I, III, VI, and VII and altered interaction with collagen fibers and integrins affecting cell adhesion. However, the role of other extracellular matrix components, such as proteoglycans, remains unclear. Whether changes in the properties of skin from patients with SSc result from alterations in the metabolism of dermatan sulfate (DS) proteoglycans was examined.

Methods.—Skin was obtained from healthy persons and from affected and unaffected areas of patients with SSc. Fibroblast cultures were established, and synthesized proteoglycans were labeled with ^{3}H glucosamine and ^{35} sulfate. Hybridization with the corresponding complementary DNA (cDNA) probes was used to assess the amount of mRNA of the different DS proteoglycans.

Findings.—Cell cultures from affected and normal-appearing skin from patients with SSc showed a twofold increase in secretion of total proteoglycans. Increases were noted in the production of 2 different DS proteoglycans—aggrecan/versican fourfold and decoran twofold—in cultures of affected skin. The docorin mRNA was increased threefold. Versican mRNA levels were only slightly increased. The changes observed in cultures from the patients' normal-appearing skin were similar but less marked. In contrast, the biglycan mRNA level was reduced, and only small amounts of the product were found in SSc cultures.

Conclusion.—The substantial changes observed in DS proteoglycan metabolism distinguishes both SSc-affected skin and normal-appearing SSc skin from healthy skin. These changes may affect the organization of matrix fibers and, thus, the fibrotic process in patients with SSc.

► Systemic sclerosis is characterized by the aberrant and unregulated deposition of extracellular matrix molecules in multiple affected organs. Skin fibroblasts continue to overproduce several collagens and fibronectin when removed from the patient and propagated in vitro. This group from Lund, Sweden, has now shown that unusual quantities of the proteoglycan family known as DS are also overproduced. These consist mostly of the larger DS species called aggrecan/versican.

Slightly different patterns of overproduction are seen when patients with limited SSc are compared with patients with diffuse SSc. The overproduction is also seen in clinically normal skin of affected individuals. The differences are substantial, and proteoglycan overproduction is yet another manifestation of the activated phenotype of the SSc fibroblast. To control the overproduction of extracellular matrix is a major therapeutic goal in SSc management.

E.C. LeRoy, M.D.

Autoantibodies to Fibrillarin in Systemic Sclerosis (Scleroderma)

Arnett FC, Reveille JD, Goldstein R, et al (Univ of Texas, Health Science Ctr, Houston; Univ of Ottawa, Ont; Scripps Research Inst, La Jolla, Calif; et al)

Arthritis Rheum 39:1151–1160, 1996 4–12

Purpose.—Patients with systemic sclerosis (SSc) may have autoantibodies to nucleolar antigens in their serum. One of the nucleolar antigens targeted by these autoimmune responses is fibrillarin, a 34-35-kd basic protein of small nucleolar ribonucleoprotein (RNP) particles. Antifibrillarin antibodies have been linked to certain clinical characteristics in SSc, including diffuse skin involvement, extensive telangiectasias, and possibly more frequent muscle disease. Class II MHC alleles may have associations with specific autoantibody profiles, although there have been no studies of the HLA genes of SSc patients who produce antifibrillarin antibodies. The frequency, clinical associations, and major MHC correlations of antifibrillarin antibodies in patients with SSc were studied.

Methods.—Indirect immunofluorescence was used to screen stored sera from 335 patients with SSc for antinucleolar antibodies. Further studies for antifibrillarin antibodies were performed in patients with a primary or secondary antinucleolar antibody pattern. DNA oligotyping was performed to determine HLA class II alleles, and the results of antifibrillarin-positive patients were compared with those of patients with SSc with other autoantibodies and with normal controls.

Results.—Sera from 8% of patients showed antifibrillarin antibodies. These antibodies were found in 16% of black patients vs. 5% of white patients, and in 33% of males vs. 14% of females. Patients with cardiac, renal, or gut involvement with SSc were more likely to have antifibrillarin.

Patients with antibodies to fibrillarin were more likely to have HLA class II haplotype DRB1*1302, DQB1*0604 than race-matched controls, either normals or patients with SSc without fibrillarin antibodies. All of the patients with antibodies to fibrillarin had at least 1 of the following HLA-DQB1 alleles: *0604, *0301, *0602, and *0302. Furthermore, 62% of the patients with antibodies to fibrillarin had 2 of these alleles, which represented a significant difference from the control groups.

Conclusion.—Antibodies to the nucleolar antigen fibrillarin are relatively infrequent findings in patients with SSc. However, when antifibrillarin occurs, it is associated with severe SSc, especially in blacks and males. Antibodies to fibrillarin are also associated with a unique HLA haplotype and certain combinations of HLA-DQB1 alleles.

► Arnett and colleagues continue to define the close association between the immunogenetic (HLA) and autoimmune (antinuclear antibodies) features of patients with SSc. Of 335 patients with SSc, antifibrillarin antibodies accounted for 39% of *nucleolar* reactions and were more frequent in African Americans and in males. Even more striking, 1 or more of 4 HLA-DQ1 alleles was present in all antifibrillarin-positive patients (100%) and 60% of these patients had 2 or more of the HLA-DQB1 alleles. These compelling associations literally demand more complete biological explanations: Do the antibodies themselves induce entothelial and vascular wall changes, or do they represent the B-cell activation phase of a T cell (or fibroblast) symphony conducted by the cytokine orchestra that is profibrogenic and, ultimately, amenable to therautic harmonizing?

E.C. LeRoy, M.D.

Endothelial Cell Apoptosis Is a Primary Pathogenetic Event Underlying Skin Lesions in Avian and Human Scleroderma

Sgonc R, Gruschwitz MS, Dietrich H, et al (Univ of Innsbruck, Austria; Univ of Erlangen–Nuremberg, Germany; Univ of California, Davis)

J Clin Invest 98:785–792, 1996 4–13

Background.—Systemic sclerosis is an autoimmune disorder marked by 3 morphological changes in early skin lesions: structural and functional vascular and microvascular abnormalities, perivascular and tissue infiltration of mononuclear inflammatory cells, and increased collagenous and noncollagenous extracellular matrix molecules. Fibrotic destruction of the lungs, heart, kidneys, gastrointestinal tract, and other internal organs can occur. The etiology and pathogenesis of systemic sclerosis is unknown. The search for the cause of autoaggression requires animal models in which the disease develops spontaneously or is induced. A hereditary systemic connective tissue disease similar to systemic sclerosis in humans develops in the UCD-200/206 chicken. This animal model permits observation of the early stages of disease that are not accessible in humans. The mechanisms of degenerative skin lesions in the early stages of systemic sclerosis were identified in situ, and the targets and mechanisms of the disease process were defined in the UCD-200/206 chicken.

Methods.—Lesional skin biopsy specimens were excised from 15 patients with systemic sclerosis at different stages of disease, 9 patients with localized scleroderma, and 3 patients with keloids. The skin was analyzed for apoptosis by terminal deoxynucleotidyl transferase-mediated fluorescein isothiocyanate-deoxyuridine triphosphate nick end labeling and indirect immunofluorescence staining of cell markers with tetramethylrhodamine isothiocyanate conjugates.

Results.—In the skin of the UCD 200/206 chickens, endothelial cells were the first cells to undergo apoptosis. This process appeared to be induced by anti-endothelial cell antibodies. In human skin with fibrotic disease, apoptotic endothelial cells were detected only in early inflammatory stages of systemic sclerosis and localized scleroderma. No apoptotic cells were noted in the 8 biopsy specimens of chronic, fibrotic systemic sclerosis or in the keloid sections or skin from healthy control subjects.

Discussion.—In situ and at early stages of systemic sclerosis and scleroderma, endothelial cells undergo apoptosis contributing to other pathogenetic events in the fibrosis of these diseases. It is unclear whether inflammatory cells are involved in the induction of apoptotic processes. The use of the UCD 200/206 chicken made it possible to analyze the early stages of disease.

► The chicken model of systemic sclerosis is understudied and, thus, underappreciated. Wick and Gershwin have collaborated with others to examine the lesions of the chick and have produced important results. Previously, they characterized the inflamatory skin lesion as containing predominantly T cells of the CD8+, CD3+ type with the γ/δ T-cell receptor. In this study, they have observed apoptosis of microvascular endothelial cells colocalizing with immunoglobulin and not with T cells, which suggests that anti-endothelial cell antibodies are triggering the endothelial cell apoptosis. Similar findings are observed in human localized scleroderma and systemic sclerosis skin biopsy specimens. There is little evidence to point to how this destructive autoimmune cycle gets started, but it does place the endothelial cell squarely in the center as the autoimmune target cell, which is a concept initially introduced by Campbell et al in 1975.[1]

E.C. LeRoy, M.D.

Reference

1. Campbell PM, LeRoy EC: Pathogenesis of systemic sclerosis: A vascular hypothesis. *Semin Arthritis Rheum* 4:351–368, 1975.

Evidence of Free Radical–Mediated Injury (Isoprostane Overproduction) in Scleroderma

Stein CM, Tanner SB, Awad JA, et al (Vanderbilt Univ, Nashville, Tenn)
Arthritis Rheum 39:1146–1150, 1996 4–14

Introduction.—The pathogenesis of scleroderma may involve free radical–induced oxidative stress followed by lipid peroxidation. This hypothesis is difficult to test, however, because of the lack of reliable measures of in vivo lipid peroxidation. The F_2-isoprostanes are bioactive compounds, similar to prostaglandin F_2, which are produced in vivo by the noncyclooxygenase, free radical–catalyzed peroxidation of arachidonic acid. Previous studies have shown the F_2-isoprostanes to provide a reliable measure of lipid peroxidation in vivo. The studies were used to assess the possible link between scleroderma and enhanced oxidative stress.

Methods.—The study included 8 patients with scleroderma of varying severity, from limited disease with refractory digital ulceration or pulmonary hypertension to diffuse disease. Ten healthy controls were investigated as well. Oxidative stress was evaluated by measuring the urinary concentrations of a tetranor-dicarboxylic acid metabolite of F_2-isoprostanes (F_2IP-M) with mass spectrometry. Levels of 11-dehydro-thromboxane (TX) B_2—a stable urinary metabolite of TXA_2—were measured as well.

Results.—The mean F_2IP-M concentration was 3.41 ng/mg of creatinine in the scleroderma patients vs. 1.22 ng/mg of creatinine in the control group (Fig 1). The F_2IP-M concentration in the scleroderma patients was elevated, regardless of disease severity. Levels of F_2IP-M and 11-dehydro-TXB_2 were not correlated with each other.

Conclusion.—Levels of urinary F_2IP-M are elevated in patients with scleroderma. This finding strengthens the hypothesis that the pathogenesis of scleroderma involves free radical–induced oxidative injury. Urinary F_2IP-M may provide a useful marker of scleroderma activity and response to treatment. Further studies should examine the potential value of antioxidant therapy for scleroderma.

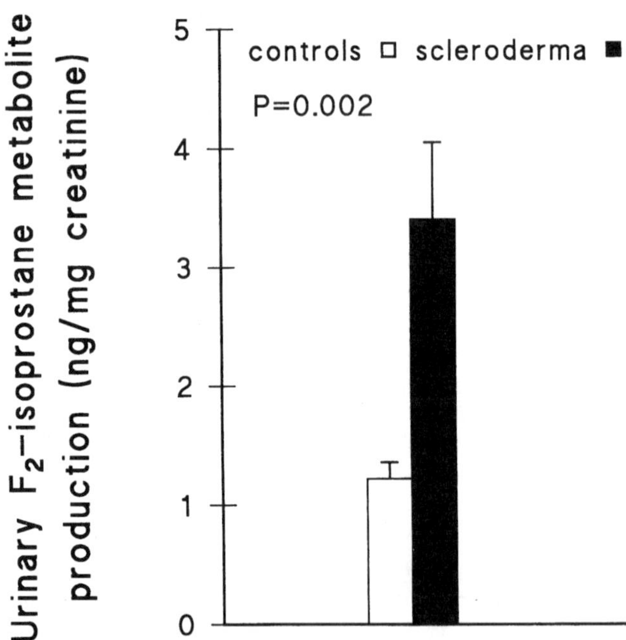

FIGURE 1.—Urinary concentrations of the stable tetranor-dicarboxylic acid urinary metabolite of F_2-isoprostanes in 8 patients with scleroderma and in 10 healthy controls. (Courtesy of Stein CM, Tanner SB, Awad JA, et al: Evidence of free radical–mediated injury [isoprostane overproduction] in scleroderma. *Arthritis Rheum* 39:1146–1150, 1996, copyright American College of Rheumatology.)

▶ Isoprostanes are derivatives of prostaglandins, which are the direct result of lipid peroxidation by free radicals of oxygen (also called reactive oxygen species). This report documents a 3-fold higher excretion of isoprostanes in the urine of 8 patients with systemic sclerosis measured by mass spectrometry. Free radicals, if not immediately neutralized by the body's antioxidant mechanisms, can injure endothelial cells and blood vessel walls and induce extracellular matrix systhesis conducive to fibrosis, the hallmark of systemic sclerosis. Even more interesting, most free radicals can be blocked by either direct (e.g., α-tocopheral [vitamin E]) or indirect (e.g., selenium to induce glutathione peroxidase) therapies of high relative safety. With a stable surrogate marker such as 24-hour urine isoprostanes, there is no reason (except for lack of a suitable funding sponsor) why a therapeutic trial should not begin.

E.C. LeRoy, M.D.

Clinical Aspects

Increased Prevalence of Systemic Sclerosis in a Native American Tribe in Oklahoma

Arnett FC, Howard RF, Tan F, et al (Univ of Texas Health Science Ctr, Houston; Choctaw Nation Hosp and Clinics, Talihina, Oklahoma; Baylor College of Medicine, Houston; et al)

Arthritis Rheum 39:1362–1370, 1996 4–15

Objective.—Although the cause of systemic sclerosis (SSc) is unknown, there is evidence that both genetic and environmental factors are involved. Recent studies have shown a strong link between certain HLA-DRB1 and/or DQB1 alleles and certain autoantibody profiles of SSc, suggesting a possible role of immune response genes in the pathogenesis or expression of SSc. A high prevalence of SSc in a tribe of Native Americans was investigated, including the results of HLA studies.

Methods.—A high prevalence of SSc was noted among the Choctaw tribe of Native Americans living in southeastern Oklahoma. This phenomenon was studied in a population of more than 21,000 Choctaws served by Indian Health Services. Twelve patients with SSc were matched to 48 controls without the disease. Various occupational, residential, and infectious exposures potentially related to SSc were investigated, together with genetic factors. HLA class I, II, and III alleles were investigated by DNA oligotypic and serologic studies.

Results.—During the 4-year study period, the prevalence of SSc among full-blooded Choctaws was at least 469/100,000, compared with 31/100,000 among non–full-blooded Choctaws (odds ratio, 15.4). All Oklahoma Choctaws had an SSc prevalence of 66/100,000, compared with 9.5/100,000 for other Native Americans in Oklahoma (Table 1).

The Choctaws with SSc were clinically similar. Most had diffuse scleroderma with pulmonary fibrosis and autoantibodies to topoisomerase I. None of the environmental exposures investigated were significantly different between patients and controls. Genetic analyses found that all of the

TABLE 1.—Estimated Prevalence of Systemic Sclerosis in Several Native American Groups

	Actual cases/ population	Estimated cases/100,000 (95% CI)	Estimated frequency
Oklahoma Choctaw			
Full-blooded	8/1,704*	469 (203–930)	1/213
Non-full-blooded	6/19,551	31 (11–68)	1/3,259
Total	14/21,255	66 (35–115)	1/1,518
Non-Oklahoma Choctaw (full-blooded)	0/4,500	—	—
Other Okalhoma Native Americans (non-Choctaw)	20/210,811	9.5 (5.8–14.6)	1/10,541

*P = 0.00001, odds ratio (OR) = 15.4; 95% confidence interval (CI) of 4.9–49.8 compared with non–full-blooded Oklahoma Choctaws. $P < 0.001$, OR = 45, 95% CI of 6.4–910 compared with non–Oklahoma full-blooded Choctaws. $P = 10^{-6}$, OR = 6.95, 95% CI of 3.3–13.7 compared with other Native Americans (non-Choctaw).

(Courtesy of Arnett FC, Howard RF, Tan F, et al: Increased prevalence of systemic sclerosis in a Native American tribe in Oklahoma. *Arthritis Rheum* 39:1362–1370, 1996, copyright American College of Rheumatology.)

SSc patients had an HLA haplotype with the alleles B35, Cw4, DRB1*1602 (DR2), DQA1*0501, and DQB1*0301 (DQ7). This haplotype was found in 54% of controls, for an odds ratio of 21.0. Study of a group of non-Oklahoma Choctaws found a high frequency of the same HLA haplotype, but no cases of SSc.

Conclusion.—Systemic sclerosis is more prevalent among full-blooded Choctaws living in Southeastern Oklahoma than among any other population group yet identified. The main risk factor for SSc in this group is an HLA haplotype that is unique to Native Americans but is not always associated with disease. Other genes and/or environmental exposures are probably involved in the development of SSc in this group.

► If you are an Oklahoma full-blooded Choctaw Indian, you have a 15-fold greater risk of SSc developing than if you are a white American. No environmental basis for this increased association has been found; however, an ancestry (traceable to 2 French brothers) identified by the haplotype B35, CW4, DRB1*1602, DQA1*0501, and DQB1*0301 seems to be the predisposing factor and diffuse disease with antitopoisomerase I autoantibodies the discernible phenotype. Further studies of the Choctaws for biological and immunogenetic explanations of the mechanisms of fibrosis are in order. If this human haplotype were stably transfected into a mouse genome, would it be sufficient to produce mouse scleroderma? It would be interesting to see.

(Unfortunately there seems to be little alternative to learning the new, sequence-specific nomenclature for human HLA alleles. Good luck!)

E.C. LeRoy, M.D.

Incidence of Systemic Sclerosis in Allegheny County, Pennsylvania: A Twenty-Year Study of Hospital-diagnosed Cases, 1963–1982
Steen VD, Oddis CV, Conte CG, et al (Georgetown Univ, Washington, DC; Univ of Pittsburgh, Pa)
Arthritis Rheum 40:441–445, 1997 4–16

Introduction.—Reports vary regarding the epidemiologic features of systemic sclerosis (SSc; scleroderma). The incidence of hospital-diagnosed SSc from 1963 to 1982 in Allegheny County, Pa, was calculated. Patterns of age-, sex-, and race-specific incidence and temporal trends during this 20-year time span were described.

Methods.—The International Classification of Diseases codes was used to search medical records for discharge diagnosis of SSc from all 35 Allegheny County hospitals for demographic data on age at diagnosis, sex, race, and location of residence; date of disease onset; and clinical information, including clinical information confirming diagnosis and disease manifestations. Age-adjusted incidence rates were determined by race and sex. Findings were expressed as new cases per million population per year, using the 1970 Allegheny County population as the standard.

Results.—The total annual incidence during the 20-year survey was 13.9 per million population (444 diagnoses of SSc). The overall incidence

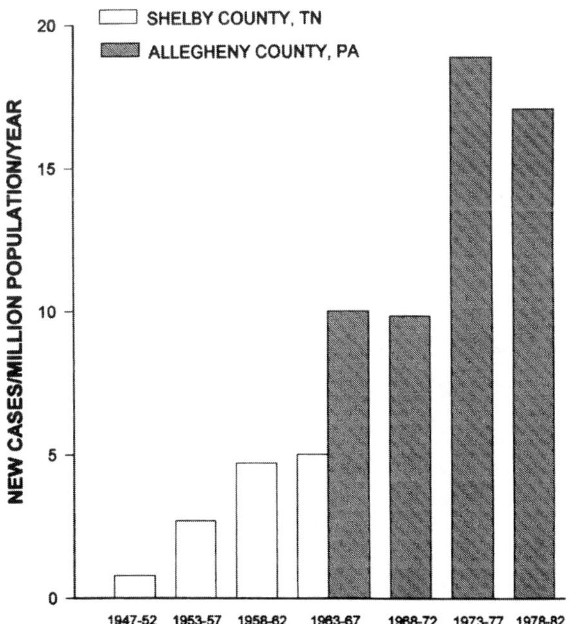

FIGURE 2.—Overall incidence of systemic sclerosis in Shelby County, Tenn (1947–1967) and Allegheny County, Pa (1963–1982). (Courtesy of Steen VD, Oddis CV, Conte CG et al: Incidence of systemic sclerosis in Allegheny County, Pennsylvania: A twenty-year study of hospital-diagnosed cases, 1963–1982. *Arthritis Rheum* 40:441–445, 1997, copyright American College of Rheumatology.)

rate doubled during 1973 to 1982, compared with 1963 to 1972 (Fig 2). The greatest increase occurred in women. At 21.2 per million population, black women had the highest incidence of SSc among women aged 15 to 24 years. The overall female-to-male incidence ratio was 3:1 (3.41 during childbearing years). Systemic sclerosis was rare in children and in men younger than age 35 years.

Conclusions.—Over time, there was a slight increase in the incidence of SSc that may be partly because of improved detection and medical record techniques. The incidence rate appears to be increasing mostly in blacks and women, especially during childbearing years.

► Medsger and his colleagues have carefully determined with precision the incidence of SSc in Allegheny County, Pa, from hospital medical records, a conservative instrument that certainly should not overestimate and, if anything, could underestimate. From these results, the incidence doubled from the 1970s to the 1980s in women but not in men. The authors propose as explanations both a greater awareness of the disease and perhaps a true increase in incidence. Because this study included patients admitted only up to 1982, it is almost time to repeat the study. We are indebted to the Pittsburgh group for these careful studies.

E.C. LeRoy, M.D.

Lung Involvement in Systemic Sclerosis (Scleroderma): Relation to Classification Based on Extent of Skin Involvement or Autoantibody Status

Kane GC, Varga J, Conant EF, et al (Thomas Jefferson Univ, Philadelphia)
Respir Med 90:223–230, 1996 4–17

Background.—For patients with systemic sclerosis (SSc), lung involvement is a major cause of morbidity and a leading cause of death. Pulmonary parenchymal or vascular involvement has been suggested to relate to other clinical features of the disease, such as skin involvement and the presence of specific autoantibodies (especially anticentromere [ACA] or anti-Scl 70 antibodies). Whether these characteristics are predictive of pulmonary parenchymal involvement in patients with SSc was retrospectively studied.

Methods.—Medical records of 72 consecutive patients with SSc who were evaluated at a scleroderma center between 1990 and 1992 were reviewed. Interstitial lung disease was diagnosed based on pulmonary function tests and chest radiographs.

Results.—Restrictive lung disease was diagnosed in 30% of patients with limited SSc and in 50% of patients with diffuse SSc. Significant interstitial disease was evident radiographically in 28% of patients with limited SSc and 32% of patients with diffuse SSc. The mean lung function did not differ according to presence or absence of anti-Scl 70 antibody, but it did differ significantly according to presence or absence of ACA (Table

TABLE 6.—Interstitial Abnormalities on Chest Radiograph According to Antibody Status

	ACA + (n=17)	ACA⁻ (n=32)	*P* value	Scl 70⁺ (n=8)	Scl 70⁻ (n=41)	*P* value
No radiographic abnormalities or radiographically insignificant abnormalities	16 (94%)	11 (34%)	<0.001	4 (50%)	23 (56%)	n.s.
Minimal	1 (6%)	6 (19%)	=0·012	1 (12%)	6 (15%)	n.s.
Significant	0 (0%)	15 (47%)	=0·002	3 (38%)	12 (29%)	n.s.

Abbreviations: ACA, anticentromere antibody; *Scl 70*, anti-Scl 70 antibody.

(Reprinted from Kane GC, Varga J, Conant EF, et al: Lung involvement in systemic sclerosis [scleroderma]: Relation to classification based on extent of skin involvement or autoantibody status. *Respir Med* 90:223–230, 1996, by permission of the publisher WB Saunders Company Limited London.)

6). Patients with ACA also showed less frequent radiographic evidence of severe interstitial disease.

Conclusion.—Skin involvement alone is only weakly predictive of restrictive lung disease, because restrictive lung disease is common in patients with either limited or diffuse SSc. However, restrictive disease appears to occur infrequently in patients with ACA. Anticentromere antibody might have a protective effect related to its association with specific major histocompatibility complex antigens.

▶ We are entering a new era in the subset classification of patients with SSc as having either limited or diffuse disease. The new era will add immunogenetic (histocompatibility leukocyte antigens) and serologic (antinuclear antibodies) parameters to the degree of skin tethering already used for this purpose. The most promising candidates for addition to the criteria are ACA, reacting with the kinetochore apparatus of the mitotic spindle. Using actively dividing HEp-2 (human laryngeal carcinoma) cells, this test is readily available.

Kane and colleagues have reviewed 72 patients with SSc and compared skin score with autoantibody status as a predictor of the presence of interstitial lung disease. The presence of ACA strongly predicted the absence of significant lung disease. In 3 patients with ACA and diffuse skin disease, 2 were free of lung involvement and the third, whose disease was an example of delayed diffuse SSc, died with interstitial lung disease and pulmonary hypertension.

It is interesting that the absence of ACA was predictive of the presence of interstital lung disease, whereas the presence of antibodies to topoisomerase I was not and skin score was only weakly predictive. The patient with ACA who is positive for SSc is usually female, often white, and negative for a history of exposure to environmental triggers of SSc (plastics, solvents, epoxies, silica). This patient must still be watched for the development of isolated pulmonary hypertension (by ECHO-Doppler) but does seem protected from the development of interstitial lung disease. In contrast, the male or nonwhite patient with SSc is usually negative for ACA, often has diffuse disease, and may have a higher risk of exposure to environmental triggers. These distinctions in the identification of subsets of SSc are useful in the individual patient to design diagnostic and therapeutic plans, especially in this era of managed care and limited reimbursement resources.

E.C. LeRoy, M.D.

Prevalence of Pulmonary Hypertension in Limited and Diffuse Scleroderma

Battle RW, Davitt MA, Cooper SM, et al (Univ of Vermont, Burlington)

Chest 110:1515–1519, 1996 4–18

Introduction.—Premortem diagnosis of pulmonary involvement in patients with limited or diffuse scleroderma (SSc) is often difficult because symptoms are often minimal, and physical examination and chest radiographs are usually normal. Doppler echocardiography has been used to detect pulmonary hypertension in patients with connective tissue disease. The prevalence of pulmonary hypertension was assessed in patients with SSc but without an existing diagnosis of pulmonary hypertension.

Methods.—Of 34 patients, 29 had limited and 5 had diffuse SSc. Patients underwent physical examination, 12-lead ECG, and 2-dimensional and Doppler echocardiography. The estimated pulmonary artery systolic pressure (PA_s) was determined using the sum of the transtricuspid gradient and the estimated right atrial pressure.

Results.—The Doppler spectral signals of tricuspid regurgitation were adequate in 33 of 34 patients. The mean calculated PA_s was 30 mm Hg (range, 15–95 mm Hg). Twelve patients (35%) had pulmonary hypertension with a mean calculated PA_s of 43 mm Hg (range, 30–95 mm Hg). Of these, 1 patient each had values of 56 and 95 mm Hg, respectively. Evidence of pulmonary hypertension was detected on physical examination alone in 2 patients, ECG alone in 1 patient, and both in 1 patient. The PA_s in these patients was 21, 31, 34, and 95 mm Hg, respectively. Of 21 patients who had chest radiographs within 1 year of evaluation, 17 had normal results, 3 had diffuse interstitial changes, and 1 had significant pulmonary fibrosis. Six of 17 patients with normal radiography results had pulmonary hypertension. Of 14 patients who had pulmonary function testing within 1 year of evaluation, 10 had abnormalities including reduced diffusing capacity, evidence of airflow obstruction, and evidence of restrictive impairment. Four patients had normal pulmonary function test results. Of 10 patients with abnormal results of pulmonary function tests, 6 did not have Doppler evidence of pulmonary hypertension.

Conclusion.—Pulmonary hypertension was detected on Doppler examination in 35% of patients with scleroderma who had no previous diagnosis of pulmonary hypertension. If the significance of pulmonary hypertension in asymptomatic patients can be clarified, it may be possible to identify and treat patients early in the disease process.

► Twelve (35%) of 34 consecutive patients with systemic sclerosis were shown to have pulmonary hypertension by noninvasive Doppler echocardiography techniques. This is a high proportion and suggests that this abnormality is frequent in both limited and diffuse SSc. Because early and mild pulmonary hypertension would appear to be more responsive to calcium channel blocker or a prostacyclin analogue therapy than is severe, late disease, surveillance of all patients with SSc for pulmonary hypertension is in order, as severe pulmonary hypertension is uniformly fatal in 2 to 3 years.

E.C. LeRoy, M.D.

Isolated Pulmonary Hypertension in Systemic Sclerosis With Diffuse Cutaneous Involvement: Association With Serum Anti-U3RNP Antibody

Sacks DG, Okano Y, Steen VD, et al (Univ of Pittsburgh, Pa; Albany Med College, NY)

J Rheumatol 23:639–642, 1996 4–19

Introduction.—Many patients with systemic sclerosis (SSc)—both the diffuse cutaneous (dc) and limited cutaneous (lc) forms—have lung involvement and pulmonary fibrosis. However, previous reports suggest that mainly patients with lcSSc have isolated pulmonary hypertension (PHT). A group of patients with dcSSc and IPHT was studied.

Methods.—Fourteen patients with dcSSc and IPHT were examined at the authors' department from 1975 to 1992. All patients underwent SSc specific serum autoantibody testing methods. The clinical, laboratory, and natural history findings of patients with dcSSc and IPHT were compared

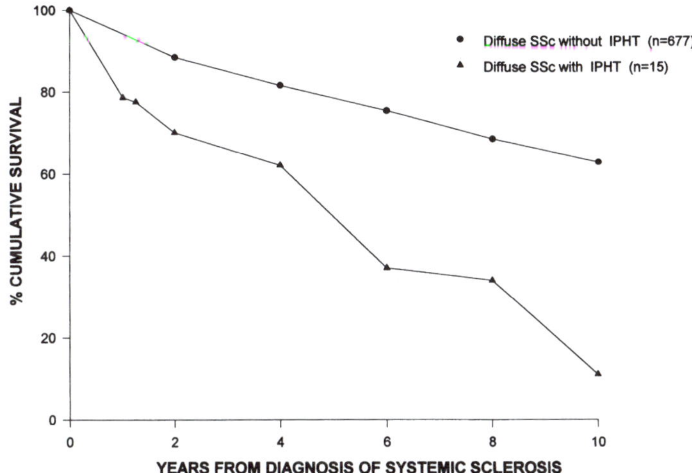

FIGURE 1.—Cumulative survival from diagnosis of systemic sclerosis (*SSc*) in patients with diffuse cutaneous SSc with (n = 15) or without (n = 677) isolated pulmonary hypertension (*IPHT*). Patients with IPHT have significantly decreased survival ($P < 0.001$), compared with others with diffuse cutaneous SSc. (Courtesy of Sacks DG, Okano Y, Steen VD, et al: Isolated pulmonary hypertension in systemic sclerosis with diffuse cutaneous involvement: Association with serum anti-U3RNP antibody. *J Rheumatol* 23:639–642, 1996.)

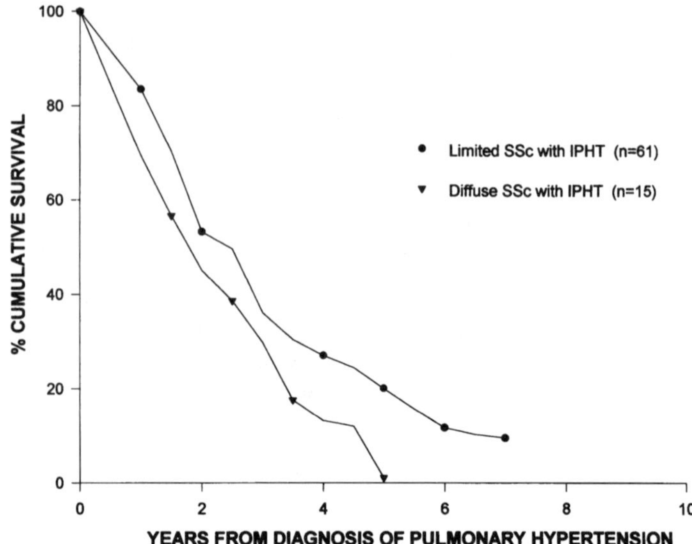

FIGURE 2.—Percentage of cumulative survival from diagnosis of isolated pulmonary hypertension (*IPHT*) in patients with limited cutaneous systemic sclerosis (*SSc*) with IPHT (n = 61) compared with patients with diffuse cutaneous SSc with IPHT (n =15). Both groups have very poor survival. (Courtesy of Sacks DG, Okano Y, Steen VD, et al: Isolated pulmonary hypertension in systemic sclerosis with diffuse cutaneous involvement: Association with serum anti-U3RNP antibody. *J Rheumatol* 23:639–642, 1996.)

with those of 60 patients with lcSSC and IPHT and 677 patients with dcSSc and no pulmonary hypertension.

Findings.—The 14 patients with dcSSc and IPHT represented 2% of all patients with dcSSc, whereas 10% of patients with lcSSc seen during the same period were found to have IPHT. Among patients with either form of SSc, those with and without IPHT were similar in terms of age, race, sex, or cutaneous manifestations. The chest radiographs of patients with dcSSc IPHT showed few or no signs of pulmonary interstitial fibrosis. The DLCO was measured in 12 patients with dcSSc IPHT—the mean value was 50% of predicted, which was comparable to the values of lcSSc patients. Five of the 14 patients with dcSSc had a history of "sclerodermal renal crisis." Immunoprecipitation testing from serum anti-U3RNP antibody was positive in 46% of patients in the dcSSc IPHT group, compared with only 6% of patients with dcSSc without IPHT. Survival was significantly better for patients with dcSSc without IPHT than for those with IPHT (Fig 1). The initial symptom of pulmonary hypertension was usually exertional dyspnea. Most patients with IPHT, regardless of what form of SSc they had, died within 2 years after that time (Fig 2).

Conclusion.—In patients with the dc form of SSc, severe and fatal IPHT can develop. Approximately half of the patients with dcSSc with IPHT will have serum anti-U3RNP antibody. Survival is poor for all patients with SSc and IPHT. All patients with SSc with diffuse cutaneous involvement and a marked decrease in DLCO but little or no pulmonary interstitial fibrosis should be considered at risk for IPHT.

► This excellent retrospective study of large numbers of patients with scleroderma (SSc) shows the following:

1. Pulmonary hypertension does occur in patients with diffuse SSc.
2. In patients with diffuse SSc, anti-U3RNP autoantibodies are found in half of the subset who had pulmonary hypertension.
3. Whether in diffuse or limited SSc, pulmonary hypertension is usually lethal in 2 years.

Even though only 1 in 4 patients with diffuse SSc and U3RNP autoantibodies has pulmonary hypertension, all patients with diffuse SSc and U3RNP should be observed carefully, with tests including ECHO-Doppler ultrasound, for this potentially lethal vascular feature.

E.C. LeRoy, M.D.

Cardiorespiratory Responses to Incremental Exercise in Patients With Systemic Sclerosis

Schwaiblmair M, Behr J, Fruhmann G (Univ of Munich, Germany)

Chest 110:1520–1525, 1996 4–20

Background.—Pulmonary abnormalities are found histologically in patients with systemic sclerosis (SSc), despite normal findings on chest radiography and/or conventional pulmonary function. Cardiopulmonary exercise testing was used in an attempt to detect the early features of lung involvement in patients with progressive SSc.

Methods.—Seventy-eight patients meeting criteria for SSc were included. Forty-four were classified as having limited cutaneous SSc and 34 as having diffuse cutaneous SSc.

Findings.—Diffusing capacity was significantly reduced (to 65% of that predicted) only in patients with diffuse cutaneous SSc. Those with lung involvement had significantly decreased exercise capacity (to 54% of that predicted) and oxygen uptake (to 70% of that predicted). In addition, functional dead space ventilation was increased and alveolar-arterial oxygen difference widened during exercise. Fifteen percent of the patients with normal single-breath diffusing capacity for carbon monoxide had an increased dead space–to-tidal volume ratio on cardiopulmonary exercise testing (Fig 1).

Conclusion.—Patients with SSc and apparent normal pulmonary function may have occult pulmonary impairment. Cardiopulmonary exercise testing may be useful for detecting such impairment. Resting data have limitations in predicting abnormalities during exercise in patients with SSc.

► By stimulating an organ's function, one can determine reserve capacity. Exercise does this for both the ventilatory and perfusion aspects of lung function. As demonstrated by this careful study of 78 patients with SSc (44 limited, 34 diffuse) by the Munich pulmonary group, exercise testing detected the only abnormalities of function noted in one out of every seven patients. Figure 1 shows 9 (11%) of 78 patients with increased A-a gradients

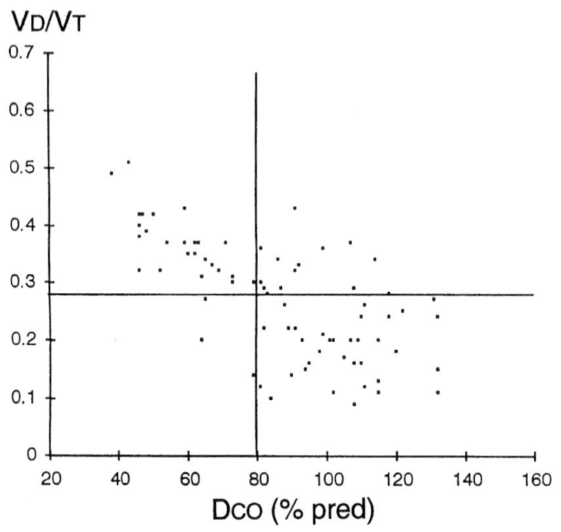

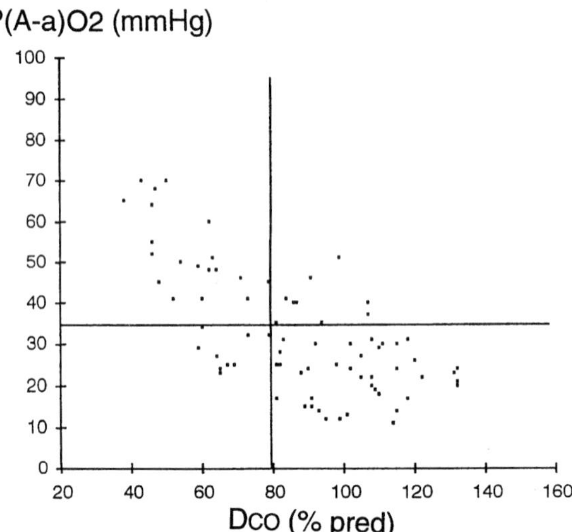

FIGURE 1.—Correlation between resting diffusing capacity of carbon monoxide (*Dco*) (percent of predicted) and physiologic dead space ventilation (*VD/VT*) and alveolar-arterial oxygen pressure difference (*P (A-a)O_2*) (mm Hg) in 78 patients with systemic sclerosis. The horizontal and vertical lines indicate the upper 95% confidence limit of normal values. (Courtesy of Schwaiblmair M, Behr J, Fruhmann G: Cardiorespiratory responses to incremental exercise in patients with systemic sclerosis. *Chest* 110:1520–1525, 1996.)

who had normal diffusion, as well as ventilation, studies (see the upper right quadrant of the right side of Fig 1). Also, 15% of patients had abnormally increased physiologic dead space/tidal volume ratios, detected only by exercise (see the upper right of the left side of Fig 1).

Thus, exercise testing can identify early lung abnormalities in 10% to 15% of patients with SSc, with the preponderance of those found to be abnormal being patients with diffuse SSc. Presently, the prefibrotic pulmonary state of alveolitis is being detected by high resolution chest tomography and/or bronchoalveolar lavage—expensive or invasive techniques. Perhaps exercise testing of the patient with diffuse SSc could be predictive and cost effective in the early detection of interstitial lung disease.

E.C. LeRoy, M.D.

Comprehensive Noninvasive Assessment of Cardiac Involvement in Limited Systemic Sclerosis

Candell-Riera J, Armadans-Gil L, Simeón C-P, et al (Hosp Gen Universitari Vall d'Hebron, Barcelona)

Arthritis Rheum 39:1138–1145, 1996 4–21

Introduction.—Primary cardiac involvement in SSc is seen as pericardial or myocardial abnormalities. Necropsy studies have reported pericardial involvement in 33% to 72% of patients; myocardial disease, in 12% to 89% of patients. Echocardiographic studies have shown that patients with SSc commonly have cardiovascular abnormalities, even when cardiovascular symptoms are not present. Diastolic function abnormalities in patients with SSc have been shown by Doppler echocardiography and radionuclide ventriculography. Radionuclide perfusion studies with thallium-201 or positron emission tomography have revealed perfusion defects that may have been caused by local coronary spasms. Most of these studies were of patients with diffuse forms of SSc. Limited SSc has a better prognosis and is found in up to 80% of such patients. To noninvasively assess cardiovascular abnormalities, echocardiographic and scintigraphic studies were done in patients with limited systemic sclerosis (SSc).

Methods.—Doppler echocardiography and thallium-201 scintigraphy were done in 63 consecutive patients with limited SSc. These procedures were done after a cold-stress test and radionuclide ventriculography.

Results.—A significantly higher rate of abnormal left-diastolic and right-diastolic function parameters, thickening of papillary muscles, and mild mitral regurgitation were seen in patients with limited SSc than in control patients (Table 2). In 9 patients, systolic pulmonary arterial hypertension was found. In 11 patients, pericardial effusion was found. An ischemic response on the thallium cold-stress scan was detected in 64% of patients. In 57% of patients with primary Raynaud's phenomenon, an ischemic response also was noted.

Discussion.—The high rate of mild mitral regurgitation in these patients with limited SSc was similar to results reported by others. In the patients in the current study, this was not associated with age or mitral annular calcification, but with mitral subvalvular thickening. This association has not previously been reported and may explain the mitral regurgitation. Doppler echocardiography also detected significant involvement of the diastolic function parameters of the right and left ventricles. A significant rate of cardiovascular abnormalities was found with noninvasive methods

TABLE 2.—Clinical Data and Abnormal Findings for Controls and Patients With Limited Systemic Sclerosis

Parameter	Controls (n = 40), no. (%)	Limited SSc (n = 63), no. (%)	P*
Pericardial effusion	0	11(18)	0.0149†
Subvalvular mitral thickening	6 (15)	29 (46)	0.0031‡
Mitral annulus calcification	1 (3)	8 (13)	0.1478†
Mitral regurgitation	3 (8)	31 (49)	<0.0001‡
Tricuspid regurgitation	5 (13)	19 (30)	0.0774
Pulmonary arterial hypertension	0	9 (14)	0.0114

*By chi-square test (1 *df*), except where indicated.
†Fisher's exact test.
‡Statistical significance after adjustment for multiple comparisons.
(Courtesy of Candell-Riera J, Armadans-Gil L, Simeón C-P, et al: Comprehensive noninvasive assessment of cardiac involvement in limited systemic sclerosis. *Arthritis Rheum* 39:1138–1145, 1996, copyright American College of Rheumatology.)

in these patients, but primary cardiac involvement did not seem to have a striking impact on the disease.

▶ There remains a significant number of sudden deaths in patients with SSc—deaths that are largely unexplained. Because most patients with SSc have the limited (limited cutaneous) subset, and because these patients have 40 or more years of life after initial diagnosis, the prospective, noninvasive cardiovascular evaluation of 63 patients from Barcelona with limited SSc could provide useful information. This is especially true because a direct comparison is made with 58 patients with primary Raynaud's phenomenon. These groups should be valuable for long-term survival and follow-up clinical evaluation.

Follensbee, Stein and Medsger noted that thallium scintigraphy detected myocardial perfusion abnormalities in more than 90% of patients with diffuse SSc and that this test, when abnormal, predicted a shortened survival.[1] In the present Barcelona study, thallium scans after cold and Doppler echocardiography were more sensitive than thallium scans or scans after exercise (so-called stress thallium scans) in detecting a large proportion of myocardial wall, subvalvular, and ventricular diastolic abnormalities in largely asymptomatic individuals. These abnormalities, including subvalvular thickening as an explanation for mild mitral regurgitation, were clinically unimportant at the time detected. The crucial question is, are they of prognostic significance? In limited SSc, 30- and 40-year data from the onset of first symptoms (the patients were studied 17 and 7 years after diagnosis, respectively) would be most important. I hope that these Barcelona patients can be followed up for such evaluation.

There is 1 major caveat in this type of nonetheless-promising study. In this and other control series applying the number of noninvasive cardiologic techniques used and thus amassing large quantities of data, the frequency of the type of subclinical "abnormalities" found here varies from 20% (this study) to as high as 50% in "healthy" individuals; thus, the prognostic implications of these findings in all of us remains to be determined.

E.C. LeRoy, M.D.

Reference

1. Follansbee WP, Curtiss EI, Medsger TA, Jr, et al: Physiologic abnormalities of cardiac function in progressive systemic sclerosis with diffuse scleroderma. *N Engl J Med* 310:142–148, 1984.

Thallium Perfusion Defects Predict Subsequent Cardiac Dysfunction in Patients With Systemic Sclerosis

Steen VD, Follansbee WP, Conte CG, et al (Univ of Pittsburgh, Pa)

Arthritis Rheum 39:677–681, 1996 4–22

Background.—The most life-threatening developments of systemic sclerosis (SSc) are cardiac and renal complications. Cardiac problems can occur at any time during the course of the disease, but only skeletal myositis has been identified as a risk factor for serious cardiac events. A follow-up study of patients who underwent thallium perfusion scans assessed whether thallium perfusion defects were predictive of cardiac disease or death.

Patients and Methods.—The 48 consecutive patients underwent a radionuclide myocardial function study in 1982 and 1983. Each also had laboratory evaluation for organ-system involvement, an ECG, a chest radiograph, planar exercise thallium scintigrams, and an exercise radionuclide ventriculogram study. Perfusion defects were expressed as a defect score (DS) for each patient. Data were available for all 48 patients during 1991–1992 follow-up.

Results.—At the time of the initial study, patients with SSc had a mean age of 51 years and a mean disease duration of 8.2 years; 77% were women and 54% had diffuse cutaneous involvement. Abnormal thallium scintigram findings were present in 34 patients. In this group, 26 had fixed perfusion defects and 10 had exercise-induced defects (2 had both). Symptomatic heart disease was present in 7 patients at the initial study and developed in 8 more during follow-up. Defect scores were significantly greater in patients with diffuse scleroderma than in those within limited scleroderma (mean 3.5 vs. 1.4). A high initial DS was significantly associated with ECG abnormalities and reduced left ventricular ejection fraction throughout the course of illness. Compared with a low DS (less than 1.6), a high DS was significantly associated with higher rates of symptomatic heart disease (56% vs. 26%) and of death from any cause during follow-up (69% vs. 19%). Symptomatic heart disease also developed significantly more rapidly in those with a higher DS.

Conclusion.—Patients with SSc who have major thallium perfusion defects have a significantly increased risk of serious cardiac disease and death. In a logistic regression analysis that included 10 variables, only thallium DS was significantly independently associated with subsequent death. Identification of those at risk may allow interventions to prevent permanent myocardial damage.

► In 48 patients with SSc, 65% of whom had diffuse disease, myocardial radionuclide scans (so-called stress thallium scans) were done and assessed as showing large or small defects scores. Ten years later, 80% of those with small or no defects were alive, whereas 70% of those with large defects were dead. No other parameter of SSc provided similar predictive information. Stress thallium myocardial scans are thus an independent predictive variable for survival in the individual patient with SSc.

E.C. LeRoy, M.D.

Left Ventricular Myocardial Perfusion and Function in Systemic Sclerosis Before and After Diltiazem Treatment

Geirrsson AJ, Danielsen R, Pétursson E (Univ Hosp, Reykjavík, Iceland)

Scand J Rheumatol 25:317–320, 1996 4–23

Objective.—In patients with systemic sclerosis, vasospasm during cold exposure can effect not only the digital circulation but also the internal organs. These patients may have reversible myocardial perfusion defects during cold exposure or after exercise. The associated left ventricular dysfunction can be prevented by short-term treatment with nifedipine. The long-term benefits of calcium-channel blocker treatment in patients with sytemic sclerosis were investigated.

Methods.—Ten patients with systemic sclerosis underwent evaluation of systemic sclerosis at rest, during cold exposure, and at peak exercise. All had cardiopulmonary symptoms, consisting of shortness of breath in 7 patients and palpitations in 5. Seven patients received a mean of 11 months of treatment with diltiazem. Doppler echocardiography was done before and after treatment.

Results.—Cold provocation induced no significant change in myocardial perfusion, whereas exercise produced an average 48% increase. Myocardial isotope uptake averaged 35% higher after exercise than after cold exposure. Myocardial uptake values were unchanged after diltiazem treatment. However, Doppler echocardiography showed increased left ventricular end-diastolic diameter, fractional shortening, and left ventricular outflow tract velocity.

Conclusions.—In patients with systemic sclerosis, long-term diltiazem treatment may improve left ventricular filling and, thus, performance. It does not increase myocardial perfusion, however, whether at rest, after exercise, or during cold exposure. These patients appear to have sufficient functional reserve to meet the demands of increased oxygen consumption.

▶ Calcium-channel blockers are commonly prescribed for scleroderma, usually in an attempt to palliate symptoms of secondary Raynaud's phenomenon. There is some suggestion that intermittent vasospasm affects other vascular beds, particularly the myocardium, where it may underlie the progressive fibrotic cardiomyopathy that is the fate of many a patient with scleroderma. Furthermore, calcium-channel blockers can be shown to acutely abrogate myocardial vasospasm in some patients. It has been postulated that a long-term benefit of these agents in scleroderma may be to spare the heart the typical contraction band necrosis and scattered fibrosis.

This article is an attempt to show such benefit from exposure to diltiazem, 240 mg daily, for about a year. No important change in myocardial perfusion or cardiac anatomy could be found. There is a suggestion of enhanced left ventricular function.

Inferences that can be drawn from this study are limited by the small number of patients, the knowledge that the authors had preserved myocardial function at entry, and the notion that little change might be anticipated in a year. However, the study is reassuring, particularly because long-term calcium-channel blocker exposure may itself have cardiac toxicity.

N.M. Hadler, M.D.

Renal Vascular Damage in Systemic Sclerosis Patients Without Clinical Evidence of Nephropathy

Rivolta R, Mascagni B, Berruti V, et al (Università di Milano, Italy)

Arthritis Rheum 39:1030–1034, 1996 4–24

Background.—Two approaches have been used to evaluate vascular damage in patients with systemic sclerosis (SSc): kidney biopsy and traditional clearance techniques. Biopsy is invasive and cannot be frequently repeated, and clearance techniques are not very sensitive or accurate. The potential clinical usefulness of color-flow Doppler ultrasonography for measurement of kidney blood flow in patients with SSc was studied.

Patients and Methods.—Study participants were 25 outpatients with SSc; the median disease duration was 8 years. Nine had diffuse cutaneous SSc and 10 had limited cutaneous SSc. All had normal urinalysis results, plasma creatinine levels, and endogenous creatinine clearance. Patients and 25 normal volunteers matched for age, sex, and blood pressure were studied with color-flow Doppler ultrasonography. A resistance index (RI), based on analysis of the spectral waveform, was determined on main, interlobar, and cortical vessels.

Results.—The right and left kidneys showed no significant difference in RI, but there was a significant difference in RI between normal controls and patients with SSc and between sampling sites. Although RI values tended to decrease from the main renal artery to the interlobar artery to the kidney cortex in both groups, controls showed a significant difference between the main artery and cortical vessels. In patients with SSc, cortical vessel RI differed significantly from both interlobar and main artery val-

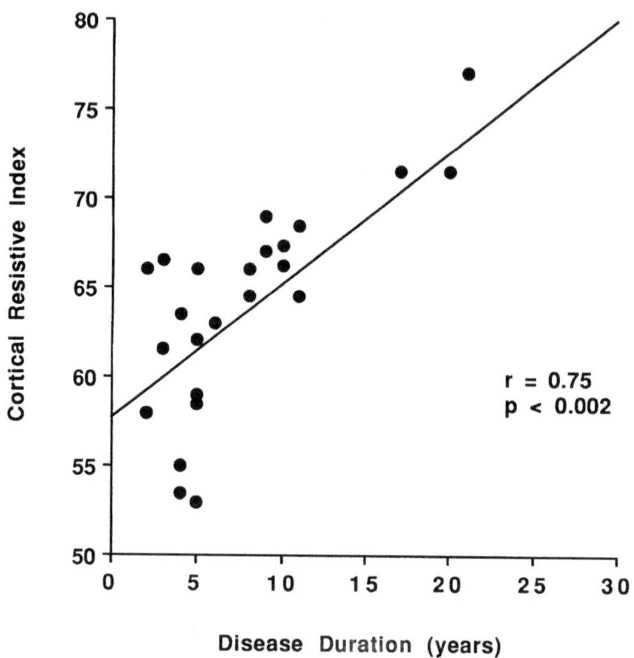

FIGURE 3.—Relation between resistance index values (×100), measured on cortical vessels, and disease duration in patients with systemic sclerosis. (Courtesy of Rivolta R, Mascagni B, Berruti V, et al: Renal vascular damage in systemic sclerosis patients without clinical evidence of nephropathy. *Arthritis Rheum* 39:1030–1034, 1996, copyright American College of Rheumatology.)

ues. There was a relationship between RI and duration of SSc, particularly when cortical vessels were measured (Fig 3). Regression analysis failed to identify a relationship between RI and creatinine clearance values.

Conclusion.—Color-flow Doppler ultrasonography, by directly exploring blood flow changes in various kidney vascular branches, is a sensitive technique for evaluating vascular damage in SSc. The noninvasive test also allows the site of vessel narrowing to be determined.

▶ Doppler ultrasonography scores again in scleroderma! Already useful in detecting pericardial effusion and pulmonary hypertension, it is now being used in the estimation of renal vascular resistance as a noninvasive measurement of "the scleroderma kidney." Kidney involvement in SSc is a multistage process. The characteristic intimal vascular scarring is insidious and progressive throughout the course of both limited and diffuse disease. When severely affected or suddenly stressed, there are acute reductions in renal perfusion in the already compromised setting of chronically decreased flow, with autoregulatory mechanisms already protecting glomerular perfusion by arcuate artery vasoconstriction and reduced renal blood flow, and a damaged endothelium less able to participate in nonthrombogenicity and local vasomotor needs. These reductions lead abruptly to thrombosis, cortical infarction, and oliguric renal failure. The big questions are whether this "scleroderma renal crisis" can be predicted and prevented.

These authors suggest that Doppler ultrasonography with color-flow technology could be helpful in selecting patients at risk. It would have been helpful to compare these flow techniques with the other predictor of renal scleroderma, microangiopathy. It is also of interest to ask whether angiotensin-converting enzyme inhibitors can prevent or reverse the reductions in flow and whether they are needed intermittently or permanently.

It is a distinctly positive occurrence that, since the introduction of captopril in 1980, far fewer cases of scleroderma renal crisis are seen. There remain, nonetheless, examples of multiple-organ failure in which renal insufficiency is a prominent part. Perhaps color-flow Doppler ultrasonography can be used in the lung, the heart, and the digestive system as well. It is also possible that the effects of angiotensin-converting enzyme inhibitors may be positive in the microcirculation in general.

E.C. LeRoy, M.D.

Investigation of Anal Function in Patients With Systemic Sclerosis

Herrick AL, Barlow JD, Bowden A, et al (Univ of Manchester, England; Hope Hosp, Salford, England)

Ann Rheum Dis 55:370–374, 1996 4–25

Objective.—Bowel function in patients with systemic sclerosis (SSc) has not been well studied. A detailed analysis of anal function was undertaken in women with SSc, with and without lower gastrointestinal symptoms.

Methods.—Anorectal manometry was done in 16 women, 14 with SSc and 2 with Raynaud's phenomenon, and in 11 healthy female controls. Seven patients had constipation, 3 had diarrhea, and 6 had no or minimal bowel symptoms. An 8-lumen polyvinylchloride water-perfused catheter was used to record mean resting pressure, maximum voluntary squeeze effort, radial asymmetry at rest, radial asymmetry during squeeze, vector volume at rest, and vector volume during squeeze. Circumferential information was gathered using a station pull-through in 1-cm steps from the rectum to the anal verge.

Results.—Mean resting pressure, maximum voluntary squeeze effort, and vector volume during squeeze were lower in patients than in controls and significantly lower in constipated patients. Radial asymmetry during squeeze was greater in constipated patients than in controls. Nine of 10 symptomatic patients had gastrointestinal reflux, gastrointestinal dysmotility, or both.

Conclusions.—Patients with SSc have anorectal dysfunction that is more significant in patients with constipation. Lower pressures, lower vector volumes, and greater squeeze asymmetry indicate subclinical dysmotility in patients with SSc.

► The lower gastrointestinal tract is as often involved as is the upper gastrointestinal tract in patients with SSc. When severe, anal canal problems can be most troublesome. Herrick and her colleagues have carefully examined the anal functional lesion in 16 patients with SSc. Mechanisms are poorly understood and treatment is unsatisfactory. When caught between the Scylla of obstipation and the Charybdis of diarrhea and fecal incontinence, management can be most vexing. Interestingly, there was frequently a history of lower abdominal and gynecologic surgery in symptomatic patients. Perhaps all elective surgery should be avoided in patients with SSc.

E.C. LeRoy, M.D.

Raynaud's Phenomenon

Vasospasm of the Nipple—A Manifestation of Raynaud's Phenomenon: Case Reports

Lawlor-Smith L, Lawlor-Smith C (Aldinga Beach, SA, Australia; Happy Valley, SA, Australia)

BMJ 314:644–645, 1997 4–26

Introduction.—Raynaud's phenomenon is much more common in women and can affect up to 22% of healthy women in the 21- to 50-year age group. Five women with Raynaud's phenomenon affecting their nipples were seen.

Patients.—Five breast-feeding women had Raynaud's phenomenon affecting their nipples (Table 1). Severe, debilitating pain was the major complaint. When breast-feeding a previous child, 3 of the women had had identical pain. During and immediately after feeds, and also in between feeds, blanching of the nipple occurred.

Results.—Nipple blanching and pain occurred after exposure to cold. In the nipples, 2 women had classical triphasic color change or Raynaud's phenomenon (white, blue, and red), whereas 2 women had white and blue color change. None of the women smoked, and 4 had nipple trauma. Poor positioning of the baby at the breast was the most common cause of nipple pain. The patients were visited by a lactation consultant for optimal positioning and attachment of the baby to the breast.

Conclusion.—Because the nipples are exposed and subject to mechanical stimulation during the breast-feeding process, breast-feeding may increase the risk of nipple vasospasm. There is the dual problem of distressing pain and the increased risk of failure of breast-feeding with Raynaud's phenomenon.

▶ Lest anyone think this a sexist selection, readers are referred to a description of penile Raynaud's phenomenon.[1]

R.S. Panush, M.D.

Reference

1. Mooradian AD, Viosca SP, Kaiser FE, et al: Penile Raynaud's phenomenon: A possible cause of erectile failure. *Am J Med* 85:748–750, 1988.

TABLE 1.—Characteristics of Women With Vasospasm of the Nipple

Case No	1	2	3	4	5
Age	28	30	32	32	30
Smoking	No	No	No	No	No
Family history	No	Father	Mother (positive antinuclear antibody)	No	No
History of Raynaud's phenomenon before first pregnancy	No	Fingers and nipples	Fingers and nipples	No	No
Birth order of index child	2	2	2	1	2
Age of child when mother's symptoms started	1 Week	3 Weeks	2 Weeks	1 Week	1 Day
Nipple vasospasm with previous baby	4 Months; breastfed for 14 months	Stopped breastfeeding at 6 weeks because of pain	Breastfed for 7 months in spite of pain	Not applicable	No
Nipple pain during pregnancy	No	No	No	No	No
Nipple trauma	No	Cracked nipples both sides	Ulcer left nipple	Blistering both sides	Cracked nipples both sides
Nipple colour change	Triphasic	Triphasic	Biphasic (white and blue)	Biphasic (white and blue)	Biphasic (white and blue)
Screening tests for secondary Raynaud's phenomenon	Negative	Positive antinuclear antibody (titre 80, pattern speckled); rheumatoid factor activity 22 (<21)	C-reactive protein 24 mg/l (<9); erythrocyte sedimentation rate 39 mm/h (1–15); mild increase in α_2 globulins	Negative	Negative

(Courtesy of Lawlor-Smith L, Lawlor-Smith C: Vasospasm of the nipple—A manifestation of Raynaud's phenomenon: Case reports. *BMJ* 314:644–645, 1997.)

Severe Raynaud's Syndrome Associated With Interferon Therapy: A Case History

Creutzig A, Freund M (Medizinische Hochschule, Hannover, Germany)
Angiology 47:185–187, 1996 4–27

Introduction.—Interferon (IFN) is a new therapy and is used to treat various diseases. Its use in hepatitis is generally limited to 6 months. Long-term use of IFN for myeloproliferative disorders has resulted in chronic side effects from lupus-like autoimmune disease in some patients. In patients with arthralgia and myalgia with high titers for antinuclear antibodies, and in patients with cryoglobulinemia, Raynaud's phenomenon has been associated with IFN therapy. In 1 case, a patient with Raynaud's phenomenon and digital artery occlusions possibly resulting from IFN treatment was studied.

Case Report.—Woman, 60, with chronic myelogenous leukemia, had been treated with IFN for 49 months. Cytarabine was added for 12 months. In the last 6 months before permanent symptoms appeared, hydroxycarbamide plus 6-mercaptopurine were added, and the dose of IFN was reduced. The patient experienced Raynaud's attacks of digits 1–3 of both hands. Her right index finger became permanently cold, cyanotic, and painful. Digital plethysmography showed completely absent pulse curves at left D1 and right D1–D3. An inhomogeneous pattern of capillaries with avascular regions and microhemorrhages were shown on nailfold microscopy. The patient also had occlusions of the deep palmar arch, both digital arteries of D2, and the radial artery of D3. Interferon treatment was discontinued, and prostaglandin and nifedipine were administered for 4 weeks. The patient experienced the Raynaud's attacks less frequently.

Discussion.—This is the first report of digital artery occlusion documented arteriographically and associated with IFN. It is unlikely that cytarabine or hydroxycarbamide caused the Raynaud's attacks. The evidence indicates that these attacks were caused by IFN therapy. Careful monitoring for Raynaud's phenomenon is necessary in patients receiving long-term therapy with IFN.

▶ This case report highlights the vasospastic complications of IFN, especially IFN-α, therapy. This patient had abnormal nailfold capillaries suggestive of vasculitis and an anticentromere antibody titer of 1:160 suggestive of connective tissue disease, so she may have a genetic predisposition to Raynaud's and digital gangrene that was augmented by IFN-α.

E.C. LeRoy, M.D.

Digital Vascular Responses to Cooling in Subjects With Cold Sensitivity, Primary Raynaud's Phenomenon, or Scleroderma Spectrum Disorders

Maricq HR, Weinrich MC, Valter I, et al (Med Univ of South Carolina, Charleston; Univ of South Carolina, Columbia)

J Rheumatol 23:2068–2078, 1996 4–28

Background.—The diagnosis of Raynaud's phenomenon (RP) is usually based on the patient's description of an attack. Researchers have tried to find more objective ways of diagnosing this disorder. Differences in digital vascular responses to cooling were defined and their utility for diagnosing RP was determined.

Methods.—Four groups of individuals were studied: 96 with primary RP, 108 with RP associated with scleroderma (SSc) spectrum disorders, 88 reporting cold sensitivity in the fingers, and 120 RP-negative controls. Digital systolic blood pressure, digital blood flow, and digital skin temperature were measured at 18° or 23°C ambient air. The effect of local finger cooling was assessed at 30°, 20°, 15°, and 10°C.

Findings.—The 4 groups were clearly differentiated by digital blood pressure responses. Blood flow and skin temperature means differed among groups but not significantly. Digital pressure responses were very sensitive and specific in distinguishing between patients with RP and controls and also between the 2 types of RP. A relative digital systolic pressure of less than 70% at local finger cooling temperatures of 15° and 10°C differentiated SSc spectrum RP from primary RP with a 97.1% sensitivity. A zero reopening pressure had a specificity of 100% at 30°C

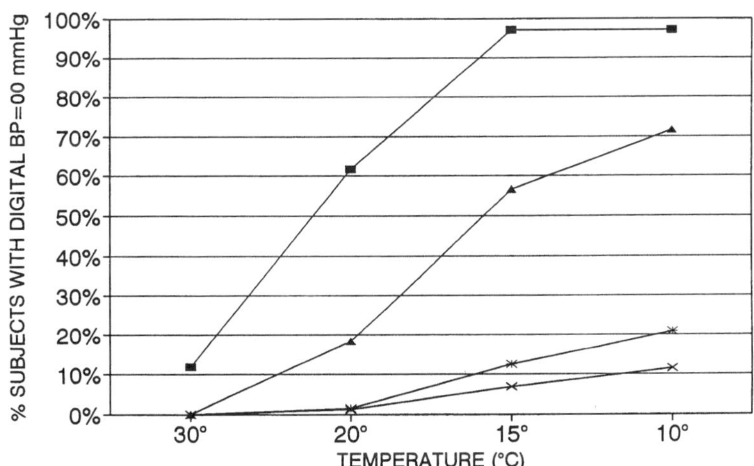

FIGURE 4.—Proportion of subjects with zero reopening pressure at different local cooling temperatures in 1 group tested at 18°C. Scleroderma spectrum Raynaud's phenomenon is designated by *black squares*; primary RP by *black triangles*; cold sensitivity by *asterisks*; controls by *Xs*. *Abbreviation: BP*, blood pressure. (Courtesy of Maricq HR, Weinrich MC, Valter I, et al: Digital vascular responses to cooling in subjects with cold sensitivity, primary Raynaud's phenomenon, or scleroderma spectrum disorders. *J Rheumatol* 23:2068–2078, 1996.

and 81.7% at 20°C in differentiating these 2 groups. Zero reopening pressures were seldom correlated with clinically visible RP (Fig 4).

Conclusion.—The digital pressure response to cooling is useful in patients with RP and those with cold sensitivity. This test is very sensitive and specific in distinguishing among groups.

▶ The digital blood pressure response to cooling was introduced 2 decades ago by Nielsen for the objective diagnosis of patients with RP. Maricq et al. have had extensive experience with this and related techniques for measuring cold-induced vasospasm. Here they show a complete separation among 3 groups of subjects: (1) controls or cold-sensitive persons who do not fulfill criteria for RP; (2) patients with primary RP; and (3) patients with SSc who have RP. By means of an elaborate protocol with pressure measurements after digital exposure to 30°, 20°, 15°, and 10°C (by circulating water at that temperature through finger cuffs), subjects could be distinguished from one another with high sensitivity and specificity. This technique should be useful in the diagnostically difficult patient suspected of having connective tissue disease and for the systematic evaluation of standard and newly introduced vasodilation and sympatholytic therapies.

E.C. LeRoy, M.D.

Treatment of Ischaemic Digital Ulcers and Prevention of Gangrene With Intravenous Iloprost in Systemic Sclerosis

Zachariae H, Halkier-Sørensen L, Bjerring P, et al (Marselisborg Hosp, Aarhus, Denmark; Univ of Aarhus, Denmark)

Acta Derm Venereol 76:236–238, 1996 4–29

Background.—Minimizing vascular damage in patients with systemic sclerosis (SSc) is important. Painful ischemic digital ulcers and gangrene have been associated with SSc. The prostacyclin-stable analogue iloprost was used successfully in patients with SSc.

Methods and Findings.—Twelve patients with SSc received iloprost 0.5–2 ng/kg/min for 6 hours from 8 to 13 days. In 2 patients, treatment stopped imminent gangrene, and healing began. One patient with severe Raynaud's phenomenon withdrew from the study after 3 days because of severe headache. Improvement was noted in the remaining 2 patients with Raynaud's phenomenon. However, a patient with vasculitis of the lower leg did not improve. Adverse effects such as headache, nausea, and flushing prevented the maximum infusion rate from being achieved in all but 5 patients. In 9 patients, digital blood flow before and after the study and plasma endothelin were assessed. No significant differences were found. However, 3 of 6 patients with healing ulcers had a marked reduction in plasma endothelin.

Conclusions.—Iloprost appears to be useful in patients with imminent gangrene and ischemic ulcers associated with SSc. The vasodilating ability of this agent may be important in the treatment of SS in general.

▶ This brief report by a respected investigator, Hugh Zachariae, and colleagues shows improvement of digital ulcers and gangrene associated with IV iloprost administration. This improvement was not associated with improvement of cutaneous resting capillary blood flow (laser Doppler). The unchanged resting blood flow measurements do not preclude a therapeutic response in blocking cold-induced vasospasm, the most consistent physiologic abnormality in patients with scleroderma. Changes in plasma endothelin levels were variable.

Although up to 8 days of 6-hour daily infusions of a medicine that gives severe headaches and flushing is unpleasant, aggressive, invasive, and expensive, if it can save digits and even lives (by its use in pulmonary hypertension) it may be worth it. [Note that trials of oral iloprost have not been consistently impressive. See the following selection, Abstract 4–30.... R.S. Panush, M.D.]

E.C. LeRoy, M.D.

Controlled Multicenter Double Blind Trial of an Oral Analog of Prostacyclin in the Treatment of Primary Raynaud's Phenomenon

Vayssairat M, and the French Microcirculation Society Multicentre Group for the Study of Vascular Acrosyndromes (Hôpital Tenon, Paris)

J Rheumatol 23:1917–1920, 1996 4–30

Purpose.—Prostaglandin I_2, given by repeated infusions, is clinically beneficial in the treatment of primary or secondary Raynaud's phenomenon (RP). Beraprost sodium is an orally given prostanoid prostaglandin I_2 analogue. It was studied for efficacy and tolerance in a large group of patients with primary RP.

Methods.—The multicenter, randomized, double-blind trial included 125 patients with primary RP who were too disabled to do their usual work. After a 2-week period of no treatment, the patients received 6 weeks of treatment with either beraprost or placebo. The beraprost group took one 20-µg tablet 3 times a day for the first 3 weeks, then 2 tablets 3 times a day for 3 weeks. The study was conducted during the winter months, and the 2 groups were matched for outdoor environmental temperatures. The effects of treatment were compared in terms of frequency and severity of RP attacks, overall disability, and the results of digital cold challenge testing.

Results.—Both groups had a significant reduction in the number of RP attacks, with no difference between groups. The percentage reduction was 34% in the placebo group and 37% in the beraprost group, with overlapping confidence intervals. Similarly, there was no significant difference in the severity of RP attacks or overall disability. Patients in the beraprost group were more likely to report headaches, but there were no severe side effects. There was no change in the results of cold tests in either group.

Conclusions.—Beraprost is no more effective than placebo in the treatment of primary RP. The results do not appear to be influenced by using too low a dose or by differences in climatic conditions. Other, although not all, trials of RP treatment also have shown a strong placebo effect.

► All of us experience digital vasospasm when we are exposed to cold or when we are anxious. Most of us are aware of this homeostatic response to the extent that our extremities are cool. For some 15% of us, in 1 population survey, we are aware to the extent that our hands seem pale or blue. For 2% to 3% of us, the color changes can seem dramatic. Whether these individuals represent the extremes of the normal response, or have abnormal vasospasm, is still debated. Nonetheless, for some of these individuals, who are otherwise well and who have no damage to their digits, the vasospasm is sufficiently bothersome or worrisome to cause them to seek care. Usually their condition is labeled "primary Raynaud's phenomenon." Some clinicians reserve this label for vasospasm that causes a discrete demarcation between the blanched distal digit and the more normal skin. Some further demand an impressive hyperemic recovery phase. The inference is that vasospasm of this magnitude is placing tissue at risk and therefore is a disease state and not a variant of normal reactivity.

For those who seek care, wise clinicians have long known that reassurance and truncal warming are the first line of intervention. However, the literature is littered with attempts at pharmaceutical interventions. There is a suggestion that a high-dose of orally administered reserpine can abrogate vasospasm, often at the price of an affective disorder. There is a suggestion that ketansarin, a serotonin antagonist, might have some role. And there are trials with iloprost, which seem promising. Iloprost is a prostacyclin congener that is a vasodilator but must be administered parenterally. Because of that, there is considerable interest in designing orally administered prostacyclin congeners for this purpose.

This article is an impressive multicenter, randomized, controlled trial of 1 such agent. The agent turned out to be no more beneficial than placebo. But the placebo worked impressively; there was about a 40% improvement in frequency, severity, and consequence of vasospastic attacks. Long live the wise clinicians!

N.M. Hadler, M.D.

5 Vasculitis, Systemic Rheumatic Diseases, and Other Related Disorders

Introduction

The vasculitides resist insight. They are rare so that even referral centers are hard pressed to accumulate an experience that might generalize. The inflammations are heterogeneous, even within the classification of the day, making generalization even more difficult. But they play such havoc with the lives of the afflicted patients that we must grasp for any therapeutic straw. Prednisone has been the mainstay; there is currently no better way to squelch the symptoms of inflammation. However, it is clear that corticosteroids accomplish little, if anything, in abrogating tissue damage from the primary vasculitis process. And it is certain that corticosteroid has obligate toxicities that are dose-, duration-, and host-predicated and can be a match for the morbidity and mortality of any systemic diseases. No wonder therapeutic substitutes have long been considered a holy grail.

This year, methotrexate was tested as the savior. It was tested in polymyalgia rheumatica where the median duration of the disease approaches three years, and the population afflicted is least likely to escape the major morbidities of Cushing's syndrome regardless of the dose or duration. The results are inconsistent at best. They are not dramatic in relapsing polychondritis. Even in RA, where the common wisdom holds otherwise, methotrexate has proven disappointing.

This point is perhaps the most telling of this chapter. However, there is a potpourri of intellectual tidbits here for the savoring.

Nortin M. Hadler, M.D.

Lead Article

► Variability. Unpredictability. Overlap. Remission. Migration. These are all terms with which rheumatologists and their patients live. If rheumatic diseases are "entities," why don't they conform? Finally, we are generating the insights to answer such a question. The following paper is a landmark in that regard.

Giant cell arteritis is a pathologic diagnosis, a synonym for temporal arteritis. However, for some patients the arteritis is subclinical and polymyalgia rheumatica predominates. For others, the painful temporal arteries are all that one can discern. Are these two diseases or a "spectrum?" And if they're a "spectrum," why? How?

The answer related to the pathophysiology of arteritis. Damage to the elasticum in the presence of infiltrating round and giant cells is *sine qua non*. But the extra-arteritic manifestations seem to relate to the quality of this inflammation. In some settings, cytokines are generated that exert solely local effects. But in other patients, cytokines are generated that correlate with distant illness. We need to understand the rules that govern this heterogeneity. Then we can approach therapy with incisiveness rather than with prednisone.

R.S. Panush, M.D.

Disease Patterns and Tissue Cytokine Profiles in Giant Cell Arteritis

Weyand CM, Tetzlaff N, Björnsson J, et al (Mayo Clinic and Found, Rochester, Minn)

Arthritis Rheum 40:19–26, 1997 5–1

Background.—Although giant cell arteritis (GCA) exhibits a defined tissue tropism, its presentation includes a wide spectrum of clinical manifestations. Whether this clinical heterogeneity is associated with different patterns in the tissue-specific inflammatory response was investigated.

Methods.—Twenty-three patients with typical histomorphological findings of GCA were studied. Inflammatory responses in temporal artery biopsy specimens were assessed by semiquantification of cytokine mRNA transcripts using reverse transcriptase-polymerase chain reaction and oligonucleotide hybridization with cytokine-specific probes. Clinical patterns were then correlated with the tissue cytokine profiles (Table 1).

Findings.—Inflammatory cytokine expression was observed in all temporal artery tissues. Different inflammatory patterns were distinguished by in situ synthesis of interleukin-2 (IL-2), interferon-γ (IFNγ), and IL-1β mRNA, but not IL-10 or IL-12 mRNA. These patterns were associated with clinical manifestations of the disease. Patients with ischemic symptoms typically had higher expression of IFNγ mRNA and IL-1β mRNA concentrations. Fever was associated with lower copy numbers of IFNγ. Giant-cell formation in the granulomatous infiltrates was correlated with

TABLE 1.—Clinical Characteristics of Patients With Giant-cell Arteritis

Characteristic	
No. of patients	23
No. of females/males	14/9
Median age (range), years	72 (63–85)
Jaw claudication and/or visual abnormalities, % patients	57
Fever, % patients	48
Polymyalgia rheumatica, % patients	57
Giant cell formation in the inflammatory infiltrates, % patients	61

(Courtesy of Weyand CM, Tetzlaff N, Björnsson J, et al: Disease patterns and tissue cytokine profiles in giant cell arteritis. *Arthritis Rheum* 40:19–26, 1997, copyright American College of Rheumatology.)

the local synthesis of IFNγ mRNA. Tissue from patients with polymyalgia rheumatica (PMR) as well as GCA showed higher levels of IL-2 mRNA transcripts (Fig 2).

Conclusion.—Variations in the clinical presentation of GCA were associated with cytokine mRNA expression in the affected temporal arteries. These patterns were distinguished by differences in the effector functions of tissue-infiltrating T cells. The patterns were characterized by the predominance of local ischemic symptoms or systemic involvement or the co-occurrence of polymyalgia rheumatica.

► The clinical spectrum associated with GCA is puzzling in its breadth and more puzzling in that not all patients are similarly affected. Some manifestations can be ascribed directly to the inflamed arteries, which are at risk for occlusion; localized tenderness (temporal arteritis, caput medusae, etc.) and ischemia (jaw claudication, infarction of the ocular disc) are examples. Other manifestations (fever, polymyalgia, severe proximal gelling [morning stiffness]) are not so readily explained. It has been postulated that the magnitude of the local inflammation and the magnitude of the more distant and systemic manifestations might be a consequence of separate properties of the inflammatory process in the arteries. This study is a test of that hypothesis.

The clinical characteristics of the 23 patients in this study are presented in Table 1. All had undergone biopsies documenting temporal arteritis. The messenger RNA was extracted from the biopsy tissue and the number of cytokine-specific mRNA copies quantified. For the predominantly macrophage-associated cytokines (IL-1β, IL-10, IL-12), the number of copies was adjusted for the number of genes coding the macrophage structural protein β-actin. The T cell-derived cytokines, IL-2 and IFNγ, were adjusted for the quantiy of T cell-receptor sequences. As exemplified in the Figure, patterns of cytokine production are emerging that correspond to clinical presentations.

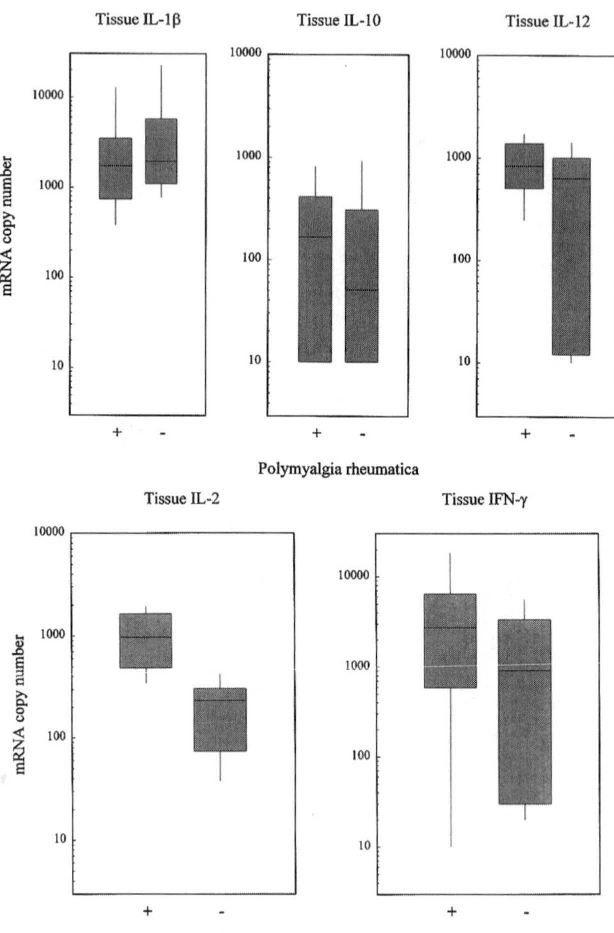

FIGURE 2.—In situ cytokine production in patients with giant-cell arteritis with symptoms of polymyalgia rheumatica (PMR). Patients with giant-cell arteritis were grouped according to the presence (+)(r = 13) or absence (−) (n = 10) of PMR symptoms. Patients with PMR symptoms were characterized by a higher production of IL-2 mRNA in the tissue (P = 0.001). Production of IFN-γ (P = 0.29), Il-1β (P = 0.38), IL-10 (P = 0.89), and IL-12 (P = 0.23) did not differ between the 2 patient groups. *Abbreviations*: *IL*, interleukin; *IFN*, interferon. (Courtesy of Weyand CM, Tetzlaff N, Björnsson J, et al: Disease patterns and tissue cytokine profiles in giant cell arteritis. *Arthritis Rheum* 40:19–26, 1997, copyright American College of Rheumatology.)

This is an exciting approach to studying the pathophysiology of GCA that may facilitate the design of specific therapeutic interventions. It is also an approach relevant to other inflammatory disorders.

N.M. Hadler, M.D.

Systemic Vasculitides

Development and Initial Validation of the Vasculitis Damage Index for the Standardized Clinical Assessment of Damage in the Systemic Vasculitides

Exley AR, Bacon PA, Luqmani RA, et al (Univ of Birmingham, England)

Arthritis Rheum 40:371–380, 1997 5–2

Purpose.—Since the systemic vasculitides are chronic relapsing diseases, it is essential to evaluate the quality of survival. Rather than just mortality, outcome evaluation must include a global assessment of disease severity. The development and validation of a standardized clinical assessment of patients with systemic vasculitides, the Vasculitis Damage Index (VDI), is reported.

Methods.—Principles for assessing damage in the systemic vasculitides were obtained through a nominal group approach. The study definition of damage was irreversible changes resulting from scarring. Once the principles were agreed on, they were developed into the VDI. The instrument included an extensive list of items of damage in different body systems, including the skin; renal, ear, nose, and throat; ocular; pulmonary; cardiovascular; musculoskeletal; peripheral vascular; and neuropsychiatric systems, as well as a category of other damage. All damage was scored as present or absent. Guidelines for use and a glossary were developed as well. The validity, reliability, and feasibility of this instrument were assessed.

Results.—At last observation, the median VDI score of 100 surviving patients with systemic vasculitis was 3. Analysis of patients with Wegener's granulomatosis found a median score of 7 for 12 nonsurvivors vs. 4 for 12 survivors. In 100 patients with systemic vasculitis, the median VDI score increased by a median of 3 from baseline to last observation (median interval 5 years). Comparison with other indices showed that the VDI assessed more items and was more sensitive to change than the Systemic Necrotizing Vasculitis Damage Index and the Systemic Lupus International Cooperating Clinics/American College of Rheumatology (SLICC/ACR) Damage Index. With training, raters were able to produce moderately consistent damage scores using the VDI. At the assessment visit, clinicians were able to complete the VDI score sheet within 5 minutes.

Conclusions.—The development and validation of the VDI for clinical assessment of damage in patients with systemic vasculitides are reported. This instrument appears to be a sensitive, reproducible, comprehensive, and usable clinical tool. The authors call for further study to validate and test the VDI in patients with specific forms of vasculitis. With further validation, the VDI should be useful in comparing different treatments.

► This is another clinical scale for a rare but important group of diseases. Such scales are useful as standardization initiatives, mnemonics, and quantitative important clinical states. Witness how APGAR, with much less psychometric testing, changed neonatology! The VDI is more sensitive than SLICC/ACR damage index developed for systemic lupus erythematosus. The former concept and instrument are a logical extension of SLICC and could replace it. The authors show that reproducible scoring, like all clinical schemes, requires training.

M.H. Liang, M.D., M.P.H.

Pathogenic Role of Anti-endothelial Cell Antibodies in Vasculitis: An Idiotypic Experimental Model

Damianovich M, Gilburd B, George J, et al (Sheba Med Ctr, Tel Hashomer, Israel; Tel Aviv Univ, Israel; Univ of Milan, Italy)

J Immunol 156:4946–4951, 1996 5–3

Background.—The finding of antibodies (Abs) directed against a heterogeneous family of endothelial cell-membrane proteins has been reported in patients with various autoimmune diseases associated with vasculitis. Thus, the presence of anti-endothelial cell Abs (AECA) in the sera of such patients may be a marker for vascular damage or vasculitis. However, the association of AECA with clinical manifestations, their in vitro binding to target cells, and their cytotoxic potential provide only indirect evidence for their clinical significance and pathogenetic role in autoimmune vasculitis and associated disorders. An experimental model for the induction of autoimmune diseases by idiotypic manipulation was used in the current study to obtain direct evidence of the pathogenicity of AECA.

Methods and Findings.—To induce AECA and autoimmune vasculitis in the murine model, AECA derived from the plasma of a patient with Wegener's granulomatosis was used. Immunoglobulin was purified by absorption on a proteinase-3 affinity column, leading to the depletion of anti-neutrophil cytoplasmic Ab activity. The absorbed IgG fraction showed a high AECA titer, evidenced by a cyto–enzyme-linked immunosorbent assay against unfixed human umbilical vein endothelial cells. Three months after active immunization with the purified AECA, endogenous AECA but not Abs to proteinase-3, cardiolipin, or DNA developed in the mice. Histologic assessment of the lungs and kidneys showed lymphoid cell infiltration surrounding arterioles and venules and deposition of Igs at the outer part of the blood vessel walls.

Conclusions.—This experimental model of vasculitis has provided the first direct evidence of the pathogenicity of AECA. From these findings AECA and anti-neutrophil cytoplasmic Abs can be inferred to represent 2 distinct pathogenic groups of autoantibodies.

▶ We have known about the idiotype network for decades, thanks to the genius of the Nobel Prize winner Jerne. The concept is as follows: the binding site of any antibody is a unique configuration; otherwise, binding would not be specific for a particular antigenic structure, an epitope. The unique configuration that is the binding site is called an idiotype. If you immunize with an Ab, the host is faced with a novel structure, that Ab's binding site, and should be able to respond with an Ab to the immunizing idiotype. There are 2 predictions for the structure of this anti-idiotype's binding site: it should be complementary to the immunizing Ab's idiotype, and it is an immunizing structure as well that will evoke an anti-anti-idiotype Ab response. This anti-anti-idiotype Ab's binding site should be complementary to that of the anti-idiotype and therefore should recognize the same epitope that the first antibody recognized.

Here is why all of this is relevant. Let us assume you have a patient with Wegener's granulomatosis with high titer of anti-proteinase 3 and of anti-endothelial cell Abs. Could the anti-endothelial Abs have pathogenetic potential independent of the anti-proteinase 3 Ab? To answer the question, you can adsorb the anti-proteinase 3 Abs out of a sample of the patient's serum and immunize several inbred mice with the IgG that remains and others with normal human IgG. Three months later, some of the mice that were immunized with the patient's adsorbed IgG are producing high titers of Ab to human endothelial cells and are developing histopathologic features of vasculitis. Clearly, these few mice have made an anti-anti-idiotype with autoimmune consequences.

That is the experiment described in this article. Other workers have developed similar systems in which immunizing can perturb the network with salutory results. Maybe some day we will attempt that in our patients.

N.M. Hadler, M.D.

Systemic Vasculitis and Myelodysplastic Syndromes

Philippe B, Couderc L-J, Droz D, et al (Université Paris Ouest, Suresnes; Hôpital Necker, Paris; Hopital La Pitié Salpétrière, Paris)

Arthritis Rheum 40:179–182, 1997 5–4

Background.—Myelodysplastic syndromes (MDS), characterized by cytopenia and the histologic features of hematopoietic dysplasia, have rarely been associated with cutaneous vasculitides. Two patients with systemic vasculitis were seen.

Case 1.—Man, 68, sought attention for pruritic erythematous papules on his back, shoulders, neck, and head. Skin biopsy demonstrated a perivascular cellular infiltrate consisting of small lymphocytes and histiocytes in the dermis. Infiltration of the capillary vessel walls without leukocytoclasia was observed. Significant laboratory findings included mild anemia, with a hemoglobin level of 93 g/L. Findings on bone marrow aspiration were consistent with refractory anemia with excess blasts. The patient's cutaneous lesions regressed within 3 days of red blood transfusion and the initiation of prednisolone, 40 mg/day. One year later, the patient reported an enlarged testis and blood in the urine. There were no cutaneous lesions, but biopsy of the epididymis showed characteristic interstitial lesions of vasculitis. Transjugular renal biopsy showed extensive polymorphic interstitial cellular infiltration consisting of lymphocytes, plasma cells, polymorphonuclear cells, and eosinophils. Interstitial bleeding was noted in the medulla. The glomeruli were ischemic, and epithelial necrosis was noted in the tubules. Interstitial plasma cells containing IgA and C3 deposits in the vessels were documented. After treatment with hemodialysis and prednisone, the testis appeared normal. Several relapses of the cutaneous vasculitis occurred in the first year of prednisone tapering. Treatment with danazol was begun, which enabled the prednisone dose to be reduced to 20 mg/day.

Case 2.—Man, 27, had a 3-year history of dyspnea. Previous radiologic studies had shown diffuse bilateral interstitial infiltrates. After other tests were performed, an open lung biopsy was done, revealing neutrophil polymorphonuclear foci and small lymphocytes with destruction of small vessel walls. The patient's dyspnea worsened 15 days after lung biopsy. Diffuse bilateral alveolar and interstitial opacites were seen radiographically at this time. Arterial blood gases showed mild hypoxemia, but the patient's religious beliefs precluded blood transfusion. Intravenous methylprednisolone and oral prednisone treatment was begun. His condition improved, along with the pulmonary opacity, and he was discharged on a regimen of 40 mg of prednisone per day.

Conclusions.—Vasculitis may develop before or after a diagnosis of hematologic disorder. Treatment with high-dose corticosteroids appears to be effective.

Varicella Zoster Virus, a Cause of Waxing and Waning Vasculitis: The *New England Journal of Medicine* Case 5—1995 Revisited

Gilden DH, Kleinschmidt-DeMasters BK, Wellish M, et al (Univ of Colorado, Denver; Harvard Med School, Boston; Univ of Liege, Belgium)
Neurology 47:1441–1446, 1996 5–5

Background.—In a recent issue of *The New England Journal of Medicine*, the case report of a man with an ill-defined fatal vasculitis involving the CNS was published as a clinicopathologic exercise. The pathologic material from that patient was re-examined and described.

Patient and Findings.—The patient was a 73-year-old immunocompetent man in whom headache, fever, mental status changes, and focal deficit developed. Although this patient lived for 314 days after symptom onset, the pattern of his neurologic symptoms and signs was acute-subacute during his initial 20 days in the hospital. Studies revealed a persistent mixed pleocytosis of white blood cells, predominantly mononuclear, and red blood cells. Multiple superficial and deep infarcts were observed in central gray and white matter and brain stem on brain MR images.

Cerebral angiography demonstrated focal narrowing in the internal carotid, anterior, and middle cerebral arteries. Cerebral spinal fluid showed antibody to varicella zoster virus (VZV). At autopsy, multiple brain infarcts were observed, caused by an unclassifiable arteritis with multinucleated giant cells.

The current investigators searched for VZV because of the patient's constellation of clinical and radiologic features, although he was previously immunocompetent and had no cutaneous signs of herpesvirus infection during his long illness. Polymerase chain reaction and immunocytochemistry were used in the brain and in multiple large cerebral arteries. In 3 of 5 cerebral arteries, re-examination revealed both VZV DNA and VZV-specific antigen but not herpes simplex virus or cytomegalovirus DNA or herpes simplex virus or cytomegalovirus-specific antigen. The inflammatory response, disruption of the internal elastic lamina, and detection of viral antigen were patchy from one artery to another and within a given artery.

Conclusion.—When both the central and peripheral nervous systems are involved, focal narrowing is present in large arteries, brain imaging reveals infarction in gray and white matter, and white matter is disproportionately involved in patients with vasculitis, clinicians should search for VZV. The diagnosis does not require the presence of zosteriform rash.

▶ So-called primary CNS vasculitis is a challenging clinical construct. It is a rare cause of a destructive multifocal process suspected on imaging studies and confirmed by histopathology. Usually there are no extracranial manifestations. By definition, there is no demonstrable cause. It's the last, the diagnosis of exclusion, that is anxiety-provoking for all clinicians caring for a patient with such a devastating and usually relentless process.

Such a patient was the topic of a clinicopathologic conference in the *New England Journal of Medicine* in 1995. The physicians involved were not satisfied with "unclassifiable arteritis with multinucleated giant cells" as the final diagnosis at autopsy. They restudied the tissue and demonstrated VZV DNA by polymerase chain reaction and specific antigen by immunocytochemistry in some of the arteries. Could this be a complication of the patient's terminal, course which involved immunosuppressant therapy complicated by a number of infections? After all, VZV encephalitis in the absence of rash has seldom been documented. Is that because it has not been sought so assiduously? Maybe this patient should have received acyclovir instead of cyclophosphamide?

N.M. Hadler, M.D.

Minocycline Induced Arthritis Associated With Fever, Livedo Reticularis, and pANCA

Elkayam O, Yaron M, Caspi D (Tel Aviv Univ, Israel)

Ann Rheum Dis 55:769–771, 1996 5–6

Introduction.—The semisynthetic tetracycline minocycline is used in patients with various infections or acne vulgaris. Although this drug has several different adverse effects, few rheumatic effects have been described. Three patients had a similar pattern of minocycline-induced arthritis.

Patients.—The patients, all women, were aged 19–22 years. All had used minocycline for prolonged periods for the treatment of acne. All had recently started taking the drug again after 1–2 years of not taking it. Within a few weeks of taking minocycline, marked pyrexia, arthritis/arthralgia, and livedo reticularis developed in all 3 patients. Laboratory studies showed elevated levels of serum perinuclear anticytoplasmic antibodies and antimyeloperoxidase antibody. When minocycline treatment was stopped, the symptoms resolved; when the treatment was given again, the symptoms returned. Anti-myeloperoxidase autoantibodies decreased gradually during remission.

Conclusions.—Minocycline can cause a characteristic vasculitic reaction characterized by fever, fatigue, polyarthritis, and livedo reticularis. This reaction is associated with positive immunofluorescent p-perinuclear anticytoplasmic antibodies and anti-myeloperoxidase antibody. Many young women take minocycline for acne, sometimes without adequate medical supervision. Physicians should be aware of this complication. The reaction usually resolves when the patient stops taking the drug.

▶ Chronic low-dose minocycline therapy is an option for acne vulgaris and RA. The latter indication is bolstered by 2 sizable long-term trials suggesting that the slight benefit was justified because the agent was so well tolerated. However, given this indication, the existence of a rheumatic toxicity needs recognition. Fever and livedo reticularis are unusual in RA; now minocycline needs to be added to the differential diagnosis should it develop in a patient with RA. Unfortunately, the perinuclear anticytoplasmic antibodies are less useful in the setting of RA, where they are a well-described epiphenomenon.

N.M. Hadler, M.D.

Factors Associated With the Development of Vasculitis in Rheumatoid Arthritis: Results of a Case–Control Study

Voskuyl AE, Zwinderman AH, Westedt ML, et al (Univ Hosp, Leiden, The Netherlands; Bronovo Hosp, The Hague, The Netherlands)

Ann Rheum Dis 55:190–192, 1996 5–7

Background.—Vascular inflammation of small and medium vessels, associated with skin rash, cutaneous ulcerations, neuropathy, constitutional symptoms, and abnormalities of visceral organs, is a complication of RA termed rheumatoid vasculitis (RV). The demographic and clinical variables in patients with RA that correlated with RV were examined.

Methods.—Records from between 1980 and 1993 were reviewed in a case–control study. Demographic and clinical data were compared between 138 patients with RA who had no indications of vasculitis and 69 patients contemporaneously given diagnosis of RA and RV (confirmed histologically in 96%).

Results.—After adjustment for other variables, variables associated with the development of RV were (in order of association strength) increased concentration of rheumatoid factor, joint erosions, D-penicillamine treatment at any time, nail-fold lesions, other extra-articular features, subcutaneous nodules, male sex, number of previously prescribed disease-modifying antirheumatic drugs, and treatment with azathioprine at any time. In a second analysis, corticosteroid treatment was related to the development of RV only when given at the time of the diagnosis of RV.

Conclusions.—Development of RV appears by virtue of the variables identified to be associated with the male sex, extra-articular features, and a severe course of RA. It may be a manifestation of severe RA as opposed to a separate disease entity. The strong association of RV with increased rheumatoid factor concentration may relate to deposition of immune complexes in vessel walls.

▶ The field of rheumatology is the keeper of the great medical tradition of exacting clinical descriptions. Most of us who have been around for a while might argue that there is little left to describe. If we have a concern, it might be that the experience of those who publish their descriptions is confounded by preconceived notions; they are more likely to publish the confounded, challenging, and extraordinary and consider all else of too little interest to the readership. For instance, take RV. Rheumatology has taught for 2 generations that there may be 2 forms of vascular inflammation capable of causing necrotic lesions in RA: leukocytoclastic angiitis and a variant of polyarteritis nodosa. Furthermore, both seem to afflict patients whose RA is more severe in general and may afflict men more than one would predict.

The Leiden rheumatology unit is one of the most prominent and respected in Europe. This paper is a retrospective case–control chart analysis of a sizable population of patients labeled as having RV between 1980 and 1993 and patients with RA chosen so that they were evaluated in the same year as each of the patients with RV. The manifestations that led to the labeling "vasculitis" and the underlying pathologic features are not detailed. When patients with both RA and RV and those without are compared, the teachings of 2 generations of rheumatologists are born out. It's reassuring.

N.M. Hadler, M.D.

Cervical Epidural Analgesia for Management of Pain Associated With Digital Vasculitis Secondary to Rheumatoid Arthritis

Green CR, de Rosayro AM (Univ of Michigan, Ann Arbor)

Reg Anesth 22:188–191, 1997 5–8

Introduction.—Progressive digital vasculitis secondary to RA and high circulating rheumatoid factors may produce ischemia, necrosis, pain, and gangrene of extremities and digits: it can be debilitating. Described is a patient with RA and digital vasculitis with concurrent ischemia in whom cervical epidural analgesia was used as an adjunct to medical therapy.

> *Case Report.*—Woman, 54, with a history of severe RA, was seen for increasing pain and paresthesias of her left hand. She did not respond to increases in prednisone from 5 to 30 mg daily. Physical examination revealed brown spots in her nail beds, blue ischemic fingertips with areas of dermal necrosis, ulnar deviation of the digits, and swan neck deformity. Her white blood cell count, hematocrit, and platelet counts were 13,900/mm^3, 37.6%, and 392,000/mm^3, respectively. Her prednisone dose was increased to 40 mg twice daily and she received methotrexate 15 mg orally every week, diclofenac 75 mg twice daily, and acetaminophen 300 mg with codeine 30 mg 4 times daily. Thrombosis was suspected when immunoglobulins G and M were positive and heparin therapy was given on hospitalization day 2. On day 5, the patient still had not responded to treatment and was given meperidine for analgesia. Angiography indicated severe occlusive vasculitis beyond the head of the metacarpals. Cervical epidural analgesia with bupivacaine produced pain relief and greatly diminished symptoms.

Conclusion.—Cervical epidural analgesia was used successfully in conjunction with medical treatment to decrease pain and other symptoms in a patient with digital vasculitis secondary to RA.

▶ Painful digital ischemia is a diabolical complication of a number of rheumatic diseases. The underlying pathophysiology usually relates to damage of microcirculatory structures either from vasculitis or endothelial proliferation, as seems to be the hallmark of scleroderma. There may be complicating vasospasm. Management usually targets the pathophysiology or presumptive pathophysiology and relies on analgesics for pain control. The result, all too often, is a patient whose ischemia is not clearly improved but whose course is always complicated by toxicities of both classes of drug.

Modern anesthesiology offers options for pain control that obviate most analgesic toxicities and are effective in palliation—so effective that clinicians might feel less desperate and eschew empirical trials of agents of dubious benefit in the rheumatic diseases when not in crisis and therefore of dubious benefit for the ischemic events. With patience and palliation, the natural history of these lesions is remittancy, although they can leave much destruction in their wake. Regional blocks with longer-acting local anesthetics can serve this goal. This article describes the use of epidural analgesia to this end.

N.M. Hadler, M.D.

Molecular Analysis of HLA-DR Polymorphism in Polymyalgia Rheumatica

Guerne P-A, and the Swiss Group for Research on HLA in Polymyalgia Rheumatica (Univ Hosp, Geneva; et al)

J Rheumatol 24:671–676, 1997 5–9

Introduction.—The etiology of polymyalgia rheumatica (PMR) is not known, but it may be mediated by immune mechanisms. The condition is closely related to giant cell arteritis (GCA). There is increasing evidence that genetic factors are involved in both PMR and GCA. It may be that HLA class II antigens are involved in genetic factors that could influence the expression of these diseases. The possible associations of HLA-DRB1 alleles with PMR were compared in controls and patients with RA in a multicenter trial.

Methods.—One hundred patients with PMR with and without signs of GCA and 200 controls who were bone marrow donors underwent HLA-DR genetic typing. Microtiter oligotyping and DR4 subtypes were analyzed by dot blot hybridization with sequence-specific oligonucleotides or by polymerase chain reaction sequence-specific primers.

Results.—There was an increase in DR4 and DR1 in PMR, compared with controls (36% vs. 30% and 19% vs. 12%, respectively). The frequencies of all RA-associated DR4 and DR1 subtypes were also increased in PMR. The frequency of the HLA-DRβ1 70–74 shared motif was significantly higher in PMR than in controls, but lower than in RA. This epitope was increased in PMR at double dose, but not significantly. It was markedly augmented in RA. The frequency of clinical signs of GCA were increased in patients with the shared epitope. The frequency of the HLA-DRβ1 DRYF 28–31 motif was the same in PMR and in controls.

Conclusion.—It is possible that PMR is associated with the HLA-DRβ1 70–74 shared epitope. This association would be weaker for PMR than for RA, especially with the shared epitope at double dose. There was no association between the HLA-DRβ1 DRYF 28–31 motif and PMR.

▶ This is the largest study of HLA-DR associations in PMR and helps reconcile previous discrepant reports on the link between DR1 and PMR. Polymyalgia rheumatica is seen with polyarthritis, and there are those who believe it to be on a spectrum with RA. At a molecular level, at least, the overlap between PMR and RA is also seen.

M.H. Liang, M.D., M.P.H.

The Use of Methotrexate in Polymyalgia Rheumatica

Feinberg HL, Sherman JD, Schrepferman CG, et al (Ashland Arthritis Ctr, Ky)
J Rheumatol 23:1550–1552, 1996 5–10

Background.—The usual treatment for polymyalgia rheumatica (PMR) is corticosteroids. However, because of the problems associated with steroid treatment, it would be useful to have some form of steroid-sparing therapy. Methotrexate (MTX) may be useful in the treatment of patients with PMR and probable or definite giant cell arteritis. Its use was investigated in PMR patients without complicating giant cell arteritis.

Methods.—The study included 43 patients with PMR without accompanying giant cell arteritis. All received 3 months of treatment with MTX at a dose of 7.5 mg/week. If there was no response, the dose was increased to 10 mg/week and then to 12.5 mg/week. The patients continued taking prednisone throughout the MTX treatment period. The study criteria for disease control were a normal erythrocyte sedimentation rate and no pain during examination.

Results.—Thirty-nine patients completed the 9-month study on a total daily MTX dose of 12.5 mg/week. None of the patients met the criteria for disease control, and none was able to reduce the dose of prednisone. Some patients did have a drop in erythrocyte to sedimentation rate, but there was no accompanying clinical improvement.

Conclusions.—Methotrexate does not appear to be an effective treatment for patients with PMR without accompanying giant cell arteritis. Other steroid-sparing treatments for PMR should be sought. Further study is needed to see if MTX is helpful in PMR patients with giant cell arteritis.

► MTX has been steroid sparing in almost every disease entity studied including asthma, inflammatory bowel disease, and RA. In cases of PMR without giant cell arteritis, most patients can be treated satisfactorily with less than 10–15 mg of prednisone per day. This study attempted to focus on a group of patients who had complications from steroids or who are "not adequately" controlled with greater than 20 mg of prednisone. These inclusion criteria suggest that a highly select and perhaps unusual group of patients were studied and this open-ended study showed no benefit, clinically or statistically, from treatment with MTX up to 12.5 mg/week. One wonders what would have occurred in the usual type of patient and with a longer follow-up.

M.H. Liang, M.D., M.P.H.

Methotrexate in Polymyalgia Rheumatica: Preliminary Results of an Open, Randomized Study

Ferraccioli G, Salaffi F, de Vita S, et al (Univ of Ancona, Italy)

J Rheumatol 23:624–628, 1996 5–11

Background.—Recommended treatment for polymyalgia rheumatica (PMR), which affects the elderly, consists of low-dose steroids for 18 months to 2 years. However, even low steroid doses may have adverse effects in the elderly. Methotrexate (MTX) has been used increasingly as a steroid-sparing drug in patients with chronic inflammatory diseases. The effects of MTX plus prednisone were compared with those of prednisone alone in patients with PMR.

Methods.—Twenty-four patients with recent-onset PMR were enrolled in a randomized, prospective, yearlong trial. Treatment given was MTX, 10 mg, IM plus prednisone every week or prednisone alone. An attempt to discontinue prednisone was made after 6 months.

Findings.—After 1 year of treatment, all patients were in clinical remission. Acute-phase reactants were in the normal range in both treatment groups. Six patients in the combined treatment group were no longer taking steroids, compared with none in the prednisone-only group. The amount of prednisone taken differed significantly between groups. Also, bone mineral density was reduced significantly in the prednisone-only group but not in the combined treatment group.

Conclusions.—The use of MTX allowed these patients to take much less prednisone to control PMR. There was no loss of efficacy. The use of MTX also resulted in bone sparing in these elderly patients, who were at increased risk for osteoporotic fractures.

Can Methotrexate Be Used as a Steroid Sparing Agent in the Treatment of Polymyalgia Rheumatica and Giant Cell Arteritis?

van der Veen MJ, Dinant HJ, van Booma-Frankfort C, et al (Univ Hosp Utrecht, The Netherlands; St Antonius Hosp, Nieuwegein, The Netherlands; Diakonessen Hosp, Utrecht, The Netherlands; et al)

Ann Rheum Dis 55:218–223, 1996 5–12

Background.—Polymyalgia rheumatica is characterized by neck, shoulder, or hip pain and stiffness that persist for a month or longer. Because this syndrome occurs in older individuals, a steroid-sparing agent would be useful in its treatment. The steroid-sparing effects of methotrexate (MTX) in patients with polymyalgia rheumatica and giant-cell arteritis (GCA) were studied in a double-blind, placebo-controlled trial.

Methods.—Forty patients were included. Six also had clinical symptoms of GCA. A temporal artery biopsy specimen was available from 37 patients; 6 of them showed GCA. Three of the 6 patients with clinical signs of GCA had positive results from biopsy specimens. Treatment for all patients was begun with prednisone, 20 mg/day, regardless of clinical signs and biopsy results. This was then supplemented in a blinded fashion with a weekly capsule containing MTX 7.5 mg or placebo. When clinical symptoms disappeared and the erythrocyte sedimentation rate and/or C-reactive protein level normalized, the prednisone dose was reduced. Twenty-one patients were followed up for 2 years or at least 1 year after the medication was discontinued.

Findings.—The MTX and placebo groups did not differ in time to remission, duration of remission, number of relapses, or cumulative prednisone doses. The mean daily prednisone dose was decreased by half after 21 weeks. Forty percent of the patients could stop prednisone treatment within 2 years. The median duration of steroid therapy was 47.5 weeks, ranging from 3 to 104 weeks. There were no serious complications from GCA.

Conclusions.—With a rapid steroid-tapering regimen, the mean daily prednisone dose in these patients could be decreased by 50% in 21 weeks. Within 2 years, prednisone therapy could be stopped altogether in 40% of the patients. Methotrexate had no steroid-sparing effect at a dosage of 7.5 mg/wk.

► Polymyalgia rheumatica is a syndrome diagnosis. It subsumes a population of individuals older than 55 years with severe proximal muscular pain, with tenderness and stiffness with marked gelling (morning exacerbation), a normocytic normochromic anemia, and an erythrocyte sedimentation rate over 55 mm/hr. There is no other feature to the syndrome except for exquisite palliation from prednisone in daily doses less than 15 mg (and often much less). Generally these are elderly patients who would be dreadfully ill were it not for steroid therapy. The rub is that the median duration of this self-limited illness is measured in years! Thus, the trade-off for steroid-induced palliation is the likelihood of Cushing's syndrome, which can be catastrophic in this population. Fortunately, most patients respond to very low doses (less than 10 mg every day) so that the trade-off is tolerable. Occasionally a patient requires much more for years. In such an instance, a steroid-sparing alternative would be a godsend.

There have been anecdotes suggesting that MTX might represent such an alternative. The 2 articles (Abstracts 5–11 and 5–12) tested that inference, reaching opposite conclusions.

Van der Veen et al. (Abstract 5–12) orchestrated a multicenter randomized, placebo-controlled study in 40 patients (6 with documented GCA) of the addition of a weekly dose of 7.5 mg MTX (given orally) to their standard steroid regimen. The steroid regimen entailed an initial dose of prednisone of 20 mg/day with rapid taper as long as symptoms and erythrocyte sedimentation rate remained suppressed. Methotrexate had no benefit in this setting; the mean daily prednisone dose was reduced by 50% within 6 months and 40% of patients were no longer receiving the agent within 2 years.

Ferraccioli et al. undertook a randomized controlled trial in 24 patients followed up for 1 year. All patients initially received 15 mg/day and tapered off over 6 months unless symptoms recredesced. Half received MTX 10 mg

IM weekly. At 1 year all patients were in remission with normal sedimentation rates. However, 6 of the 12 receiving MTX had also stopped receiving steroids; none of those receiving the placebo were.

I have no ready explanation for these discordant results. Perhaps the difference reflects the difference in MTX dosing. Perhaps it is nothing more than randomization error. Such is clinical investigation.

N.M. Hadler, M.D.

Eosinophilic Fasciitis

Increased Expression of Transforming Growth Factor-β1, Fibronectin, and Types I, III, and VI Collagen Genes in Fascial Fibroblasts From Patients With Diffuse Fasciitis With Eosinophilia

Kähäri L, Jiménez SA (Thomas Jefferson Univ, Philadelphia)

J Rheumatol 23:482–486, 1996 5–13

Objective.—Patients with diffuse fasciitis with eosinophilia (DFE) have cutaneous fibrosis with characteristic "orange-peel"-like induration, sometimes with extremity swelling and joint contracture. Histologic examination shows severe fascial fibrosis and sometimes tissue infiltration with eosinophils. The reasons for the excessive collections of connective tissue in the fascia are unknown. It is also unclear whether there are any differences between the fascial and adjacent dermal fibroblasts. Expression of the genes for transforming growth factor-β1 (TGF-β1) and various extracellular matrix proteins from fascial and dermal fibroblasts were assessed in patients with DFE.

Methods.—Fibroblasts from the dermis and fascia of clinically active lesions were obtained and cultured from 3 patients with DFE. Biosynthetic studies using ^{14}C-proline and Northern and dot blot hybridization using specific cDNA were done to assess collagen production and levels of messenger RNA for fibronectin, α1(I) procollagen, α1(III) procollagen, and the 3 chains of type VI collagen. Also, Northern hybridization using human TGF-β cDNA was done to assess expression of the gene encoding TGF-β1.

Results.—Biosynthesis of collagen was up to 4.6 times greater in fascial fibroblasts than in dermal fibroblasts from the same patient. Steady-state levels of fibronectin messenger RNA were up to 8.5 times greater in the fascial fibroblasts, and steady-state messenger RNA levels for α1(I), α1(III), and α3(VI) collagens were up to 3.9 times greater. The fascial fibroblasts also expressed a much higher level of TGF-β cDNA (Fig 2).

Conclusion.—In patients with DFE, the fibroblasts found in fascia show significantly greater expression of genes for several extracellular matrix proteins than the fibroblasts found in adjacent dermis. The fascial fibroblasts also express markedly higher levels of TGF-β1 messenger RNA,

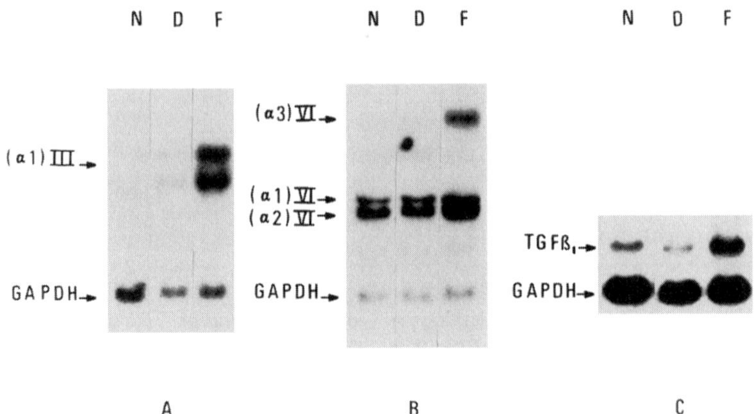

FIGURE 2.—Autoradiograms of Northern blot analyses of total RNA from dermal and fascial fibroblasts from patients with diffuse fasciitis with eosinophilia hybridized with human cDNA for α1(III), α1(VI), α3(VI) collagens and transforming growth factor (*TGF*) β1. **A,** hybridization with human α1(III) procollagen cDNA. **B,** hybridization with human α1(VI), α2(VI), and α3 (VI) collagen cDNA. **C,** hybridization with human TGF-β1 cDNA. All filters were hybridized simultaneously with rat glyceraldehyde phosphate dehydrogenase cDNA to correct for variations in the amounts of total RNA electrophoresed in each lane. **A,** case 1. **B,** case 3. **C,** case 2. (Courtesy of Kähäri L, Jiménez SA: Increased expression of transforming growth factor-β1, fibronectin, and types I, III, and VI collagen genes in fascial fibroblasts from patients with diffuse fasciitis with eosinophilia. *J Rheumatol* 23:482–486, 1996.)

suggesting that TGF-β1 may play a key role in the development of fibrosis in DFE.

▶ Although TGF-β1 is considered a major player in the profibrogenic cytokine cascade, perhaps along with connective tissue growth factor, when studied in the experimental animal, direct demonstration of TGF-β1 in human fibrotic lesions has been all too infrequent. Kähäri and Jiménez have found by Northern blot analysis of cultured fibroblastic cell strains from the fascia and dermis of patients with DFE, that TGF-β1 messenger RNA can be shown in increased quantity in affected fascial fibroblasts. We need to learn more about how to alter the expression of TGF-β and the profibrogenic cytokine cascade.

E.C. LeRoy, M.D.

Behçet's Syndrome

Systemic Levels of the T Cell Regulatory Cytokines IL-10 and IL-12 in Behçet's Disease: Soluble TNFR-75 as a Biological Marker of Disease Activity

Turan B, Gallati H, Erdi H, et al (Univ Hosp, Zürich, Switzerland; Behçet Ctr, Ankara, Turkey)

J Rheumatol 24:128–132, 1997 5–14

Introduction.—Behçet's disease (BD) is a chronic, multisystemic, immunoinflammatory disease characterized by recurrent oral and genital ulcers; ocular lesions; skin manifestations; arthritis; and vascular, intestinal, and neurologic involvement. Clinical and laboratory features suggest a pathogenic role of T lymphocytes. The levels of interleukin (IL)-10 and IL-12 were analyzed in patients with BD to determine the value of cytokines and cytokine antagonists as biological markers of disease activity.

Methods.—Using immunologic methods, sera/plasma samples of 66 consecutive patients with BD were evaluated for the presence of IL-2R, IL-6, tumor necrosis factor (TNF)-α, soluble TNF receptor (sTNFR)-55, sTNFR-75, IL-10, and IL-12. Other laboratory measures included erythrocyte sedimentation rate and C-reactive protein. Patients with inactive, mildly active, and active disease were designated as groups I, II, and III, respectively. History and clinical data were recorded to correlate cytokine levels with clinical markers of disease activity.

Results.—There were 18, 36, and 12 patients in groups I, II, and III, respectively. Interleukin-10 was increased in 42 plasma samples (64%). There was no significant difference between the percentage of samples

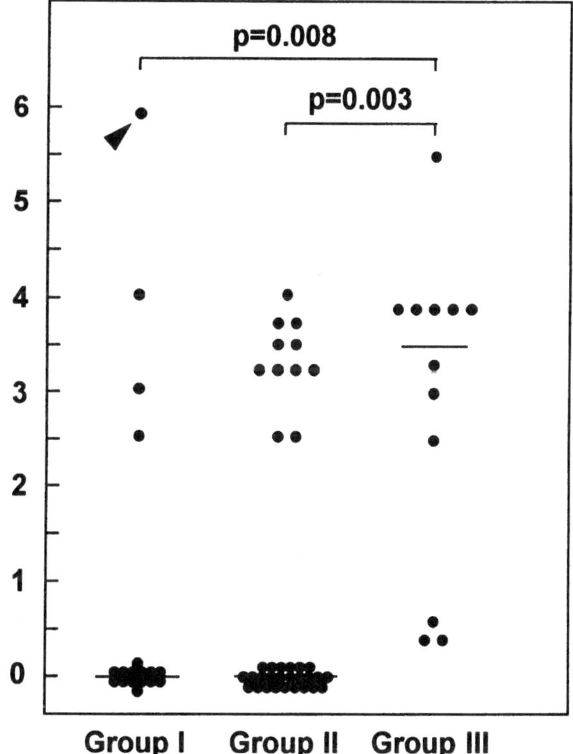

FIGURE 1.—Median soluble tumor necrosis factor receptor–75 plasma levels. A significant difference between inactive (group I) and active (group III) disease and between mildly active (group II) and active disease was found. The difference between inactive and mildly active disease was not significant. (*Arrowhead* marks patient who had acute bronchopulmonary infection at the time of venipuncture.) (Courtesy of Turan B, Gallati H, Erdi H, et al: Systemic levels of the T cell regulatory cytokines IL-10 and IL-12 in Behçet's disease: soluble TNFR-75 as a biological marker of disease activity. *J Rheumatol* 24:128–132, 1997.)

containing IL-10 and the median levels of IL-10 of the 3 patient groups. Nine patients had detectable IL-12: 1 group-I patient (5%), 3 group-II patients (8%), and 5 group-III patients (41%). There was a significant correlation between IL-12 and disease activity in group-I and -III patients. Patients with active and mildly active disease had significantly higher erythrocyte sedimentation rate, compared with patients with inactive disease. The median C-reactive protein levels were significantly higher in group III than group I. There were significant differences in STNFR-75 levels between group-I and -III patients and group-II and -III patients (Fig 1).

Conclusion.—The findings of elevated IL-10 plasma levels independent of disease activity in most patients and correlation of IL-12 plasma levels with disease activity in patients with BD suggest a pathogenic role of a Th-1-type immune response in active disease. The correlation of sTNFR-75 levels with disease activity suggest that sTNFR-75 may be useful as a biological marker of disease activity in BD.

▶ By the combined expertise of rheumatologists and dermatologists from Ankara and Zurich and by using both a United States and Israeli scoring system for disease activity, 66 patients with BD were studied for circulating levels of T-cell cytokines. Using a combination of erythrocyte sedimentation rate, C-reactive protein, IL-12, and sTNFR-75, patients with inactive, mildly active, and active disease could be distinguished from one another. These determinations are, thus, more likely to be useful in management than in initial diagnosis, and they support the case for forming centers to study and treat diseases as uncommon and indolent as BD.

E.C. LeRoy, M.D.

Behçet's Disease Associated With Myelodysplastic Syndromes

Ohno E, Ohtsuka E, Watanabe K, et al (Oita Med Univ, Japan)

Cancer 79:262–268, 1997 5–15

Background.—Rarely, Behçet's disease has been associated with myelodysplastic syndromes (MDS). Increased production of reactive oxygen species (ROS) by neutrophils is important in the development of Behçet's disease. However, reduced production of ROS by neutrophils has often been found in patients with MDS. The role of ROS production in 1 patient with Behçet's disease and MDS was investigated, and the pertinent literature was reviewed.

Methods and Findings.—The patient was a 34-year-old Japanese woman with refractory anemia and trisomy 8. Luminol-enhanced chemiluminescence (CL) assay was used to study ROS production by neutrophils. Neutrophils were obtained during the active phase of Behçet's disease. An increased CL response was observed. In addition, serum from the patient increased CL emission of neutrophils from healthy volunteers. Another 10 patients with Behçet's disease associated with MDS have been reported to date in the literature. Cytogenetic analysis of bone marrow cells had been performed in 9 of these patients, 7 of whom were found to have trisomy 8.

Conclusion.—Trisomy 8 appears to predispose patients with MDS to Behçet's disease. Increased ROS production by neutrophils may be correlated with the diverse clinical findings in this disorder. Neutrophils were activated directly by serum factors in the current study.

Myopathies

Interrelationship of Major Histocompatibility Complex Class II Alleles and Autoantibodies in Four Ethnic Groups With Various Forms of Myositis

Arnett FC, Targoff IN, Mimori T, et al (Univ of Texas Health Sciences Ctr, Houston; Univ of Oklahoma, Oklahoma City; Keio Univ, Tokyo)

Arthritis Rheum 39:1507–1518, 1996 5–16

Background.—Polymyositis (PM) and dermatomyositis (DM) are idiopathic inflammatory myopathies suspected to be of autoimmune origin. Although familial aggregation is rare, studies have shown increased frequencies of certain major histocompatibility complex (MHC) alleles associated with myositis. The interrelationships among myositis subsets, autoantibodies, and MHC class-II alleles across ethnic lines were examined, and genetic susceptibility to myositis was localized within the MHC class-II region.

Methods.—Participating in the study were 224 patients with various myositis syndromes (89 were white; 89, black; 25, Hispanic; and 21, Asian). Myositis-specific autoantibodies (MSA) were determined, and MHC class II alleles were detected by DNA oligotyping.

Results.—Although anti-Jo-1 (histidyl-tRNA synthetase) and other MSAs were equally distributed among the races, they occurred more often in patients with PM than in those with other myositis syndromes. Frequencies of MSAs correlated negatively with anti-U1 RNP and positively with anti-Ro (SS-A, the single most common autoantibody in patients with myositis). White patients with myositis, particularly those with PM or with MSAs, showed increased frequencies of the HLA-*DRB1*0301* (DR3), *DQA1*0501*, and *DQB1*0201* (DQ2) alleles (and haplotype). Only frequencies of the HLA-*DQA1*0501* and *DQA1*0401* alleles were increased in the other ethnic groups, except for the Asian group. The presence of these latter 2 alleles was significantly associated with anti-Jo-1, anti–PL-12, and other MSAs relative both to myositis patients without MSAs and to healthy, ethnically matched controls. The HLA-*DQA1*0102* and **0103* alleles predominated among MSA-positive patients negative for *DQA1*0501* and *DQA1*0401*. Polymyositis, but not DM or myositis overall, appeared negatively correlated with the HLA-DR2 alleles, (*DRB1*1501* and **1503*).

Conclusions.—These data suggest that considerable genetic heterogeneity exists among patients with myositis syndromes, possibly in part because of ethnic differences in MHC alleles. Environmental triggers and geographic patterns may also contribute. However, a significant proportion of patients with myositis syndromes, specifically those with particular anti-tRNA synthetase antibodies, express selected HLA alleles of the *DQA1* locus, especially *DQA1*0501*.

▶ In patients with myositis, the presence of myositis-specific autoantibodies has been linked to HLA-*DQA1*0501* or *0401* with a respectable odds ratio of 6.5 in whites, blacks, and Hispanics, but not in Asian patients with myositis. The strong association between immunogenetic markers and disease-selective antoantibody levels, but not necessarily clinical symptoms, also extends to other diseases, such as scleroderma.

E.C. LeRoy, M.D.

Novel Autoantibodies Against Muscle-Cell Membrane Proteins in Patients With Myositis

Stuhlmüller B, Jerez R, Hausdorf G, et al (Humboldt Univ, Berlin; Friedrich Alexander Univ, Erlangen, Germany; Ludwig Maximillian Univ, Munich; et al)
Arthritis Rheum 39:1860–1868, 1996 5–17

Purpose.—Previous studies suggest that autoimmune mechanisms play a role in the inflammatory myopathies, such as polymyositis (PM) and dermatomyositis (DM). All antibodies studied so far are directed against intracellular antigens that are found in every type of cell, and thus are unlikely to play a pathogenetic role. However, cell surface antigens on muscle cells could play a key role in inducing muscle cell damage. Patients with inflammatory myopathies were studied in an attempt to find autoantibodies against muscle cell-specific surface membrane antigens.

Methods.—The study analyzed sera from 141 patients with various rheumatic and nonrheumatic diseases. The latter group included 12 patients with cardiomyopathies, 25 patients with other muscular diseases, and 14 patients who had had major surgery or had other noninflammatory diseases. Twenty serum samples from healthy patients were studied as well. Serial dilutions with nonfixed or fixed cells were prepared for testing with a cell enzyme-linked immunosorbent assay (cell ELISA) using the human rhabdomyosarcoma cell line TE-671.

Results.—Nonfixed cell ELISA yielded positive results in 71% of patients with PM, compared to 15% of patients with DM, 18% with systemic sclerosis, 15% with systemic lupus erythematosus, and 7% with rheumatoid arthritis. There were no positive responses in sera from healthy controls or from patients with nonrheumatic diseases. The positive sera showed no reaction when other cell lines, including chondrosarcoma, bladder carcinoma, and pancreas carcinoma cells and human foreskin fibroblasts, were used as substrates. Flow cytometry and immunofluorescence studies confirmed the results of the nonfixed cell ELISA. One third of the sera from patients with PM showed a strong 50-kd protein band on plasma membrane preparations from TE-671 muscle cells.

Conclusions.—Autoantibodies against muscle-cell surface antigens are detectable in the sera of most patients with PM, DM, and certain other rheumatic diseases. Autoantibodies against these molecules, which are found in the muscle-cell surface membrane, could play a key pathogenetic role in the development of treatment for PM. This concept is consistent with the good results achieved with IgG treatment in patients with inflammatory myopathies.

▶ Myositis-specific antibodies are found in about ⅓ of patients with inflammatory myopathies although antibodies against myosin and myoglobin can be detected in the vast majority. This study searches for antibodies against muscle cell-specific surface membrane antigens in patients with inflammatory myopathies and from patients with other rheumatic and muscular disorders. In most patients with PM and DM, autoantibodies against muscle cells surface antigens were detected. They could play a major role in the pathogenesis of these inflammatory myopathies. The search for the elusive autoimmune mechnisms continues. This, like other correlative studies, does not prove causality since the antibodies might be the result of cell damage rather than the cause. Nevertheless, it's an interesting observation and needs further study.

M.H. Liang, M.D., M.P.H.

Bronchiolitis Obliterans Organizing Pneumonia as the First Manifestation of Polymyositis

Fata F, Rathore R, Schiff C, et al (Maimonides Med Ctr, Brooklyn, NY; State Univ of New York, Brooklyn)

South Med J 90:227–230, 1997 5–18

Introduction.—Causes of bronchiolitis obliterans organizing pneumonia (BOOP) include inhalation of toxic fumes, AIDS, respiratory infections, bone marrow or heart-lung transplantation, and idiopathic factors. Its pathogenesis is not known. The disease has been associated with RA, systemic lupus erythematosus, Sjögren's syndrome, and certain drugs (penicillamine, cocaine, gold, and amiodarone). It is rare that BOOP precedes or co-exists with polymyositis. The second known report of BOOP preceding polymyositis was presented.

Case Report.—Man, 51, was hospitalized with a 3-week history of fever, nonproductive cough, and shortness of breath. Bilateral basal interstitial infiltrates were observed on chest radiographs. Findings of an open lung biopsy were consistent with BOOP. The patient responded to prednisone therapy but was seen again in 8 weeks for fever, cough, and weakness of the arms and legs. He had not been compliant in regard to taking the complete course of prednisone. Elevations were detected in creatine kinase (CK), the macrophage inflammatory protein (MIP-1), and tumor necrosis factor α (TNF-α). The anti–Jo-1 antibody was not detected. A biopsy specimen from the quadriceps femoris muscle was compatible with polymyositis. The patient was afebrile, his dyspnea resolved, the pulmonary infiltrates decreased, and muscle strength improved after a second course of corticosteroid therapy. There were significant decreases in CK, MIP-1, and TNF-α after therapy.

Conclusion.—Patients with idiopathic BOOP should be observed for development of connective tissue disorders. It is not known whether elevations in MIP-1 and TNF-α are predictive of the development of polymyositis in patients with BOOP, but this question deserves further evaluation.

▶ The link between interstitial pneumonitis and connective tissue diseases has been known for years. This case of BOOP preceding polymyositis suggests that MIP-1 and TNF-α may predict which patients with BOOP will develop polymyositis; they may also be useful in following patients. These findings need prospective data.

M.H. Liang, M.D., M.P.H.

Polychronditis

Steroid Sparing Effect of Methotrexate in Relapsing Polychondritis

Park J, Gowin KM, Schumacher HR Jr (Univ of Pennsylvania, Philadelphia; Philadelphia Veterans Affairs Med Ctr)

J Rheumatol 23:937–938, 1996 5–19

Background.—Relapsing polychondritis, a rare inflammatory disorder causing recurrent inflammatory reactions in the cartilaginous structures, often worsens with the tapering of prednisone. Three patients with biopsy-proved relapsing polychondritis benefited from methotrexate as a steroid-sparing agent in the treatment of auricular chondritis.

Case 1.—Woman, 54, had recurrent swelling of the helix. She responded well to prednisone, 25 mg/day. Dapsone, 100 mg/day, was given to facilitate prednisone dose tapering, but her inflammation increased. Dapsone was stopped, and methotrexate, 7.5 mg/week, was initiated, with a gradual increase to 20 mg/week. Slight transient increases of the prednisone dose improved intermittent redness and tenderness of the helices during this period. Prednisone was eventually discontinued, and her ears remain asymptomatic with methotrexate, 15 mg/week.

Case 2.—Man, 73, had recurrent swelling of the helix and required 40 mg of prednisone per day to improve ear erythema and tenderness. This patient subsequently had right eye episcleritis as well. A methotrexate dose of 5 mg/week was begun, with a gradual increase to 15 mg/week. Transient prednisone dose increases controlled symptom exacerbations. After discontinuation of prednisone, he did well with methotrexate 10 mg/week, until a recurrence of symptoms on the helix necessitated an increase to 12.5 mg/week and a temporary reinstitution of prednisone, 20 mg/day.

Case 3.—Man, 42, had recurrent swelling of the helix, a long-standing history of diffuse psoriasis, and a 5-month history of right knee joint arthritis with effusion. When swelling and pain occurred in both ears, his dose of sulfasalazine was increased, but with no effect. This medication was stopped, and methotrexate, 7.5 mg/week, was begun. The dose was gradually increased to 22.5 mg/week. His chondritis resolved completely, although his arthritis and psoriasis were not completely controlled.

Conclusion.—This is the first report of the value of methotrexate as a steroid-sparing or avoiding agent in patients with relapsing polychondritis, at least for auricular chondritis. Methotrexate may be useful as an adjunct in patients in whom dapsone is ineffective.

▶ Relapsing polychondritis is a rare, dramatic, intermittent, and remittent inflammatory disorder that targets cartilage in a peculiar distribution; auricular, nasal, and tracheal cartilaginous inflammation are hallmarks. Palliation with steroids is the first line of therapy. However, it is not clear in this disorder, or in any other inflammatory rheumatic disease, that the palliation attendant to steroid exposure is accompanied by a decrement in tissue destruction or that the palliation has a reasonable risk/benefit ratio in the long term. Because of these last concerns, there is a quest for a substitute or synergistic long-term intervention that has less obligate toxicity.

In the case of relapsing polychondritis, such a quest is confounded by the intermittency of the natural history; by the rarity of the condition; by the multiorgan involvement that is part of the syndrome (ocular, articular, and cochlear/vestibular involvement are common features); and by the fact that polychondritis is often confounded by other rheumatic, inflammatory, and neoplastic diseases. We have to settle for anecdotes, hoping that some real insight that generalizes will emerge. Dapsone treatment and immunosuppression with cyclophosphamide, azathioprine, and cyclosporin A have inconsistent track records. This report adds methotrexate to the list of candidates again, but with limited success, if any at all. The 3 patients described had no recurrences of the major manifestation they suffered, namely, auricular inflammation.

N.M. Hadler, M.D.

6 Osteoarthritis, Crystal-related Arthropathies, Osteoporosis, Infectious Arthritides

Introduction

If I were starting a rheumatology fellowship today, I'd think seriously about studying osteoarthritis (OA). In my day it was fashionable to investigate the immunology of RA or systemic lupus erythematosus, or other effete problems of limited societal importance. OA is certainly common and will only become more prevalent as our population ages. And new insights about the genetics and biology of OA are exciting. Our therapeutic approaches, too, are beginning to expand and diversify. OA is now clearly an interesting and important problem.

Richard S. Panush, M.D.

Osteoarthritis

EPIDEMIOLOGY

The Association of Obesity With Osteoarthritis of the Hand and Knee in Women: A Twin Study

Cicuttini FM, Baker JR, Spector TD (St Thomas' Hosp, London; Guys' and St Thomas' Trust, London)

J Rheumatol 23:1221–1226, 1996 6–1

Objective.—Obesity is a preventable risk factor for osteoarthritis (OA), the most common cause of disability and knee and hip replacement in developed countries. Both genetic and environmental factors may play a role in the development of the disease. The results of a study of the association of obesity with OA at various sites in middle-aged twins are presented.

Methods.—Interviews were conducted with 158 identical and 171 fraternal twins, age 48 to 70, to ascertain arthritis and joint symptoms. Radiographs were obtained of hands and knees and evaluated independently by 2 blinded observers. Disease was graded and classified. Weight, smoking history, physical activity, and use of hormone replacement use were determined.

Results.—Twins with tibiofemoral joint (TFJ) osteophytes, patellofemoral joint (PFJ) osteophytes, or carpometacarpal (CMC) osteophytes were, respectively, 3.75, 3.05, and 3.06 kg heavier than their siblings. Twins with PFJ space narrowing were 4.73 kg heavier than their siblings. There were no weight differences in twins wherein 1 of the pair had OA of the distal interphalangeal (DIP) or proximal interphalangeal joint (PIP). The risk for developing OA osteophytes per kg of increased weight was 1.14 for patients with TFJ osteophytes, 1.32 for those with PFJ osteophytes, and 1.10 for those with CMC osteophytes. The risk for developing PFJ narrowing was 1.15 per kg of increased weight.

Conclusion.—Obesity is an important risk factor for developing TFJ, PFJ, and CMC OA. Because each 1-kg increase in body weight increases the risk of OA by 9 to 14%, weight reduction is an important preventive measure for OA.

▶ Studies on the epidemiology of osteoarthritis are difficult to do, and the condition, onset, and progression are difficult to define. Findings of osteoarthritis are not well correlated with the symptoms; OA in different sites may not have common risk factors. This well-done twin study from the United Kingdom confirms the importance of obesity in radiographic findings of osteoarthritis at the tibial femoral and patellofemoral joints and CMC joints of the hand. No effect was found at the DIP and PIP joints. In an effort to see whether OA may have decreased physical activity and therefore increased weight, a group of asymptomatic twins were studied and the analyses showed similar results. The key question is whether intervention for obesity in younger life affects the outcome of disease defined radiographically.

M.H. Liang, M.D., M.P.H.

Risk of Osteoarthritis Associated With Long-term Weight-bearing Sports: A Radiologic Survey of the Hips and Knees in Female Ex-athletes and Population Controls

Spector TD, Harris PA, Hart DJ, et al (St Thomas Hosp, London; Royal Natl Orthopaedic Hosp, Stanmore, England; Whipps Cross Hosp, London)
Arthritis Rheum 39:988–995, 1996 6–2

Background.—Increased physical activity is being widely encouraged to decrease the incidence of cardiovascular disease and osteoporosis. However, the risks associated with excessive sports activity are not clear. The risk of osteoarthritis (OA) of the hip and knee from long-term weight-bearing sports activity in ex-elite athletes and the general population was determined.

Methods.—Eighty-one female ex-elite athletes aged 40–65 years were included in the retrospective cohort study. Sixty-seven women had been middle- and long-distance runners, and 14 had been tennis players. Nine hundred seventy-seven women matched for age comprised a control group. Osteoarthritis was defined with the use of radiologic evidence of joint space narrowing and osteophytosis in the hip joints, patellofemoral (PF) joints, and tibiofemoral (TF) joints.

Findings.—The ex-athletes had higher rates of radiologic OA at all sites. This association was stronger after adjustment for height and weight differences. It was strongest for the presence of osteophytes at the TF joints, PF joints, narrowing at the PF joints, femoral osteophytes, and hip joint narrowing and weakest for narrowing at the TF joints. Within the ex-athlete group, no clear risk factors could be identified, although the tennis players tended to have more osteophytes at the TF joints and hip, whereas the runners had more PF joint disease. A subgroup of 22 women in the control group who had participated in long-term vigorous weight-bearing exercise had OA risks comparable to those of the ex-athletes. The ex-athletes had comparable rates of symptom reporting but greater pain thresholds than controls as determined with the use of calibrated dolorimeter.

Conclusions.—Vigorous weight-bearing sports activity in women increases the risk of radiologic OA of the knees and hips by two- to three-fold. Duration rather than frequency of training appears to be important.

Relationship of Running to Musculoskeletal Pain With Age

Fries JF, Singh G, Morfeld D, et al (Stanford Univ, Calif)

Arthritis Rheum 39:64–72, 1996 6–3

Background.—As the population ages, it is important to identify risk factors associated with musculoskeletal disability, pain, and stiffness to try to reduce the magnitude of this problem. The possible association between long-distance running over many years and increased musculoskeletal pain was investigated in a longitudinal study.

Methods.—Four hundred twelve members of a runners' club and 289 community control subjects were followed up prospectively for 6 years. All subjects were 53–75 years of age at the time of study enrollment. The subjects were also classified as ever-runners (n = 488) and never-runners (n = 211).

Findings.—The running club group had slightly less musculoskeletal pain than the controls. The difference between groups was significant for women but not men. Among men, mean adjusted pain scores for members of the runners' club were 18.3; for controls, 20.2; for ever-runners, 18.6; and for never-runners, 20.3. Among women, the mean adjusted pain

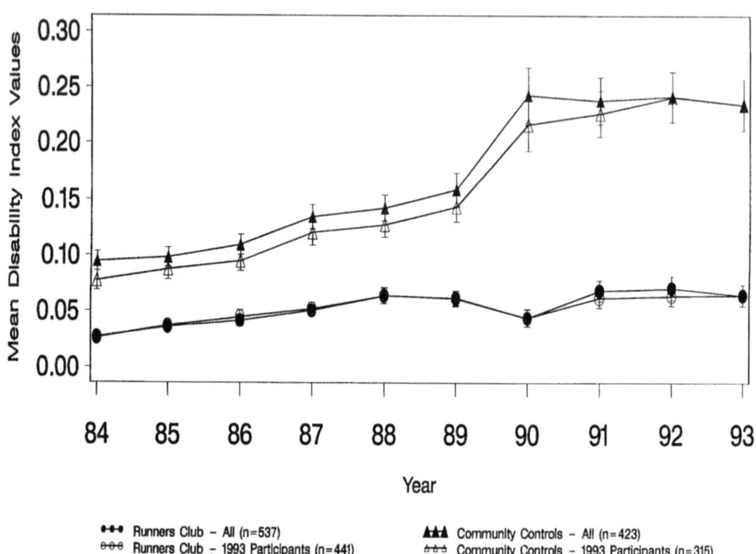

FIGURE 4.—Disability index (Health Assessment Questionnaire scores, 0–3 scale) from 1984 to 1993, by running group status. Data are presented for subjects for whom data were available in 1993, as well as for all subjects at all periods. *Filled circles*, all runners' club members (n = 537); *open circles*, runners' club members remaining in the study in 1993 (n = 441); *filled triangles*, all community controls (n = 423); *open triangles*, community controls remaining in the study in 1993 (n = 315). Runners' club members demonstrate greatly reduced disability levels, with a tendency for the differences to widen over time. These results are consistent whether all data from all participants or only those participating in 1993 are considered. Values are the mean ± SEM. (Courtesy of Fries JF, Singh G, Morfeld D, et al: Relationship of running to musculoskeletal pain with age. *Arthritis Rheum* 39:64–72, 1996, copyright American College of Rheumatology.)

scores for members of the runners club were 17.5; for controls, 22.8; for ever-runners, 17.2; and for never-runners, 23.7. After 9 years of observation, disability developed in runners' club members at a rate of one third that in the controls. Fifty-one study participants died during follow-up—41 in the control group and 10 in the runners' club (Fig 4).

Conclusions.—Vigorous running during the course of many years is not associated with increased musculoskeletal pain with age. Running may be associated with a moderate reduction in such pain, especially in women.

► I was feeling pretty good about completing the Boston Marathon last April—it was the 100th anniversary and an extraordinary celebration. If only I wasn't stiff and sore and exhausted—then I read the article by Tim Spector et al. (Abstract 6–2). It disturbed me. It appeared to contradict the consensus that running need not be deleterious to joints, as had been reported in previous YEAR BOOKS. But this report is retrospective, used radiographic criteria for OA not clinical findings, and examined certain former women elite athletes. I would be cautious about extrapolating, or generalizing about, the significance of noting some cartilaginous narrowing or, particularly, osteophytes in this population. I have long worried about the risk of OA and/or disability from running. These data do not cheer me, but I would interpret them in context and circumspectly.

The work of Jim Fries et al. (Abstract 6–3) reflects longitudinal observations of men and women running and exercising recreationally, has been validated independently, and expands previous reports. And it is more to my liking! These authors reasoned that predisposition to OA in recreational runners might be preceded by increasing pain and stiffness. However, data from this study showed no progressive increase in these symptoms in runners, as in their previous studies, supporting the contention that recreational runners need not be predisposed to OA. I hope I'm not!

I also like the model for OA (Fig 1 in the original article), which revises many of our traditional concepts.

R.S. Panush, M.D.

Biology

Synovial Membrane Inflammation and Cytokine Production in Patients With Early Osteoarthritis

Smith M, Triantafillou S, Parker A, et al (Repatriation Gen Hosp, Daw Park, Australia)

J Rheumatol 24:365–371, 1997 6–4

Introduction.—Despite several studies reporting inflammatory changes in the synovial membranes of patients with osteoarthritis, which can be indistinguishable from those seen in patients with RA, the relevance of inflammatory changes in the synovial membranes of patients with osteoarthritis is controversial. At various stages in the development of osteoarthritis, synovial membrane histopathology and cytokine content were examined.

Methods.—The knees of 63 patients who complained of unexplained knee pain or who were having joint replacement surgery were sampled for synovial membrane at the time of arthroscopy. The synovial membranes were evaluated for the thickness of lining layer, vascularity, and inflammatory cell infiltrated. In situ hybridization with biotin-labeled riboprobes and immunohistochemistry was used to determine production of interleukin-1α, interleukin-1β, tumor necrosis factor-α, and interleukin-1 receptor antagonist at the mRNA and protein levels in a subset of 20 patients.

Results.—In synovial membranes of patients with all grades of osteoarthritis, there was evidence of thickening of the lining layer, increased vascularity, and inflammatory cell infiltration. Patients with advanced grades of osteoarthritis had the most marked changes seen in synovial tissue. Irrespective of the degree of articular cartilage damage, all patients with osteoarthritis had production of interleukin 1-α, interleukin 1-β, and tumor necrosis factor-α in their synovial membranes. With increasing grades of osteoarthritis, there was a decrease in the ratio of interleukin-l receptor antagonist to interleukin-1 α and 1-β,

Conclusion.—Patients with early osteoarthritis had chronic inflammatory changes with production of proinflammatory cytokines in synovial membranes. In patients at the time of joint replacement surgery, the most severe changes, which resembled those seen in RA, were seen. The production of cytokines may contribute to the pathogenesis of osteoarthritis, resulting from low-grade synovitis.

► These observations may be important. They suggest a role for inflammatory processes, mediated by mononuclear cell infiltration and cytokine elaboration, in early osteoarthritis. Might this imply that supportive, mechanical, and analgesic therapy for osteoarthritis may be insufficient?

R.S. Panush, M.D.

Pain Mechanisms in Osteoarthritis of the Knee: Effect of Intraarticular Anesthetic

Creamer P, Hunt M, Dieppe P (Bristol Royal Infirmary, England)
J Rheumatol 23:1031–1036, 1996 6–5

Introduction.—Pain is the major symptom of osteoarthritis (OA) but, for several reasons, has proven difficult to study. The mechanism of OA pain is uncertain, but may involve pain-sensitive structures located within or in intimate contact with the inner surface of the joint. If this is so, then intra-articular anesthetic injection should eliminate the pain. This intervention was tested in a study of the mechanisms of pain in knee OA.

Methods.—The single-blind study included 20 patients with symptomatic OA of both knees. Each patient underwent intra-articular injection of bupivacaine, 5 mL 0.25%, or placebo into 1 knee. The injection was given in the most painful knee, as indicated by the patient. A 100 mm visual analog scale (VAS) was used to measure pain in both knees at 1 hr, 24 hr, and 7 days after the injection. The pain was also described using terms from the McGill pain questionnaire.

Results.—Within 1 hr, the median pain score in knees injected with bupivacaine fell from 61.5 to 0 mm. The median change in VAS scores was a 45.5 mm decrease with local anesthetic versus a 3.5 mm increase with placebo. Six of 10 knees injected with bupivacaine were completely pain free at 1 hr. Pain scores also declined in the noninjected knees. The drop in VAS scores for the contralateral knees was somewhat greater in patients receiving local anesthetic injection, but not significantly so. Pain scores remained lower than baseline for 7 days after local anesthetic injection, but the difference from placebo was not significant. McGill scores for all categories of pain were reduced with bupivacaine injection but not placebo injection.

Conclusions.—Intra-articular injection of local anesthetic significantly reduces—and sometimes eliminates—knee pain in patients with OA. This supports the hypothesis that knee pain in OA is related to structures in contact with the intra-articular surface. Interventions on one knee can also affect pain perception in the other knee. Cautious use of local anesthetic could provide useful insight into the mechanisms of pain in OA and its impact on other factors involved in knee disease.

▶ This is such a simple and elegant study that one wonders why it hasn't been done before. The authors review the putative mechanisms by which OA causes pain: no one knows for sure what they are. In this study, patients with bilateral symptomatic OA knee received placebo or intra-articular bupivacaine and the findings suggest that pain comes from pain sensitive structures within or in intimate contact with the inner surface of the joint. Indeed, pain perception fell to 0 in 6 of 10 injected knees with the anesthetic agent, a remarkable finding for those experienced in using such agents. The other striking observation was that pain in the contralateral knee also changed, though not as dramatically as the knee getting the anesthetic agent.

M.H. Liang, M.D., M.P.H.

Clinical Aspects

Relation of Dietary Intake and Serum Levels of Vitamin D to Progression of Osteoarthritis of the Knee Among Participants in the Framingham Study

McAlindon TE, Felson DT, Zhang Y, et al (Boston Univ; Tufts Univ, Boston; Brigham and Women's Hosp, Boston)

Ann Intern Med 125:353–359, 1996 6–6

Objective.—The changes in bone that contribute to the osteoarthritic process are poorly understood, although a decrease in bone mineral density is suspected of playing a role in the skeletal degeneration that characterizes the disease. Because low levels of vitamin D may contribute to disease progression, the relationship between the deficiency of vitamin D in diet and serum and the progression of osteoarthritis of the knee was examined in a prospective observational study.

Methods.—Vitamin D intake and serum levels were assessed from answers to a questionnaire in a group of participants in the Framingham study who had knee radiographs taken between 1983 and 1985 (n = 18) and between 1992 and 1993 (n = 22). Two radiologists and a rheumatologist scored radiographs for global severity of osteoarthritis on a scale of 0–4, using a modification of the Kellgren and Lawrence scale, and for the presence of joint narrowing and osteophyte formation on a scale of 1–3.

Results.—When the 556 participants were elevated, osteoarthritis was found in 75 knees and was progressive in 62 knees. There was a correlation (r = 0.24) between dietary vitamin D intake and serum vitamin D levels. Participants were stratified into 3 groups based on vitamin D intake and on serum vitamin D levels. Participants in the middle and lower third for intake and serum levels had 3 times the risk of progression as the upper level group. The lower levels groups also had an increased risk of loss of cartilage and osteophyte growth. Development of osteoarthritis of the knee was not related to vitamin D intake or to serum vitamin D levels.

Conclusions.—Individuals with low dietary vitamin D intake and low serum levels of vitamin D are at increased risk of progression of osteoarthritis of the knee. Additional studies of the relationship of prevention of osteoarthritis of the knee are needed.

▶ These interesting observations support the novel, emerging, and important theme that vitamin D, indeed bone density, influences the evolution of osteoarthritis.[1] This has significant public health and preventive implications.

R.S. Panush, M.D.

Reference

1. Nevitt MC, Lane NE, Scott JC, et al: Radiographic osteoarthritis of the hip and bone mineral density. *Arthritis Rheum* 38:907–916, 1995. (1997 Year Book of Rheumatology, p 256.)

Crystal-related Arthropathies

Inhibition and Prevention of Monosodium Urate Monohydrate Crystal-Induced Acute Inflammation in Vivo by Transforming Growth Factor β1

Lioté F, Prudhommeaux F, Schiltz C, et al (Université Paris VII, Hôpital Lariboisière, Paris; Hôpital Necker, Paris)

Arthritis Rheum 39:1192–1198, 1996 6–7

Objective.—The self-limiting nature of gouty inflammation is poorly understood, although there is some evidence that natural cytokine inhibitors can block acute and chronic inflammation. Because in vitro studies have demonstrated that transforming growth factor β (TGFβ) has anti-inflammatory properties, the ability of a single local injection of TGFβ1 to prevent and inhibit monosodium urate monohydrate (MSU) crystal–induced acute inflammation was tested in the rat subcutaneous synovium-like air pouch model.

Methods.—Six days after air pouches were produced in 139 male Sprague-Dawley rats, inflammation was induced by injecting approximately 5 mg of synthetic MSU crystals into the pouch. Group A (n = 44) received MSU crystals only; group B (n = 8) received MSU crystals plus 100 or 500 pg ultrapure human TGFβ1 (UPTGFβ1) 1 hour after injection of MSU crystals; group C (n = 41) received MSU crystals plus 10–100 pg carrier-free recombinant human TGFβ1 (rHuTGFβ1) 1 hour after injection of MSU crystals; group D (n = 8) received MSU crystals plus rHuTGFβ1 (preincubated with specific anti-TGBβ polyclonal antibodies) and anti-TGFβ antibodies 1 hour after injection of MSU crystals; group E (n = 8) received TGFβ1 only; group F (n = 8) received anti-TGFβ antibodies only; group G (n = 16) received saline vehicle; and group H (n = 6) received crystals and rHuTGFβ1 injected simultaneously. White blood cell counts in the exudate were determined at 6, 24, 48, and 72 hours after MSU injection.

Results.—The UPTGFβ1 and rHuTGFβ1 significantly reduced inflammation and showed a dose-response effect. The TGFβ1 plus MSU crystals also reduced inflammation. At 5 hours rHuTGFβ1 inhibited inflammation at doses as low as 10 pg, and at 100 pg reduced white blood cell count more than 90%. The inhibitory effect of rHuTGFβ1 was significantly reversed by preincubation. Percentage of monocytes was significantly reduced and percentage of polymorphonuclear cells was significantly increased after rHuTGFβ1 was injected at hour 6.

Conclusion.—Injected TGFβ1 appears to limit and reverse MSU crystal–induced acute inflammation in gouty attacks. These results merit further study.

▶ Why episodes of crystal-induced arthritis are self-limited and resolve spontaneously is puzzling. Perhaps insight into this process would help us better understand (and treat) other inflammatory states that perpetuate. The effects of TGFβ1 in these experiments were impressive. Could it be modulation of protease activation, hydrogen peroxide production, neutrophil phagocytosis, endothelial function, angiogenesis, adhesion molecules, or something else? The answer might be important.

R.S. Panush, M.D.

Gouty Arthritis in Nodal Osteoarthritis

Fam AG, Stein J, Rubenstein J (Univ of Toronto)

J Rheumatol 23:684–689, 1996 6–8

Objective.—The clinical features and factors associated with the development of gouty arthritis in finger joints affected with nodal osteoarthritis (OA) were reviewed.

Methods.—Nodal OA and urate crystal documented gouty arthritis of the fingers (distal and proximal interphalangeal [DIP and PIP] joints) were diagnosed in 32 patients (11 men) aged 52–88 years between 1986 and 1994. A complete blood count, urinalysis, rheumatoid factor, antinuclear antibody test, serum creatinine, pre- and posttreatment serum urate, and pretreatment 24-hour urinary urate excretion were performed. Synovial fluid and material aspirated from tophi were examined for monosodium urate crystal using compensated polarized light microscopy. Findings of 2 independent investigators were compared statistically.

Results.—The average duration of gout was 10 years for men and was 6.2 years for women. Seven men and 14 women had gouty arthritis and/or tophi in feet, olecranon bursae, and knees in addition to fingers. Eleven patients had gouty arthritis in fingers only. Twenty-nine patients had tophi of DIP and/or PIP joints, 9 had tophi only, and 20 had tophi associated with episodes of acute gouty inflammation (Fig 1). Three patients had no tophi. Serum urate averaged 614.9 μmol/L for women and 585.6 μmol/L

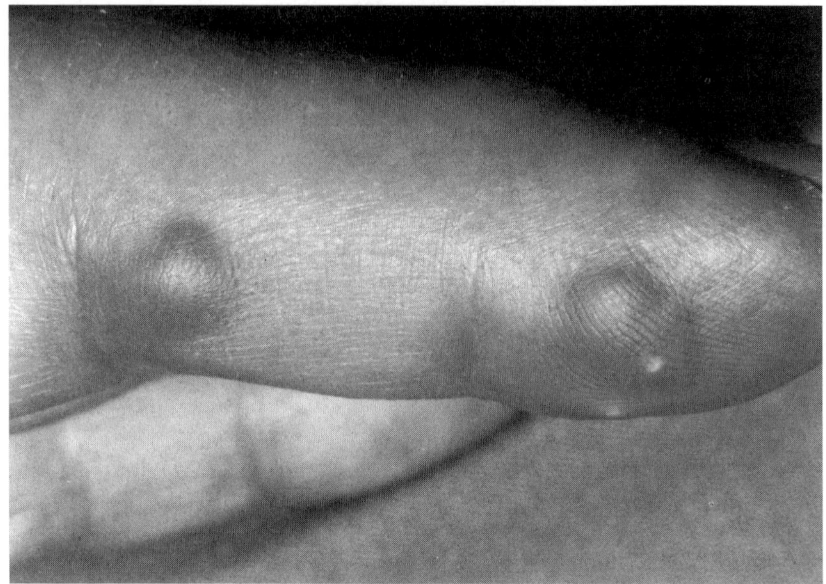

FIGURE 1.—Fingerpad intradermal tophi with gouty inflammation. (Courtesy of Fam AG, Stein J, Rubenstein J: Gouty arthritis in nodal osteoarthritis. *J Rheumatol* 23:684–689, 1996).

for men. Patients demonstrated a number of factors associated with the development of gout including diuretic use (81%), renal failure (59%), hypertension (66%), alcoholism (22%), prophylactic use of low-dose aspirin (20%), and a family history (16%).

Conclusion.—Gout may worsen joint problems in patients with nodal OA and should be considered in the differential diagnosis for older women patients with renal insufficiency, hypertension, diuretic use, and alcoholism, and using low-dose aspirin.

▶ This and another report[1] emphasize that the occurrence of gout in nodal OA is not uncommon. We recently had such a patient in the hospital whose gout was not appreciated by the primary care physician or resident and whose initial therapy was inappropriate. Recognition is obviously important for correct diagnosis and treatment.

Others identified intraarticular tophi in the knee by CT imaging,[2] tophi in the patella, and bi- or tripartite bones,[3] and concurrent gout and tuberculous arthritis.[4]

R.S. Panush, M.D.

References

1. Foldes K, Petersilge CA, Weisman MH, et al: Nodal osteoarthritis and gout: A report of four new cases. *Skeletal Radiol* 25:421–424, 1996.
2. Gerster JC, Landry M, Duvoisin B, et al: Computed tomography of the knee joint as an indicator of intraarticular tophi in gout. *Arthritis Rheum* 39:1406–1409, 1996.

3. Reber P, Crevoisier X, Noesberger B: Unusual localisation of tophaceous gout. A report of four cases and review of the literature. *Arch Orthop Trauma Surg* 115:297–299, 1996.
4. Lorenzo JP, Csuka ME, Derfus BA, et al: Concurrent gout and *mycobacterium tuberculosis* arthritis. *J Rheumatol* 24:184–186, 1997.

Idiopathic Destructive Arthropathies: Clinical, Light, and Electron Microscopic Studies

Zakaoui L, Schumacher HR Jr, Rothfuss S, et al (Univ of Tunis, Tunisia; Univ of Pennsylvania, Philadelphia; Veterans Affairs Med Ctr, Philadelphia)
J Clin Rheumatol 2:9–17, 1996 6–9

Objective.—Idiopathic destructive arthritis (IDA) affects the shoulder, hip, and knee joints. Other joints can also be affected in older individuals. The features of the syndrome in older patients, mainly women, were reviewed.

Methods.—Clinical and radiologic features were recorded for 20 patients (4 men) aged 67–89 years with IDA. Patients with avascular necrosis, Paget's disease, chronic renal failure, neuropathic joints, hemochromatosis, endocrine disorders, and chondrocalcinosis were excluded. Synovial fluid samples from all patients were examined for leukocyte counts, apatite crystals, and calcium.

Results.—Most patients had pain on use and reduced range of motion. Six patients had received intra-articular steroid injections. All patients took nonsteroidal anti-inflammatory drugs. Six patients had IDA of the knee, 16 had IDA of the shoulder, and 6 had smaller joints affected. All patients had severe cartilage loss and some bone loss. Eleven patients had significant destruction of juxta-articular bone, 8 had mild osteophytosis, and 13 had mild, local sclerosis. Most patients had bloody or clear synovial effusions. Seven patients had positive apatite tests, and 9 had calcium pyrophosphate dihydrate crystals on electron microscopy. Other x-ray patterns could not be identified.

Conclusion.—Crystals in synovial fluid contribute to the joint destruction in IDA in ways that are still not clear.

▶ This is a nice preview of this topic. The propensity of certain crystalline arthropathies to become destructive and of others to resolve is trying to teach us something.

R.S. Panush, M.D.

Uric Acid Lowering Effect of Oxipurinol Sodium in Hyperuricemic Patients: Therapeutic Equivalence to Allopurinol

Walter-Sack I, de Vries JX, Ernst B, et al (Univ of Heidelberg, Germany; Technical Univ of Dresden, Germany; Univ of Hamburg, Germany)
J Rheumatol 23:498–501, 1996 6–10

Objective.—Oxipurinol does not produce free radicals when metabolized as does allopurinol. Because new formulations of oxipurinol have improved its absorption from the gastrointestinal tract, its bioavailability as compared with that of allopurinol differs by only 25%. The uric acid lowering effect, tolerability, and safety of once daily oxipurinol compared with equimolar dosages of allopurinol were tested in hyperuricemic patients.

Methods.—In a multicenter, double-blind, crossover trial, 99 male hyperuricemic patients (average age, 53.4 years) were randomly assigned to receive either allopurinol/ oxipurinol (A/O, n = 51) or oxipurinol/allopurinol (O/A, n = 48) in amounts equivalent to 300 mg of allopurinol. Drugs were administered for 10 days to the first 9 patients and for 14 days to the remaining patients. Plasma uric acid and steady state concentrations of both drugs were measured at baseline and 24 hours after the end of each treatment arm. Safety and effectiveness were determined.

Results.—Baseline plasma uric acid concentrations were 8.3 mg/dL for the A/O group and 8.7 mg/dL for the O/A group. At crossover, the plasma uric acid concentrations for 47 A/O patients were 5.4 mg/dL after the allopurinol arm, increasing to 5.7 mg/dL after the oxipurinol arm. At crossover for the O/A group, plasma uric acid concentrations were 6.0 after the oxipurinol arm and 5.6 after the allopurinol arm. The equimolar dose-equivalent reductions of 3.0 mg/dL for allopurinol and 2.6 mg/dL for oxipurinol were significantly different. The mean total oxipurinol concentrations of 9.24 µg/dL after the allopurinol arm and 9.9 µg/dL were not significantly different. The incidence of adverse events was similar between groups, and all adverse events were mild or moderate.

Conclusion.—Oxipurinol is safe and effective as a uric acid lowering agent for hyperuricemic patients, and can be substituted for allopurinol in these patients and possibly in patients treated with allopurinol for other disorders.

▶ This study tells us that oxypurinol and allopurinol were virtually equivalent in hypouricemic effect and tolerability. This information is pertinent to the management of the patient who is allergic to allopurinol. Although some allopurinol-allergic individuals will have cross-reactive allergy to oxypurinol, oxypurinol will be an attractive alternative for the others.

R.S. Panush, M.D.

Osteoporosis

Use of Oral Corticosteroids in the Community and the Prevention of Secondary Osteoporosis: A Cross Sectional Study

Walsh LJ, Wong CA, Pringle M, et al (City Hosp, Nottingham, England; Queen's Med Centre, Nottingham, England)
BMJ 313:344–346, 1996 6–11

Objective.—More than 5.5 million prescriptions for systemic corticosteroids were written in 1993 in the United Kingdom. The prevalence of continuous use of oral steroids and conditions for which they are prescribed, including prevention of osteoporosis, was investigated.

Methods.—A 4-year cross-sectional retrospective survey of continuous use of oral corticosteroid was conducted in 65,786 patients (52% female) in 8 general practices in central and southern Nottinghamshire. "Continuous use" was defined as at least 3 months.

Results.—A total of 303 patients (65% female) aged 12–94 years were continuous users of oral corticosteroids, and 97% took an average of 8 mg/day of prednisolone. The average duration of treatment was 3 years. Corticosteroids were prescribed for RA (23%), polymyalgia rheumatica (22%), and asthma or chronic obstructive airway disease (19%). Only 10% of women older than 45 years and taking oral corticosteroids were also taking hormone replacement therapy.

Conclusion.—This review shows that 250,000 people in the United Kingdom are taking oral corticosteroids continuously, though most are not addressing prevention of osteoporosis.

► Disturbing. But not really surprising. Last year at our own institution we found that none of 100 consecutive inpatients started on corticosteroids received any intervention relating to osteoporosis.[1] And as I write this, I have just received the preprint of the October 1996 *ACR News* story about the American College of Rheumatology guidelines for steroid-induced osteoporosis, which appeared in-full in the November issues of *Arthritis and Rheumatism*. Our attention to this is long overdue.

R.S. Panush, M.D.

Reference

1. Pensabeni-Jasper T, Panush RS: Corticosteriod usage: Observations at a community hospital. *Am J Med Sci* 311:234–239, 1996.

► The diagnosis and treatment of osteoporosis has been advanced significantly by the widely applied techniques of bone mass approximation through the use of the bone densitometer and the new availability of drugs to decrease bone loss (Abstracts 6–12 through 6–16). These include the development of new modalities of therapeutic delivery for salmon calcitonin and the development of new bisphosphonates. Both of these drugs inhibit bone resorption, although there is some evidence in vitro and in vivo that at least alendronate may have some indirect effects on bone formation as well.

Rheumatologists also learned at a recent American College of Rheumatology meeting that by using a highly sensitive and specific calcitonin receptor, it can be shown that many cells busy resorbing bone at the margin of the pannus in the joint of the rheumatoid patient are osteoclasts. In addition, through the efforts of many investigators worldwide, we know that alendronate and probably other bisphosphonates inhibit the activity of the osteoclast and probably also inhibit the recruitment of new osteoclasts to arrive at the bone surface. In osteoporosis, this is clinically important in those patients who have low bone mass with or without fractures.

Alendronate has been shown to be effective at decreasing the incidence of vertebral fractures and nonvertebral fractures without any effect on mineralization. This is in contrast to the effects of etidronate, another bisphosphonate marketed by a different company, which also decreases osteoclast activity. Unfortunately, etidronate also has other effects such as dose-related inhibition of bone mineralization, and thus can clinically worsen bone pain. Newer dosage regimens such as 14 days of therapy with less than 5 mg/kg per 24 hours of etidronate on an empty stomach followed by 11 weeks off of therapy, have decreased the problems with mineralization and have also been effective in decreasing vertebral fractures in patients with osteoporosis. In addition, both alendronate and etidronate therapy increase bone mineral density; however, more important is a clinically observed decrease in fractures.

Unfortunately, some preliminary studies have not shown bisphosphonate therapy to be useful in treating RA, even though the osteoclast has been shown to be an important cell pathologically participating in bone resorption in the inflamed joints of patients with rheumatoid arthritis. These studies were less than 3 months in duration, whereas the studies in osteoporosis have needed to be carried out over 5 or more years to show important sustained clinical differences. Perhaps we shall have to do the same in examining the effects of these drugs in rheumatoid arthritis.

L.S. Simon, M.D.

Oral Alendronate Induces Progressive Increases in Bone Mass of the Spine, Hip, and Total Body Over 3 Years in Postmenopausal Women With Osteoporosis

Devogelaer JP, Broll H, Correa-Rotter R, et al (Cliniques Universitaires St Luc, Bruxelles, Belgium; Kaiser Franz Josef-Hosp, Vienna; Instituto Nacional de la Nutricion Salvador Zubiran, Tlalpan, Mexico; et al)
Bone 18:141–150, 1996 6–12

Background.—Alendronate sodium (ALN) is a potent aminobisphosphonate drug used for the treatment of osteoporosis. It has no significant potential to induce osteomalacia, and leads to the formation of normal-quality bone. In dosages of 5–40 mg/day, oral ALN leads to significantly increased bone mineral density (BMD) in postmenopausal women. A 3-year randomized trial of oral ALN for postmenopausal women with osteoporosis was reported.

Methods.—A total of 516 postmenopausal women from 19 centers around the world were studied. The women, ranging in age from 45 to 80 years, all had a spine BMD at least 2.5 SD below the mean for young, premenopausal women. They were randomly selected to receive either placebo or 1 of 3 regimens of ALN: 5 or 10 mg/day for 3 years, or 20 mg/day for 2 years plus 5 mg/day for the third year. All women took calcium supplements, 500 mg/day. Bone mineral density at the lumbar spine, proximal femur, distal forearm, and total body were measured by dual-energy x-ray absorptiometry.

Results.—In the placebo group, BMD decreased by 0.6% at the spine, 0.7% at the femoral neck, and 0.4% at the trochanter over 3 years. In contrast, all 3 ALN-treated groups had significant increases in BMD. In the spine, BMD increased by 5.4% in the 5-mg ALN group, 7.4% in the 10-mg ALN group, and 8.4% in the 20/5 mg ALN group. Alendronate increased BMD by 3.5%, 5.5%, and 4.3% at the femoral neck and by 5.1%, 7.2%, and 7.2% at the trochanter, respectively. The 5-mg dose of ALN was therefore less effective than the 2 higher doses. All 3 ALN groups had continued increases in BMD during the 3-year study period, with the 10-mg group achieving the greatest gains during the third year. Treatment with ALN reduced bone turnover to a new steady-state level, as shown by changes in biochemical markers. Oral ALN was safe and generally well tolerated.

Conclusions.—Oral ALN is a promising treatment for osteoporosis in postmenopausal women, with the potential to reduce fracture risk. Given in an oral dose of 10 mg/day for 3 years, ALN produces significant and progressive increases in BMD. Its safety profile is comparable to that of placebo.

Prevention of Nonvertebral Fractures by Alendronate: A Meta-analysis

Karpf DB, for the Alendronate Osteoporosis Treatment Study Groups (Merck Research Labs, Rahway, NJ; et al)

JAMA 277:1159–1164, 1997 6–13

Introduction.—The most common disease of bone that affects up to 40% of postmenopausal women is osteoporosis, resulting in 1.5 million fractures in the United States each year. Most of the morbidity, mortality, and cost associated with the disease results from nonvertebral fractures, particularly those involving the hip. The rate of bone turnover has been normalized and the bone mineral density has been shown to increase significantly with treatment with alendronate. In postmenopausal women with osteoporosis, the effect of treatment with alendronate sodium, a potent aminobisphosphonate, was evaluated by studying the incidence of nonvertebral fractures.

Methods.—Date of 5 prospective, placebo-controlled, randomized alendronate trials of at least 2 years' duration were reviewed. They included women with osteoporosis who were postmenopausal at least 4 years and ranged in age between 42 and 85 years. The women had lumbar spine bone mineral density that was at least 2.0 SD below the mean for young adult women, as measured using dual-energy x-ray absorptiometry. The women were randomly allocated to treatment with alendronate at a dose higher than 1 mg per day or to placebo for at least 2 years.

Results.—Sixty women had nonvertebral fractures in the placebo group of 590 women during 1,347 patient-years at risk. The overall rate in this group was 4.45 women with fractures per 100 patient-years at risk. There were 73 women of 1,012 in the alendronate group who had nonvertebral fractures during 2,240 patient-years-at risk. Their overall rate was 3.26 women with fractures per 100 patient-years at risk. In the placebo group, after 3 years, the estimated cumulative incidence of nonvertebral fractures was 12.6%, whereas in the alendronate group, it was 9%. At each major site of osteoporotic fracture, including the hip and wrist, and across each of the studies, a reduction in risk with alendronate treatment was consistent.

Conclusion.—Treatment with alendronate reduces the risk of nonvertebral fractures over at least 3 years in postmenopausal women with osteoporosis.

Effect of Three Years of Oral Alendronate Treatment in Postmenopausal Women With Osteoporosis

Tucci JR, for the U.S. Alendronate Phase III Osteoporosis Treatment Study Group (Roger Williams Hosp, Providence, RI; et al)

Am J Med 101:488–501, 1996 6–14

Background.—Oral alendronate sodium specifically inhibits bone resorption mediated by osteoclasts. The efficacy and safety of this potent agent in postmenopausal women with osteoporosis were investigated.

Methods.—Four hundred seventy-eight women were enrolled in the 3-year, randomized, double-blind, multicenter trial. The women received alendronate, 5 or 10 mg/day for 3 years or 20 mg/day for 2 years followed by 5 mg/day for 1 year (20/5), or placebo. In addition, all received 500 mg of supplemental calcium daily.

Findings.—After 3 years of treatment, alendronate, 10 mg, induced substantial increases in bone mineral density (BMD) at the lumbar spine, femoral neck, and trochanter. Bone mineral density at these sites declined in the women receiving placebo. The progressive increases were significant in the second and third years. Alendronate, 10 mg, also increased total body BMD. Although it prevented loss at the one-third forearm site, it did not increase BMD. The efficacy of alendronate 20/5 was not greater than that of the 10 mg dose. Alendronate, 5 mg, was significantly less effective than 10 mg at all sites. Bone turnover declined to a stable nadir during 3 months for resorption markers and during 6 months for formation markers. In alendronate recipients, mean loss of stature was reduced by 41%. Abdominal pain was reported by women given active treatment but was usually mild and resolved with continued treatment.

Conclusions.—Alendronate appears to be an important advance in the treatment of postmenopausal women with osteoporosis. It is a highly effective treatment with a safety profile comparable to that of placebo.

Randomised Trial of Effect of Alendronate on Risk of Fracture in Women With Existing Vertebral Fractures

Black DM, for the Fracture Intervention Trial Research Group (Univ of California San Francisco; et al)

Lancet 348:1535–1541, 1996 6–15

Objective.—Although studies have shown that alendronate reduces the risk of vertebral fracture in women with low bone mineral density (BMD) by increasing BMD, its effect on nonvertebral fractures was not convincingly determined. The double-blind Fracture Intervention Trial was designed to assess the effect of alendronate on vertebral and nonvertebral fractures in postmenopausal women with low BMD and at least 1 vertebral fracture at recruitment.

Methods.—Either placebo (n = 1,005) or 5 mg daily of alendronate (n = 1,022), increased to 10 mg daily at 24 months, was administered to 2,207 postmenopausal women age 55 to 81 for at least 2 years. All the women had a femoral neck BMD of $\leq$ 0.68 g/cm^2 and at least 1 vertebral fracture. None of the women had taken estrogen or calcitonin within the last 6 months. Lateral spine radiographs were obtained at baseline, 24 months, and 36 months. New vertebral and nonvertebral fractures were confirmed radiographically, vertebral height was calculated. Patients were monitored for an average of 2.9 years.

Results.—Compared with placebo, alendronate significantly increased average bone mass and BMD and significantly decreased the risk of new vertebral fractures. Alendronate patients lost significantly less vertebral height in 36 months than the placebo patients did (6.1 mm vs. 9.3 mm). Similar numbers of women in both groups discontinued the medication because of adverse effects. Alendronate patients had significantly fewer hip and wrist fractures than placebo patients did.

Conclusion.—Alendronate significantly reduces the risk of vertebral and nonvertebral fractures in postmenopausal women with low BMD and existing vertebral fractures.

Alendronate Stimulation of Nocturnal Parathyroid Hormone Secretion: A Mechanism to Explain the Continued Improvement in Bone Mineral Density Accompanying Alendronate Therapy

Greenspan SL, Holland S, Maitland-Ramsey L, et al (Harvard Med School, Boston; Beth Israel Hosp, Boston; Merck Research Labs, Rahway, NJ)

Proc Assoc Am Physicians 108:230–238, 1996 6–16

Introduction.—Antiresorptive therapy for osteoporosis seeks to slow or halt bone loss. However, the resultant increase in bone mineral density is usually temporary, with a plateau at 1 year. The antiresorptive agent alendronate permits continued increases in bone mineral density, with steady improvement through the second and third years of treatment. One possible explanation for this effect is an exaggerated nocturnal increase in parathyroid hormone (PTH), acting as an anabolic agent. Diurnal variation in PTH and markers of bone turnover were measured in elderly women taking alendronate or placebo.

Methods.—Thirty-eight elderly women who were participating in a randomized, controlled trial of alendronate for the treatment of femoral osteoporosis were studied. All women had been receiving a stable dose of alendronate (25 patients) or placebo (13 patients) for 12–15 months. During a 24-hour period, blood samples were obtained for measurement of day-night levels and diurnal variation of PTH, serum calcium, ionized calcium, osteocalcin as a marker of bone formation, and N-telopeptide cross-links as a marker of bone resorption.

Results.—After 12 months of treatment, women in the alendronate group had a mean 4.6% increase in bone density in the spine and a 2.7% increase in the femoral neck (compared with a 2.2% increase in the spine and a 0.2% decrease in the femoral neck for the placebo group). The alendronate group had a mean nocturnal PTH level that was 21% higher than in the placebo group (39 pg/mL vs. 32 pg/mL) and a mean nocturnal serum calcium level that was 3% lower (8.7 mb/dL vs. 9.0 mg/dL). There was no significant difference in daytime PTH level. Osteocalcin was 38% lower and N-telopeptide cross-links were 50% lower in the women taking alendronate. Both groups showed significant diurnal variations of PTH, serum calcium, and osteocalcin.

Conclusions.—One year of treatment with alendronate leads to significantly increased bone mineral density and nocturnal PTH levels in postmenopausal women with osteoporosis. These changes occur along with reduced nocturnal serum calcium levels and markers of bone turnover, with preservation of diurnal variation. Bone formation may be stimulated by the nocturnal increase in PTH, consistent with the anabolic effect of low-dose intermittent PTH treatment. This could explain the continued improvement in bone mineral density after more than 1 year of alendronate therapy.

▶ Unfortunately, not everything about the use of alendronate has been positive. Clearly, with the media blitz that has ensued regarding the use of alendronate to treat and prevent postmenopausal osteoporosis, there are increasing numbers of women and men who are prescribed this bisphosphonate. On the one hand this is a good thing, for there is ample evidence demonstrating that this drug will decrease bone loss over time through inhibition of bone resorption while not inhibiting bone formation or mineralization. This leads to clear-cut improvements in bone mineral density as measured by densitometry. However, there has been continued concern that there will be problems with daily use of this drug.

One problem that has arisen, probably because of the nature of the chemical compound itself, is the development of esophageal ulceration and has led to a stringent protocol for prescribed use of the drug (Abstracts 6–17 and 6–18). This drug now needs to be taken on an empty stomach, first thing in the morning with at least 8 oz of water, with the patient remaining either standing or sitting but not lying down for at least 30 minutes. After this the patient may eat, but the patient is still discouraged from lying down. This protocol has been daunting for some patients. In addition, there is some concern specifically within the rheumatology community that the combination of alendronate with classic nonsteroidal anti-inflammatory drug (NSAID) therapy might lead to an epidemic of esophageal lesions. This has not been borne out in large clinical trials as of yet.

L.S. Simon, M.D.

Esophagitis Associated With the Use of Alendronate

de Groen PC, Lubbe DF, Hirsch LJ, et al (Mayo Clinic and Found, Rochester, Minn; Merck Research Labs, Rahway, NJ; Univ of South Florida, Tampa)
N Engl J Med 335:1016–1021, 1996 6–17

Background.—Alendronate, used to treat osteoporosis in postmenopausal women and Paget's disease of the bone, is an aminobisphosphonate and selective inhibitor of osteoclast-mediated bone resorption that can irritate the upper gastrointestinal mucosa. The adverse esophageal effects reported to Merck, the manufacturer of alendronate, were reviewed, and 3 new affected patients described.

Methods and Findings.—A total of 1,213 reports of adverse effects had been received as of March 1996 from among an estimated 475,000 patients given the drug worldwide. In 199 patients, adverse effects were related to the esophagus. In 51 patients, including the 3 current ones, the adverse effects were considered serious or severe. Thirty-two patients needed to be hospitalized, and 2 were temporarily disabled. Endoscopic examinations revealed chemical esophagitis with erosions or ulcerations and exudative inflammation, accompanied by thickening of the esophageal wall. Bleeding was rare. Stomach and duodenal involvement were uncommon. Esophagitis appeared to be associated with swallowing alendronate with little or no water, lying down during or after ingestion, continuing alendronate use after symptom onset, and having pre-existing esophageal disorders.

Conclusions.—In some patients, alendronate can cause chemical esophagitis, including severe ulcerations. The risk of this complication may be reduced by drinking 6–8 oz of water when taking the tablet, taking it in the morning after getting up, remaining upright for at least 30 min afterwards, and stopping medication immediately if esophageal symptoms occur.

A New Probable Increasing Cause of Esophageal Ulceration: Alendronate

Colina RE, Smith M, Kikendall JW, et al (Walter Reed Army Med Ctr, Washington, DC)

Am J Gastroenterol 92:704–706, 1997 6–18

Objective.—The bisphosphonate drug alendronate is used to inhibit bone resorption in postmenopausal women with osteoporosis. Clinical studies have shown low rates of gastrointestinal tract adverse effects. However, there have been increasing reports of esophageal complications, including esophageal ulcers. A patient in whom esophageal ulcerations developed during treatment with alendronate was described.

> *Case.*—Woman, 38, with systemic lupus erythematosus, was taking 10 mg of sodium alendronate for prevention of glucocorticoid-related osteoporosis. She was also taking prednisone, 10 mg daily and azathioprine, 100 mg daily. Two weeks after starting alendronate, she sought medical attention for retrosternal pain and severe odynophagia. Endoscopy of the upper gastrointestinal tract revealed 2 large, deep ulcers at the gastroesophageal junction. Biopsy specimens showed necroinflammatory debris and acute esophagitis, but no organisms. An enzyme-linked immunosorbent assay (ELISA) for HIV was negative. Within 1 week after cessation of alendronate therapy, the patient's symptoms resolved. The ulcers were completely healed on follow-up endoscopy at 1 month.

Discussion.—A broad range of alendronate-induced esophageal injuries has been reported, from mild esophagitis to severe erosive injury and ulcers. Such esophageal complications are likely to become more common as alendronate gains in popularity. These complications may result from taking alendronate with little water, taking it at bedtime, or lying down after taking it.

Infectious Arthritis

Addition of Corticosteroids to Antibiotic Treatment Ameliorates the Course of Experimental *Staphylococcus aureus* Arthritis

Sakiniene E, Bremell T, Tarkowski A (Univ of Gothenburg, Sweden)

Arthritis Rheum 39:1596–1605, 1996 6–19

Objective.—The most common cause of bacterial arthritis is *Staphylococcus aureus*. The disease continues to progress even after bacteria are

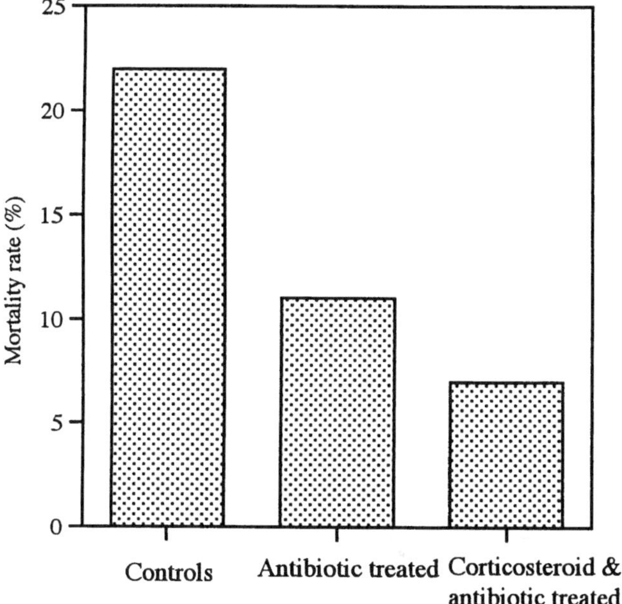

FIGURE 2.—Mortality rate in Swiss mice injected with an arthritogenic dose of *Staphylococcus aureus* strain LS-1 and treated with antibiotics (n = 27), corticosteroids and antibiotics (n = 29), or not treated (controls; n = 27). (Courtesy of Sakiniene E, Bremell T, Tarkowski A: Addition of corticosteroids to antibiotic treatment ameliorates the course of experimental *Staphylococcus aureus* arthritis. *Arthritis Rheum* 39:1596–1605, 1996, copyright American College of Rheumatology.)

eradicated. Because CD4 T lymphocytes have been implicated in the functional damage that occurs even after the infection has been treated, corticosteroids may be effective in treating the disease. The effect of combined antimicrobial and corticosteroid therapy in the management of *S. aureus*–induced arthritis in the mouse was presented.

Methods.—Mice injected with *S. aureus* were evaluated for arthritic symptoms; scored on a 0–3 scale for the appearance of each limb; and treated with cloxacillin (n = 27), cloxacillin and dexamethasone sodium phosphate (n = 29), or not treated (n = 29) on day 3 after infection. Serum and bacterial isolates were examined when the mice were killed on day 14.

Results.—Symptoms of arthritis developed in 70% of mice 3 days after infection. The frequency of arthritis on day 14 was 22% in the cloxacillin-corticosteroid group, 48% in the cloxacillin group, and 81% in the control group. Severity of arthritis and mortality rates were similarly distributed (Fig 2). The incidence of synovitis was lower in the cloxacillin group and significantly lower in the cloxacillin-corticosteroid group (Fig 3). There was a 3-fold decrease in macrophages and a 10-fold decrease in CD4-positive cells in the cloxacillin-corticosteroid group compared with the other 2 groups. Antibiotic treatment significantly decreased polyclonal B cell activation. Serum levels of interferon-γ were decreased by 4-fold in the cloxacillin group and by 15-fold in the cloxacillin-corticosteroid group.

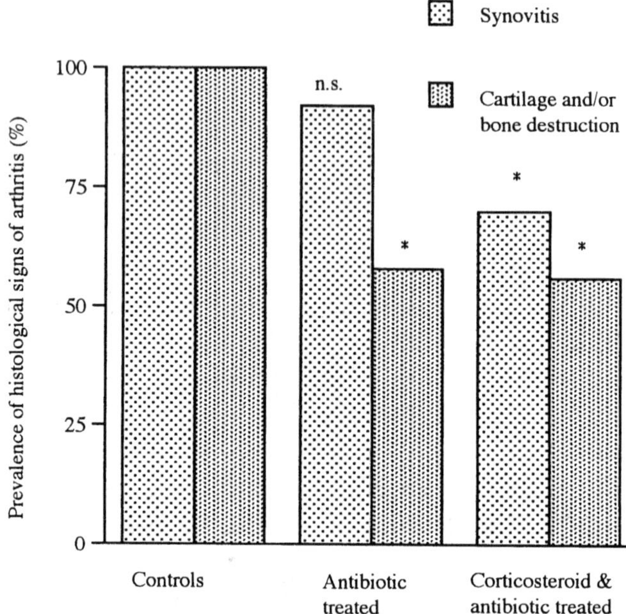

FIGURE 3.—Effect of antibiotic treatment vs. corticosteroid and antibiotic treatment on the frequency of synovitis and cartilage or bone destruction (n = 21–27 mice per group). Histopathologic examination was performed after routine fixation, decalcification, paraffin embedding, and tissue sectioning of joints. The joints were examined by a blinded observer for synovial hypertrophy, defined as synovial membrane thickness of more than 2 cell layers, and cartilage–subchondral bone destruction. $^*P \leq 0.05$ vs. controls. *Abbreviation: n.s.*, not significant. (Courtesy of Sakiniene E, Bremell T, Tarkowski A: Addition of corticosteroids to antibiotic treatment ameliorates the course of experimental *Staphylococcus aureus* arthritis. *Arthritis Rheum* 39:1596–1605, 1996, copyright American College of Rheumatology.)

Serum NO_3^- levels and the number of polymorphonuclear cells were significantly decreased in both treatment groups. Administration of corticosteroids decreased the number of CD4-positive T lymphocytes by 4-fold and immunoglobulin-positive B lymphocytes by 10-fold in naive mice and significantly reduced T-cell proliferation in vitro.

Conclusion.—By decreasing production of T and B lymphocytes, interferon-γ, and macrophages, corticosteroids improve the results of antibiotic treatment of *S. aureus*–induced arthritis.

▶ Provocative. The data were impressive (see Figs 2 and 3). As residents, more than a few years ago, we were taught that steroids mask everything but death. We would never risk using them in a patient with even the possibility of infection. Could our traditional abhorrence to using corticosteroids in patients with infections, based on concerns of compromising protective host immune responses and facilitating infectious complications, be fallacious? These authors argue persuasively for the appropriate clinical trial.

R.S. Panush, M.D.

Tuberculous Tenosynovitis and Bursitis: Imaging Findings in 21 Cases

Jaovisidha S, Chen C, Ryu KN, et al (Veterans Affairs Med Ctr, San Diego, Calif; Univ of California, San Diego; Mahidol Univ, Bangkok, Thailand; et al)

Radiology 201:507–513, 1996 6–20

Background.—Although secondary tuberculous involvement of soft tissue from disease of the bone and joint is well recognized, primary tuberculous tenosynovitis or bursitis is rare. Tuberculous tenosynovitis or bursitis occurs in approximately 1% of patients with osteoarticular tuberculosis. The imaging features of this condition were described.

Methods.—Participating in the study were 21 patients with surgically and/or pathologically confirmed tuberculosis of the tendon sheaths (12) or bursae (9). They received various combinations of routine radiography, arthrography, CT, and MRI.

Results.—Bursitis occurred most often around the hip, particularly in the trochanteric bursa. Tenosynovitis was found most commonly in the hand and wrist. Plain radiography revealed soft-tissue swelling in all patients; 3 of 9 patients also showed calcification. Hygromatous, serofibrinous, and fungoid forms of tuberculous tenosynovitis were evident with CT and MRI. These imaging techniques revealed 2 patterns of bursitis: distended bursae or multiple small abscesses. Communication between the affected structures could be delineated in many cases by contrast material–enhanced radiography.

Conclusions.—Complementary information is provided by the different imaging methods, and MRI provides the best evaluation of lesion extent, which is a task that was previously an indication for surgery.

▶ Twenty-one cases of tuberculous bursitis and tenosynovitis represent an impressive series. Although the imaging findings are of interest, this diagnosis should be made on clinical and microbiological observations. The incidence of tuberculosis has increased during the past decade. Tuberculosis should be considered in the evaluation of certain musculoskeletal symptoms; we have seen this diagnosis overlooked. My colleagues, Drs. Neil Kramer and Elliot Rosenstein, have presented a nice review of rheumatologic manifestations of tuberculosis.[1]

R.S. Panush, M.D.

Reference

1. Kramer N, Rosenstein ED: Rheumatologic manifestations of tuberculosis. *Bull Rheum* 46:5–8, 1997.

Lyme Disease

▶ Abstracts 6–21 through 6–26 illumine several aspects of Lyme disease. Diagnosis may be facilitated by PCR amplification of *B. burgdorferi* DNA, and synovial tissue was a richer source of material than synovial fluid. Patients with EM may have fewer and less prominent systemic symptoms than thought; elevated erythrocyte sedimentation rate (24%), tender joints (8%), swollen joints (1%), and myopathy (12%) were not common. Some patients seem to experience subjective and often vague systemic, musculoskeletal, and neurocognitive symptoms after adequate therapy; it is not clear what this represents or how to manage it. Some patients (approximately 10%) with Lyme disease will have concomitant babesiosis; because their symptoms may be more severe than with either illness alone, this possibility should be considered in moderate to severe Lyme disease. Amoxicillin (500 mg 3 times a day for 20 days) was effective for EM, and better than azithromycin. And there may be more to infectious arthritis than infection alone; the beneficial effect of anti-IL-12 on murine Lyme arthritis (and benefit of steroids for experimental infectious arthritis, see Abstract 6–19) suggest an important role of immune responses in contributing to symptoms. This could be blocked by selective (nonantimicrobial) interventions.

R.S. Panush, M.D.

Detection of *Borrelia burgdorferi* by DNA Amplification in Synovial Tissue Samples From Patients With Lyme Arthritis

Jaulhac B, Chary-Valckenaere I, Sibilia J, et al (Université Louis Pasteur, Strasbourg, France; Universitaire de Nancy, France; Hôpitaux Universitaires de Strasbourg, France)

Arthritis Rheum 39:736–745, 1996 6–21

Objective.—*Borrelia burgdorferi*, the cause of Lyme arthritis, is difficult to culture from synovial tissue. A direct diagnostic method is needed to improve the ability to detect this disease. A new polymerase chain reaction (PCR) assay for detection of *B. burgdorferi* chromosomal DNA in synovial tissue (ST) was used to compare the frequency of detection of *B. burgdorferi* chromosomal DNA in ST and synovial fluid (SF) in a prospective study of consecutive patients with Lyme arthritis.

Methods.—A PCR assay was done on DNA extracted from synovial samples obtained between February 1992 and October 1994 from 12 patients with Lyme arthritis and from 29 controls with various rheumatic diseases. The PCR products were subjected to Southern blot hybridization, and the lowest detection threshold for the amplification method was determined. Results of PCR in SF and ST were analyzed statistically.

Results.—No DNA amplification was seen in control samples. *Borrelia burgdorferi* was detected in 5 SF and 10 ST samples from the 12 patients with Lyme arthritis, but all patients had at least 1 positive result.

Conclusion.—The DNA amplification method detected chromosomal *B. burgdorferi* in all patients with Lyme arthritis but appears to be more sensitive in ST samples than in SF samples.

The Clinical Spectrum of Early Lyme Borreliosis in Patients With Culture-Confirmed Erythema Migrans

Nadelman RB, Nowakowski J, Forseter G, et al (New York Med College; Westchester County Med Ctr, Valhalla, NY)

Am J Med 100:502–508, 1996 6–22

Objective.—Erythema migrans (EM) is reported to occur in 63% of cases of Lyme borreliosis, although there are few cases of microbiological corroboration. *Borrelia burgdorferi* was isolated systematically from patients with EM, and results of a prospective study to characterize the clinical manifestations of these patients were reported.

Methods.—A skin biopsy sample or needle aspirate and a blood sample were obtained from inside the advancing margin of the primary EM in 79 patients (30 females) aged 16–76 years, attending the Lyme Disease Diagnostic Center of the Westchester County Medical Center in Westchester, New York, between June 1991 and September 1993. Specimens were cultured for *B. burgdorferi*. The relationship between EM duration and diameter of EM lesion was statistically analyzed.

Results.—Seventeen patients had several positive cultures, but only 8 blood cultures were positive for *B. burgdorferi*. Duration of EM was significantly related to the lesion diameter. Lesions were mildly pruritic in 39% of patients and mildly tender in 32%. Fourteen patients had several lesions. Symptoms were mild or nonexistent in 32%. The remaining patients most commonly experienced fatigue (54%), arthralgia (44%), myalgia (44%), headache (42%), fever or chills (39%), stiff neck (35%), and anorexia (26%). When examined patients had localized (23%) or generalized (6%) lymphadenopathy, fever (16%), and pain (9%). Abnormal hematologic results were rare, and muscle damage (as determined by creatine phosphokinase levels) was uncommon and not associated with myalgia. More than one third of patients had abnormal liver function. At the initial visit, 34% were seropositive, but by 1 month 88% were seropositive and had formed antibodies to *B. burgdorferi*. The patients in this study appeared less sick than previous EM populations.

Conclusion.—The ability to isolate *B. burgdorferi* from EM lesions should make it easy to confirm the clinical features of these patients, as associated with Lyme borreliosis, and to select the appropriate therapy.

Clinical and Neurocognitive Features of the Post Lyme Syndrome

Bujak DI, Weinstein A, Dornbush RL (New York Med College, Valhalla)

J Rheumatol 23:1392–1397, 1996 6–23

Objective.—Some patients with Lyme disease have persistent arthralgia, fatigue, and subjective memory loss despite antibiotic treatment. Whether symptoms represent chronic, residual, or function damage is unknown. Patients with post-Lyme syndrome (PLS) were compared with control patients who recovered from Lyme disease in a study that assessed clinical and emotional status by neurocognitive and psychological testing, any predisposing features, and the extent to which these patients fulfill the criteria for fibromyalgia (FM) or chronic fatigue syndrome.

Methods.—The clinical, neurocognitive, and psychological attributes and demographic and treatment data for 23 patients with PLS (65% female), aged 25–60 years, were compared statistically with information from 23 matched controls.

Results.—Time since onset of disease was 5 years for the PLS group and 6 years for the control group. Similar number of patients in each group were seropositive at follow-up. Patients with PLS tended to receive treatment later than control patients. Post-Lyme Syndrome began during initial antibiotic therapy in 44% of patients. Symptoms did not respond to antibiotic therapy. Seven patients with PLS had fibromyalgia, 3 had chronic fatigue syndrome, and 10 had symptoms of both but met insufficient criteria to be classified. Patients with PLS scored significantly lower than control patients on attention and concentration neurocognitive tests and in psychological tests for somatization, obsessive–compulsive behavior, depression, anxiety, hostility, general severity, and total positive symptoms. Patients with PLS also had significantly higher hysteria and hypochondriasis scores. Logical regression analysis showed that fatigue (49.7-fold increase) and arthralgia (31.8-fold increase) at onset were significant independent predictors of development of PLS.

Conclusion.—Patients with Lyme disease that subsequently exhibited PLS have a higher frequency of myalgia, arthralgia, fatigue, and Lyme arthritis. These patients show significantly lower scores in attention and concentration, and many have fibromyalgia or chronic fatigue syndrome.

Concurrent Lyme Disease and Babesiosis

Krause PJ, Telford SR III, Spielman A, et al (Univ of Connecticut, Farmington; Harvard School of Public Health, Boston; Tufts Univ, Boston; et al)
JAMA 275:1657–1660, 1996 6–24

Introduction.—Despite the naturally close associations between the pathogens responsible for human babesiosis and Lyme disease, only 3 episodes of coinfections have been reported in detail. The illness was severe in these patients, and 1 died. A clinic-based cohort study sought to determine whether coinfection by the agents of human babesiosis and Lyme disease would cause more severe disease than the sum of symptoms associated with either infection alone.

Methods.—Epidemiologic information was obtained from a small island community in Rhode Island and from 2 medical clinics in Connecticut. Residents in these areas are frequently exposed to the agents of Lyme disease or human babesiosis. All cases of the diseases were sought for the months of May through September from 1990 to 1994 in Block Island and from 1992 to 1994 in southeastern Connecticut. Case findings were analyzed and the results of laboratory assays reviewed for the study.

Results.—Ninety-seven (8.4%) of 1,156 serosurvey subjects were seroreactive against Lyme disease spirochete antigen and 14 (14%) were concurrently seroreactive against babesial antigen. Twenty-six (11%) of 240 patients with Lyme disease were coinfected with babesiosis. Certain symptoms were more frequent in coinfected patients than in those with Lyme disease alone. These symptoms included fatigue, headache, sweats and chills, nausea, and splenomegaly. Among patients for whom follow-up was available, symptoms continued for 3 months or longer in 13 (50%) coinfected patients vs. 7 (4%) patients with Lyme disease alone. Compared with babesial infection alone, coinfection with Lyme disease was associated with more symptoms and a more persistent episode of illness. Circulating spirochetial DNA was detected in 3 (27%) of 11 coinfected patients, 6 (5%) of 81 with Lyme disease alone, and in none of the 7 patients with babesiosis alone.

Conclusion.—Human coinfection with the agents of Lyme disease and human babesiosis is relatively common, and the symptoms that characterize both infections tend to be exacerbated in coinfected patients. In areas where both diseases have been reported, concomitant babesial infection should be considered in patients with a diagnosis of moderate to severe Lyme disease.

Azithromycin Compared With Amoxicillin in the Treatment of Erythema Migrans

Luft BJ, Dattwyler RJ, Johnson RC, et al (State Univ of New York, Stony Brook; Univ of Minnesota, Minneapolis; Kaiser Permanente, Rocky Hill, Conn; et al)
Ann Intern Med 124:785–791, 1996 6–25

Background.—Both amoxicillin and azithromycin have shown excellent activity against *Borrelia burgdorferi* in open trials. To assess the relative efficacy of the 2 agents, relief of the acute manifestations and their sequelae were compared in patients with erythema migrans treated with either a 20-day course of amoxicillin or a 7-day course of azithromycin in a large, multicenter, double-blind, randomized trial.

Methods.—Adult patients with erythema migrans were stratified by the presence or absence of flulike constititutional symptoms, then randomly assigned to treatment with either azithromycin, 500 mg once daily for 7 days, or amoxicillin, 500 mg 3 times daily for 20 days. The azithromycin group was given placebo twice daily for 7 days, then 3 times daily for the next 13 days. The patients were examined at baseline and 8, 20, 30, 90, and 180 days after treatment began. Their response was assessed by evaluating clearance of erythema migrans and relief of symptoms. Blood samples were obtained during examinations for serologic testing for *B. burgdorferi.*

Results.—Of the 217 assessable patients on day 20, a complete response was achieved by 88% of the amoxicillin group vs. 76% of the azithromycin group. All the patients treated with amoxicillin had at least a partial response within the first 20 days, whereas 3 patients treated with azithromycin had no response or worsened in the first 20 days. A complete response in the azithromycin group was more common among seropositive than seronegative patients. Relapse within 6 months occurred in 16% of the azithromycin group and only 4% of the amoxicillin group. Relapse was significantly predicted by a partial response. Adverse events occurred in 35% of the azithromycin group and 24% of the amoxicillin group.

Conclusion.—Amoxicillin was significantly more effective than azithromycin in obtaining complete resolution of erythema migrans and preventing relapse within 6 months. Further study is needed to determine the long-term efficacy of these treatments. The relationship between complete response to azithromycin therapy and humoral response to *B. burgdorferi* suggests that an early immune response may help limit early disease or that there is a synergistic association between humoral response and azithromycin.

Effect of Anti-Interleukin 12 Treatment on Murine Lyme Borreliosis

Anguita J, Persing DH, Rincón M, et al (Yale Univ, New Haven, Conn; Mayo Clinic and Found, Rochester, Minn)

J Clin Invest 97:1028–1034, 1996 6–26

Objective.—The degree of Lyme arthritis has been correlated to the production of interleukin (IL)-4 and interferon (IFN)γ in mice infected with *Borrelia burgdorferi.* Because IL-12 is an inflammation and immune response modulator, it has been postulated that using anti-IL-12 neutralizing antibodies might influence the chronic effects of Lyme disease in mice. The evolution of Lyme borreliosis in C3H mice treated with this antibody was studied.

Methods.—Hearts and joints of C3H/HeN control and treated (with anti-IL-12 monoclonal antibody [mAb]) mice infected with *B. burgdorferi* were examined microscopically, spirochetes in ear tissue were quantitated by polymerase chain reaction, T-cell restimulation was studied, and cytokine production was quantitated. Development of arthritis was assessed at 14 days (acute inflammation) and at 60 days (resolution phase).

Results.—Production of serum IgG2a and IFN-γ decreased in mice treated with anti-IL-12 mAb. No IL-4 production was detected. Antibody treatment did not affect in vivo activation of $CD4^+$ T cells, and IgG1 and IgG2b levels did not increase. More spirochetes were found in the ears of anti-IL-12 mAb-treated mice than in the ears of control mice. At day 14, anti-IL-12 mAb-treated mice had significantly less arthritis in knees and tibiotarsus than control mice. Arthritis results were similar in both groups at day 60. No differences in carditis results were observed between groups at either time point.

Conclusion.—The severity of acute but not resolution-phase arthritis is decreased in *B. burgdorferi*-infected C3H mice treated with anti-IL-12 mAb, suggesting a decrease in Th1 response. Th2 response does not appear to be affected.

Apoptosis of Fas^{high} CD4^{+} Synovial T Cells by *Borrelia*-reactive Fas-ligand^{high} $\gamma\delta$ T Cells in Lyme Arthritis

Vicent MS, Roessner K, Lynch D, et al (Univ of Vermont, Burlington; Immunex Corp, Seattle; Univ of Lausanne, Switzerland; et al)

J Exp Med 184:2109–2117, 1996 6–27

Purpose.—There is a minor subset of T lymphocytes expressing alternate γ and δ chains. The function of these $\gamma\delta$ T cells is unknown, but they occur at increased proportions at epithelial barriers, during certain infections, and at sites of chronic inflammation. Some of these T cells react to microbial products, but there is little evidence showing their responsiveness to a bacterial antigen from a naturally occurring human infection. Responsiveness of $\gamma\delta$ T cells in Lyme arthritis to *Borrelia burgdorferi* is reported.

Methods.—Studies were performed in patients with Lyme arthritis from areas endemic for Lyme disease. Studies were performed on lymphocytes isolated from the peripheral blood or synovial fluid.

Findings.—The synovial fluid lymphocytes were found to contain a large proportion of $\gamma\delta$ cells, most of which were of the Vδ1 subset. These cells showed vigorous proliferation in response to stimulation with *B. burgdorferi*, the causative spirochete of Lyme arthritis. In culture, the absolute number of CD4^{+} cells showed little change or decreased, while the number of $\gamma\delta$ cells increased to as much as 50% of the cultured synovial lymphocytes. Synovial T cell clones were found to express persistently high levels of the ligand for Fas (APO-1, CD95), compared with $\alpha\beta$ T cells. Also, the synovial $\gamma\delta$ cells induced apoptosis of Fas^{high} CD4^{+} synovial lymphocytes, in a Fas-dependent manner. A nonlytic anti-Fas antibody inhibited Jurkat cell cytolysis by $\gamma\delta$ clones.

Conclusions.—Synovial fluid $\gamma\delta$ cells from patients with Lyme arthritis show a response to *B. burgdorferi*. Experimental findings suggest that $\gamma\delta$ cells play a role in the defense against infections in humans. They also appear to play an immunoregulatory function at inflammatory sites via Fas-mediated apoptosis.

▶ These elegant studies suggest that the $\gamma\delta$ subset of T cells can be activated by antigen (in this case by *Borrelia burgdorferi*) and induce apoptosis of CD4^{+} synovial T cells expressing the Fas antigen; this process may pertain to host defense against infections as well as immunoregulatory and inflammatory events. Another recent study examined RA synovial cells and did not find a high frequency of apoptosis.[1] (Apoptosis, I have learned, is pronounced "Ay-paw-TOE-sis."[2]) Study of possible perturbations of mechanisms regulating programmed cell death in rheumatic diseases is burgeoning as we attempt to understand processes such as synovial cell hyperplasia in

RA, effects of antirheumatic drugs, fibroblast biology in scleroma, T and B cell function in lupus (and other rheumatic diseases), and lymphoproliferation in Sjögren's syndrome, among others.[2, 3, 4]

R.S. Panush, M.D.

References

1. Sugiyama M, Tsukazaki T, Yonekura A, et al: Localisation of apoptosis and expression of apoptosis related proteins in the synovium of patients with rheumatoid arthritis. *Ann Rheum Dis* 55:442–449, 1996.
2. Kuska B: You say tomato and I say tomahto: Getting a handle on pronouncing apoptosis. *J Natal Cancer Inst* 89:351, 1997.
3. Mountz JD, Wu J, Cheng J, et al: Autoimmune disease: A problem of defective apoptosis. *Arthritis Rheum* 10:1415–1420, 1994.
4. Talal N: Oncogenes, autogenes, and rheumatic diseases. *Arthritis Rheum* 37:1421–1422, 1994.

Borrelia burgdorferi DNA Is Undetectable by Polymerase Chain Reaction in Skin Lesions of Morphea, Scleroderma, or Lichen Sclerosus et Atrophicus of Patients From North America

Dillon WI, Saed GM, Fivenson DP (Henry Ford Health Sciences Ctr, Detroit)
J Am Acad Dermatol 33:617–620, 1995 6–28

Introduction.—It is not certain whether *Borrelia burgdorferi* infection is directly associated with morphea and lichen sclerosus et atrophicus (LSA). Polymerase chain reaction (PCR) was used to determine whether *B. burgdorferi* was present in archival tissue specimens from the involved skin of 20 North American patients with morphea, 10 with LSA, and 4 with scleroderma.

Methods.—Paraffin-embedded tissue blocks were obtained from lesional skin and DNA was extracted. Four sets of PCR primers were used for PCR amplification. One set of PCR primers was used for the *B. burgdorferi* flagellin gene, one was specific for European strains of *B. burgdorferi*, and another was common to both the European and American strains. Nested PCR primers were used to further amplify a subset of samples.

Results.—With the use of routine and nested PCR, *B. burgodorferi* DNA was absent in the archival skin lesions from the 20 North American patients with morphea, the 10 patients with LSA, and the 4 patients with scleroderma.

Summary.—The findings strongly suggest that there is no association of the *B. burgdorferi* spirochete with the pathophysiology of skin disease in North American patients, and they also support other reports indicating that there are varying forms of the *B. burgdorferi* strain in North America and Europe.

▶ Treatment for scleroderma, morphea, and LSA remains symptomatic and inconclusive. Thus, any hint of curative therapy is widely acclaimed, as was the identification of *Borrelia burgdorferi* in morphea lesions from European patients. This report that there is *no* evidence for spirochetal infection in these diseases is reassuring, and with negative reports also from Finland, the Netherlands, and Germany, the proclivity of European physicians to treat these diseases with IV high-dose penicillin can be questioned. Certainly such treatment is not indicated in North America.

E.C. LeRoy, M.D.

7 Regional Pain Syndromes, Non-Articular Musculoskeletal Disorders, Fibromyalgia, and Miscellaneous Topics

Introduction

These entities comprise much of office medicine and rheumatology. They are important—so much so that I've given them their own chapter in this YEAR BOOK. And included on our editorial board is a member with well-known expertise in this area, Nortin Hadler. These disorders, however, still don't have the cachet of lupus or vasculitis, and there aren't too many R01s awarded to study the molecular biology of lateral epicondylitis, so the literature is sparse and new insights few.

Richard S. Punush, M.D.

Regional Pain Syndromes and Non-Articular Musculoskeletal Disorders

Musculoskeletal Problems Among VDU Workers in a Hong Kong Bank

Yu ITS, Wong TW (Chinese Univ of Hong Kong)

Occup Med 46:275–280, 1996 7–1

Background.—A high prevalence of musculoskeletal complaints has been associated with visual display unit (VDU) work in many countries. Although VDU use is widespread in Hong Kong, no one has studied musculoskeletal discomfort among workers there. Musculoskeletal problems among VDU workers in a Hong Kong bank were investigated.

Methods and Findings.—One hundred fifty-one workers in 6 departments where VDUs were used completed a self-administered questionnaire. Thirty-one percent reported problems in the neck, 30.6% in the back, 16.5% in the shoulder, 14.9% in the hand and wrist, and 6.6% in the arm. Compared with infrequent VDU users, frequent users had significantly more musculoskeletal problems in the neck and shoulder areas. Individual musculoskeletal complaints were associated with personal factors, working posture, repetitive movements, and work station design. Problems with the back, neck, and shoulders were more strongly associated with unfavorable working postures. Repetitive movements more greatly affected the arm, hand, and wrist. Some musculoskeletal risk factors were related specifically to the nature or design of VDU work (Fig 1).

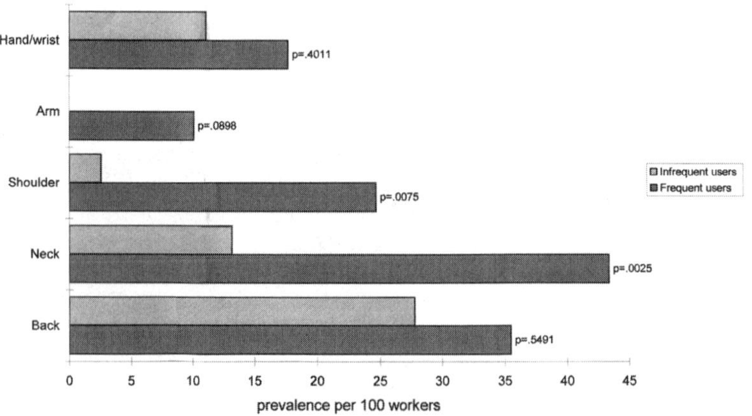

FIGURE 1.—Musculoskeletal problems among visual display unit (VDU) workers. The prevalence of musculoskeletal complaints among frequent VDU users and infrequent VDU users are shown for comparison. The *P*-values are from chi square tests comparing the prevalence among the frequent users and infrequent users for individual complaints. (Courtesy of Yu ITS, Wong TW: Musculoskeletal problems among VDU workers in a Hong Kong bank. *Occup Med* 46:275–280, 1996. Courtesy of Rapid Science Publishers, Ltd.)

Conclusion.—Musculoskeletal problems were common in this group of Hong Kong bank workers. Eliminating the identified work-related risk factors should improve the health of VDU users.

▶ Office workers, as well as factory workers, are prone to occupational symptoms and complaints when they are engaged in activities that call for concentration in a fixed body posture, especially when that posture is not a natural one. Automation and the computer age increase the physical immobility of modern office work, especially in banks where data management is paramount. This study shows the association between immobility (frequent use of VDUs) and back, neck, and shoulder, arm, hand, or wrist complaints among frequent and intense users of VDUs. Unfavorable work posture was also a factor. Ergonomics, posture training, and work-time organization were proposed as, but were not demonstrated to be, solutions.

E.C. LeRoy, M.D.

Conservative Management of Mechanical Neck Pain: Systematic Overview and Meta-analysis

Aker PD, Gross AR, Goldsmith CH, et al (Canadian Mem Chiropractic College, Toronto; McMaster Univ, Hamilton, Ont; Univ of Saskatchewan, Sask)

BMJ 313:1291–1296, 1996 7–2

Background.—Neck pain is a common symptom. Although many conservative treatments are available, there is little documentation of their relative efficacy. A systematic overview and meta-analysis of published and unpublished studies of conservative treatment for mechanical neck pain were presented.

Methods.—Studies were identified through computerized and manual searches of bibliographic databases; reference lists from primary articles; and letters to authors, agencies, foundations, and content experts. Effect sizes were determined from raw pain scores and combined using meta-analytic techniques.

Findings.—Twenty-four randomized clinical trials met selection criteria. Nine involved manual treatments; 12, physical medicine methods; 4, drug treatments; and 3, patient education. Data from 5 of the 9 trials using manual treatment could be combined. The pooled effect size 1–4 weeks after treatment was −0.6, equivalent to an improvement of 16 on a 100-point scale. Pooled estimates of effect could not be established for other interventions.

Conclusion.—There is little evidence from clinical trials to support many of the conservative treatments currently used for mechanical neck pain. In general, such treatments have not been studied thoroughly enough to determine their efficacy.

▶ This is another of those papers that are disturbing, but not surprising. We do not know how to manage neck pain. Or, at least, we do not have evidence-based data to confidently support current approaches, not unlike back pain.[1–4] Rheumatology now has an important opportunity to take a leadership role in identifying the proper approaches to these and other "non-articular" and regional musculoskeletal disorders.

R.S. Panush, M.D.

References

1. 1997 Year Book of Rheumatology, pp 292–296.
2. 1996 Year Book of Rheumatology, pp 2–7.
3. 1995 Year Book of Rheumatology, pp 239–241.
4. 1994 Year Book of Rheumatology, pp 256–258.

Trochanteric Bursitis (Greater Trochanter Pain Syndrome)

Shbeeb MI, Matteson EL (Mayo Clinic, Rochester, Minn)
Mayo Clin Proc 71:565–569, 1996 7–3

Description.—One of the most common regional pain syndromes is that of greater trochanteric pain. Although commonly referred to as "trochanteric bursitis," local heat, redness, and swelling are generally not present. The syndrome is characterized by chronic, intermittent aching pain over the lateral aspect of the hip, and it can affect any age group, although it is more common in those aged 40–60 years. Women are more commonly affected than men.

Pathogenesis.—The syndrome appears related to trauma, and in some cases it may be related to repetitive microtrauma caused by the active use of the muscles inserting on the greater trochanter with subsequent degenerative changes. Calcification in the region may be observed; bursal inflammation associated with calcified tendons is probably secondary.

Clinical Aspects.—The syndrome may be chronic or subacute; in the latter case, pain may be sharp and intense. Pain increases with certain hip movements and may be triggered by prolonged standing or lying on the affected side. In virtually all symptomatic patients, localized tenderness can be elicited over the greater trochanter. The junction of the upper thigh and greater trochanter is the area of maximal tenderness. The syndrome may be distinguished from intra-articular hip disease by the absence of pain on flexion and extension of the hip. Arthritis may be the underlying cause of pain if hip range of motion is affected. Associated conditions such as lumbar spondylosis or hip arthritis may be present. Radiographic findings are not necessarily diagnostic; clinical criteria for diagnosis have been developed but not validated.

Treatment.—The syndrome causes pain and can result in limitation of function. Various treatment modalities including local glucocorticoid injection, nonsteroidal anti-inflammatory drugs, and physical therapy have been used, but no controlled studies have compared their efficacies. The authors conducted an open observational trial in which 60% of patients treated with local injection of glucocorticoids and local analgesics reported relief of pain after a single injection.

Conclusions.—The syndrome of greater trochanteric pain is probably underdiagnosed but can be treated. When treatment and correction of possible underlying causes is not successful, patients should undergo further diagnostic assessment.

▶ This is a state-of-the-art review from the Mayo Clinic. The take-home message is that the state-of-the-art is a throwback to midcentury. There are plenty of individuals, otherwise well, who experience—and some who complain of—regional musculoskeletal pain that is aching, mechanical, and poorly localized to the anterolateral buttock. They don't have intra-articular hip disease and they don't qualify for other labels, many of which are comparable examples of orthopedic nosologic flotsam and jetsam. The diagnosis usually reflects that they do not like being poked in the buttock, particularly in spots that are posterior and superior to most bursal structures about the hip. Why label it "bursitis"? Why poke? Why inject? There are no systematic studies of the specificity of the poking or the effectiveness of injecting the site that hurts. The published observations are quite varied. It is time to place periarticular mechanical hip pain under scientific scrutiny.

N.M. Hadler, M.D.

Prognostic Value of a Hand Symptom Diagram in Surgery for Carpal Tunnel Syndrome

Bessette L, Keller RB, Lew RA, et al (Harvard Med School, Boston; Maine Med Assessment Found and Maine Health Information Ctr, Augusta)
J Rheumatol 24:726–734, 1997 7–4

Introduction.—Patients receiving benefits for carpal tunnel syndrome (CTS) under Worker's Compensation have markedly worse outcomes than other patients. It would be helpful to have reliable, simple, and inexpensive tools for prognostic stratification so that selection of optimal treatment could be improved. A hand-symptom diagram was prospectively evaluated for its ability to predict outcomes in patients undergoing surgery for CTS.

Methods.—Two-hundred two patients with CTS completed a hand-symptom diagram before and 6 months after surgery. Three symptoms were evaluated separately for each of 6 regions: pain, numbness/tingling (NT), and "other" symptoms. At 6-month follow-up, outcome was expressed as the percentage of change on the Symptom Severity Scale and Function Status Scale of the Carpal Tunnel Syndrome Assessment Questionnaire as well as patient satisfaction with the result of surgery. Thirty-seven percent of patients were receiving Worker's Compensation.

Results.—Hand-symptom drawing patterns significantly associated with greater symptom or functional improvement or more satisfaction with surgery included pain of 2 or more of the first 4 fingers, NT in finger 2, 3, and 4, "other" symptoms involving the dorsal surface of the fingers, pain of the upper palm, and pain of the lower or upper arm. Hand-symptom drawings not associated with less symptom or functional improvement or less satisfaction included NT involving the dorsum of the hand and/or wrist and NT of the arm. Hand symptom variables accounted for total explained variance in 30% of satisfaction, 14% of symptom severity, and 24% of functional status. Patients who received Worker's Compensation had more wrist pain and NT of the arm, less pain involving the arm and upper palm, worse outcomes, and less satisfaction with surgery. Drawing expansion was correlated with a low score on the short form-36 mental health subscale. Psychological impairment was not associated with poorer outcome.

Conclusion.—Symptom drawing pattern variables in patients with CTS could predict symptom and functional improvement and satisfaction 6 months after surgery.

▶ Having patients describe their experiences by drawing the distribution and quality of symptoms has been used in musculoskeletal disorders for over 20 years. This can aid diagnosis and prognosis. For example, in diagnosing back pain in patients, it can sort out patients with psychological overlap, fibromyalgia, and lumbar radiculopathy. This study uses elegant statistical methods to identify 3 pain syndromes in patients with CTS and attempts to correlate them with various outcomes. This study was done in a group of patients from Maine. It would be interesting to see whether these pain patterns are prognostically important in other populations.

M.H. Liang, M.D., M.P.H.

Fibromyalgia

Increased Rates of Fibromyalgia Following Cervical Spine Injury: A Controlled Study of 161 Cases of Traumatic Injury

Buskila D, Neumann L, Vaisberg G, et al (Soroka Med Ctr, Beer Sheva, Israel; Ben-Gurion Univ of the Negev, Beer Sheva, Israel; Univ of Kansas, Wichita; et al)

Arthritis Rheum 40:446–452, 1997 7–5

Introduction.—Evidence is insufficient to determine a causal relationship between trauma and fibromyalgia syndrome (FMS). It is possible that biomechanical disturbances in the cervical spine are important in the pathogenesis of FMS. The incidence of FMS was compared in 102 patients with neck injury and 59 patients with leg fracture (controls) attending the only regional occupational clinic in the southern part of Israel.

Methods.—Patients and controls were examined for nonarticular tenderness and the presence of FMS. Tender points were assessed by thumb palpation and tenderness thresholds were determined by dolorimetry at 9 tender sites. Patients were interviewed and Visual Analogue Scales were used to assess presence and severity of neck and FMS-related symptoms. Physical functioning and quality of life were assessed by questionnaire.

TABLE 2.—Prevalence and Severity of Symptoms in Patients With Neck Injuries and in Patients with Leg Fractures*

Symptom	Neck injuries (n = 102)	Leg fractures (n = 59)	*P*
Poor concentration	12 (12)	0 (0)	0.004
Blurred vision	13 (13)	0 (0)	0.004
Dizziness	67 (66)	0 (0)	0.001
Forgetfulness	6 (6)	0 (0)	0.231
Fatigue†	2.0 (2.7)	0.6 (1.6)	0.002
Anxiety†	0.6 (1.6)	0.1 (0.6)	0.030
Depression†	1.6 (3.0)	0.6 (1.6)	0.010
Pain†	1.7 (2.7)	0.6 (1.5)	0.004
Morning stiffness†	1.9 (2.5)	0.4 (1.4)	0.001
Global well-being†	1.9 (2.7)	0.8 (1.9)	0.007
Sleep disturbance	26 (25)	4 (7)	0.010
Headache	31 (30)	6 (10)	0.003
Paresthesias	27 (26)	6 (10)	0.010
Subjective joint swelling	17 (17)	3 (5)	0.030
IBS	4 (4)	1 (2)	0.653

*Except where otherwise indicated, values are the number (%) of patients. Symptoms were assessed 6 to 18 months after the trauma.

†Values are the mean (standard deviation) score on a scale of 0–10, where 10 = worst condition.

Abbreviation: IBS, irritable bowel syndrome.

(Courtesy of Buskila D, Neumann L, Vaisberg G, et al: Increased rates of fibromyalgia following cervical spine injury: A controlled study of 161 cases of traumatic injury. *Arthritis Rheum* 40:446–452, 1997, copyright American College of Rheumatology.)

The 1990 American College of Rheumatology criteria were used to determine diagnosis of FMS.

Results.—No patients had a diagnosis of chronic pain syndrome before trauma. After injury, 21.6% of patients with neck injury and 1.7% of controls with lower leg injuries received a diagnosis of FMS (a significant difference). Almost all symptoms were significantly more common and severe in patients with neck injuries, compared with controls (Table 2). Fibromyalgia syndrome was detected a mean of 3.2 months after injury. Patients with neck injuries and FMS had more tenderness, severe and prevalent FMS-related symptoms, lower quality of life, and impaired physical functioning than patients with neck injuries and no FMS. All patients were employed at the time of evaluation. Twenty of 102 patients with neck injuries and 24% of patients with leg fractures filed an insurance claim with the National Insurance Plan of Israel. There was no association between tendency to file a claim and presence of FMS, increased FMS symptoms, pain, or impaired functioning.

Conclusions.—Patients with neck injuries experienced FMS 13 times more frequently than those with lower extremity injury. All patients remained employed and insurance claims were not increased in patients with FMS in this cohort of Israeli workers.

▶ This study of Israeli workers with FMS points out that neck injury is 13 times more likely to lead to FMS than lower-extremity injury. In addition, in Israel very few with FMS receive disability benefits, and all in this study returned to work, which is food for thought in these litigious United States of America.

E.C. LeRoy, M.D.

Orthostatic Sympathetic Derangement in Subjects With Fibromyalgia

Martínez-Lavín M, Hermosillo AG, Mendoza C, et al (Instituto Nacional de Cardiología Ignacio Chávez, Mexico City; Hosp Gea González, Mexico City; Hosp Español, Mexico City)

J Rheumatol 24:714–718, 1997 7–6

Introduction.—It is possible that the cluster of symptoms observed with fibromyalgia (FM) may be explained by autonomic dysfunction. Modulation of the autonomic nervous system was evaluated by power of spectral analysis of heart rate in patients with FM to determine the response of the sympathetic-parasympathetic limbs to active orthostatic stress.

Methods.—Nineteen women with FM and 19 age-matched normal controls underwent high resolution electrocardiography in supine and standing positions after achieving a stable heart rate. The fast Fourier transform algorithm was used to determine spectral analysis of R-R intervals.

Results.—Analysis of the frequency domain revealed a significant difference between patients with FM and controls in the power spectral density of the low frequency band. Normal controls had an increased power spectral density when standing, compared with a discordant response observed in patients with FM.

Conclusion.—Patients with FM had an impaired sympathetic surge in response to orthostatic stress as demonstrated by power spectral analysis of heart rate variability. It is likely that dysregulation of the autonomic nervous system has a significant role in the pathogenesis of FM.

► As a clinical entity, autonomic dysfunction may be to neurology what FM is to rheumatology. In this study, disturbed sympathetic activity was measured by low frequency R-R intervals in heart rate function. This finding supports the hypothesis that FM is correlated with hypofunction of the hypothalamic-pituitary-adrenal axis and the sympathetic nervous system, but whether this is important from an etiologic viewpoint or is circumstantial will take more research.

M.H. Liang, M.D., M.P.H.

► Ah, fibromyalgia. Or perhaps better—oy, fibromyalgia. I think there is less to the following selections (Abstracts 7–7 through 7–11) than meets the eye. FM syndrome patients were still symptomatic 15 years after onset. Most felt a bit better; was this because of adaptation and development of coping mechanisms? Interestingly nearly half hadn't been to a physician in a year and the majority had tried "alternative" medical therapies. The suicides of two patients in this group of 39 patients are disturbing. Importantly, no new or different diagnoses were made. Group treatment programs, cognitive-educational treatment,[1, 2] zolpidem, ondansetron, bright light,[3] and other therapies[4] were not impressive (which has been my limited experience with zolpidem and ondansetron); aerobic exercise was only helpful over the short term.[5, 6]

For a still more critical view of FM syndrome, see Nortin Hadler's comment following Abstract 7–13.

R.S. Panush, M.D.

References

1. Vlaeyen JWS, Teeken-Gruben NJG, Goossens MEJB, et al: Cognitive-education treatment of fibromyalgia: A randomized clinical trial. I. Clinical effects. *J Rheumatol* 23:1237–1245, 1996.
2. Goossens ME, Rutten-van Mölken MP, Leidi RM, et al: Cognitive-educational treatment of fibromyalgia: A random clinical trial. II. Economic evaluation. *J Rheumatol* 23:1246–1254, 1996.
3. Pearl SJ, Lue F, MacLean AW, et al: The effects of bright light treatment on the symptoms of fibromyalgia. *J Rheumatol* 23:896–902, 1996.
4. While KP, Harth M: An analytical review of 24 controlled clinical trials for fibromyalgia syndrome (FMS). *Pain* 64:211–219, 1996.
5. Martin L, Nutting A, MacIntosh BR, et al: An exercise program in the treatment of fibromyalgia. *J Rheumatol* 23:1050–1053, 1996.
6. Wigers SH, Stiles TC, Vogel PA: Effects of aerobic exercise versus stress management treatment in fibromyalgia: A 4.5 year prospective study. *Scand J Rheum* 25:77–86, 1991.

A Prospective Long-term Study of Fibromyalgia Syndrome

Kennedy M, Felson DT (Boston Univ)

Arthritis Rheum 39:682–685, 1996 7–7

Background.—Fibromyalgia syndrome (FMS) is a common disorder with an unclear long-term prognosis. To date, most studies of the natural history of FMS have been limited. This current prospective study further documented the long-term natural history of this disorder.

Methods and Findings.—Thirty-nine patients with a history of FMS seen in an academic rheumatology referral practice were surveyed at symptom onset and observed for 10 years. Four patients had died by the follow-up reinterview. Twenty-nine of the remaining 35 patients (83%) were reinterviewed. The mean age at follow-up was 55 years. The mean symptom duration was 15.8 years. Although some fibromyalgia symptoms persisted in all patients, only about one half had seen a physician for these symptoms in the preceding year. Fifty-five percent of the patients had moderate to severe pain or stiffness; 48%, moderate to a lot of difficulty sleeping; and 59%, moderate to extreme fatigue. These results were not greatly changed from earlier surveys. Seventy-nine percent of the patients were still taking medications to control their symptoms. Sixty-six percent of the patients reported that their symptoms were a little or a lot better than at diagnosis. Regarding their FMS symptoms, 55% of the patients reported feeling well or very well. Only 7% said they were doing poorly. With the exception of sleep problems, baseline survey symptoms were poorly correlated with symptoms at 10 years.

Conclusions.—Chronic, unremitting symptoms appear to be the rule in FMS, with symptoms persisting for at least 15 years after disease onset. However, in the perception of many patients, despite continued symptoms, their overall condition improves.

The Fibromyalgia Syndrome: A Consensus Report on Fibromyalgia and Disability

Wolfe F, and the Vancouver Fibromyalgia Consensus Group (Univ of Kansas, Wichita)

J Rheumatol 23:534–539, 1996 7–8

Background.—In June 1994, the Physical Medicine Research Foundation convened a committee of experts on fibromyalgia (FM) to discuss diagnosis, testing, assessment, and prognosis. Their consensus report about FM and disability was presented.

Consensus Report.—The accepted criteria for diagnosis are generalized musculoskeletal pain and the presence of pain on palpation at 11 or more of 18 specified tender point sites. Patients with fewer than this number of tender points may be given a diagnosis of FM if they have widespread pain and many of the characteristic symptoms, such as fatigue, sleep disturbance, mood disturbance, headache, and irritable bowel symptoms. Diagnosis should be established in the context of longitudinal observation. Associated symptoms and their severity are considered, along with concurrent medical and psychiatric symptoms. The causes of FM are not well understood. To determine the relationship between FM and antecedent events that may have precipitated or aggravated it, the clinician should consider the patient's opinion as well as current and past medical and psychosocial history. In assessing FM severity and the patient's work capacity, the clinician should provide longitudinal documentation of the nature of the symptoms, including assessments of pain, functional ability, and psychosocial distress. In most patients, symptoms are chronic, vary in severity, and wax and wane. Most patients can work, although job modifications are often needed. A comprehensive treatment approach is important. Other health professionals and resources in the community for education and treatment may be included. Low-dose tricyclic therapy has been found effective in the short term. Prednisone and nonsteroidal anti-inflammatory drugs are not effective for FM. Narcotics should not be given. Graded cardiovascular fitness programs and cognitive behavioral therapy may be useful.

Group Treatment of Fibromyalgia: A 6 Month Outpatient Program
Bennett RM, Burckhardt CS, Clark SR, et al (Oregon Health Sciences Univ, Portland)
J Rheumatol 23:521–528, 1996 7–9

Background.—Patients with fibromyalgia (FM) are frequently seen in rheumatology practice. The value of a 6-month group therapy program involving allied health professionals was investigated.

Methods.—The FM group, attended by 15–25 patients, met weekly for 6 months. The sessions lasted a mean of 90 minutes and included formal lectures, group sessions emphasizing behavior modification, stress reduction techniques, strategies to improve fitness and flexibility, and support for significant others. Assessment included the fibromyalgia impact questionnaire (FIQ), the total tender point score, quality-of-life scale, questionnaires about coping strategies and attitudes toward illness, an index of aerobic conditioning, flexibility, distance walked in 6 minutes, and the Beck depression and Beck anxiety questionnaires.

Findings.—One hundred seventy patients with FM were evaluated between 1989 and 1993. One hundred four patients completed the program. By the end of 6 months, 70% of the patients had fewer than 11 tender points and a 25% improvement in the FIQ. Neither a pain profile on the Minnesota Multiphasic Personality Inventory nor major depression predicted poorer outcome. Improvement persisted in 33 patients observed for 2 years after the program. No improvement was seen in a control group of 29 patients who did not participate in the program.

Conclusions.—A group approach to the treatment of FM in an outpatient setting appears to be promising. A more formal, controlled study is needed to verify these initial findings.

The Effect of Zolpidem in Patients With Fibromyalgia: A Dose Ranging, Double Blind, Placebo Controlled, Modified Crossover Study
Moldofsky H, Lue FA, Mously C, et al (Univ of Toronto)
J Rheumatol 23:529–533, 1996 7–10

Objective.—No consistently effective treatment has been found for the disturbed sleep, fatigue, mood swings, and pain that characterize fibromyalgia (FM). Because zolpidem does not interfere with sleep patterns, a dose-ranging, double-blind, placebo-controlled, modified crossover study was designed to determine whether the drug would improve the symptoms of patients with FM.

Methods.—After a 2-week washout period, overnight polysomnography was performed for 4-night periods in 19 patients (1 male) aged 21–55 years, receiving placebo in 1 period and then randomly allocated to receive 5, 10, or 15 mg of zolpidem. Tenderness, patient global impression (PGI) of sleep improvement, daytime energy, time to fall asleep, total sleep time, dosage adequacy, and adverse events were evaluated every 4 days. Patients rated their sleep quality, pain, level of fatigue, and mood.

Results.—Sixteen patients completed the study. Although no dose of zolpidem had an effect on pain, number of tenderness points, sleep quality, morning fatigue or sleepiness, mood, or ability to concentrate, patients taking zolpidem took significantly less time to fall asleep, slept longer, did not wake as often, and had more energy during the day than did patients who took placebo. Patients rated 10 mg of zolpidem to be the correct dose. Adverse events were reported by 44%, 40%, and 54% of 5-, 10-, and 15-mg zolpidem users, respectively, and by 56% of placebo users. Headache, flulike symptoms, diarrhea, and abnormal dreaming were the most commonly reported side effects.

Conclusion.—Five to 15 mg of zolpidem helps the sleep disturbance symptoms of patients with FM, but it has no effect on pain or mood symptoms.

Pathogenetic Aspects of Responsiveness to Ondansetron (5-Hydroxytryptamine Type 3 Receptor Antagonist) in Patients With Primary Fibromyalgia Syndrome: A Preliminary Study

Hrycaj P, Stratz T, Mennet P, et al (Karol Marcinkowski Univ, Poznac, Poland; Hochrhein Inst for Rehabilitation Research, Bad Säckingen, Germany/ Rheinfelden, Switzerland)

J Rheumatol 23:1418–1423, 1996 7–11

Objective.—Because some evidence has shown that fibromyalgia (FM) symptoms are related to 5-hydroxytryptamine (5-HT) deficiency, drugs that block 5-HT receptors may be effective in treating the pain of FM. The results of an investigation of pain intensity and serum serotonin levels in patients treated with the 5-HT type 3 receptor (3R) antagonist ondansetron and the possible 5-HT-3R involvement in FM pathogenesis are reported.

Methods.—After a 1-week washout period, 21 patients were treated twice daily for 5 days with either 8 mg of ondansetron or 500 mg paracetamol in a double-blind, crossover, latin square fashion. Pain intensity was rated on a visual analog scale (VAS), and a pain score was applied. Pressure tenderness and functional symptoms were recorded. A 40% decrease in pain intensity was defined as a response. Serum serotonin measurements were performed.

Results.—Twenty patients (1 man), aged 25 to 58, finished the study. Functional symptoms, VAS, pain scores, tender point scores, headache, and average pain scores declined significantly for the ondansetron group. The tender point scores and average pain scores increased significantly and VAS and pain scores tended to increase for the paracetamol group. Eleven patients in the ondansetron group improved significantly. There were no serious side effects in the ondansetron group. Whereas serum levels of

5-HT increased significantly in nonresponders, there was no significant change for responders. Paracetamol had no effect on 5-HT serum levels.

Conclusion.—Ondansetron significantly improved the pain symptoms in half of the FM patients. Increased levels of serum 5-HT in nonresponders suggest that there may be 2 subsets of FM patients whose 5-HT-3R systems respond differently to perturbations of serotonin metabolism.

A Randomized, Double-blind Crossover Trial of Fluoxetine and Amitriptyline in the Treatment of Fibromyalgia

Goldenberg D, Mayskiy M, Mossey C, et al (Newton Wellsley Hosp, Massachusetts; New England Med Ctr, Boston)

Arthritis Rheum 39:1852–1859, 1996 7–12

Introduction.—Studies of medications for fibromyalgia have shown few drugs to be effective. In a 6-month randomized clinical trial, 21% of patients treated with amitriptyline, 12% of patients treated with cyclobenzaprine, and 0% of patients treated with placebo improved after 1 month. At 6 months, no difference in response was seen among patients taking drugs and patients taking placebo. Fluoxetine is a selective serotonin reuptake inhibitor that has resulted in improved sleep scores, but not in pain or tender point scores in an open, uncontrolled study of patients with fibromyalgia. In a double-blind, controlled trial, fluoxetine did not improve pain, fatigue, Health Assessment Questionnaire, global severity, or tender point scores. The efficacy of fluoxetine alone, amitriptyline alone, and fluoxetine and amitriptyline combined in the treatment of fibromyalgia was examined.

Methods.—There were 31 patients with fibromyalgia. All patients were white, and 90% were women. The mean patient age was 43.2 years. The study consisted of four 6-week trial periods. Patients received fluoxetine, 20 mg; amitriptyline, 25 mg; fluoxetine, 20 mg, and amitriptyline, 25 mg combined; or placebo. A physician performed a manual tender-point examination. Patients completed the Fibromyalgia Impact Questionnaire, Beck Depression Inventory scale; and visual analogue scales for pain, fatigue, sleep disturbance, feeling refreshed on awakening, and global well-being.

Results.—Of the 31 patients, 12 did not complete the study. Significant improvement was seen in patients treated with fluoxetine alone and amitriptyline alone compared with patients treated with placebo as measured by the Fibromyalgia Impact Questionnaire and visual analogue scales (Fig 1). When fluoxetine and amitriptyline were combined, the result was significantly better than with either drug alone. This improvement with combined treatment was twice that seen with either drug alone. Results were similar when the baseline value for each trial period was included as a covariate.

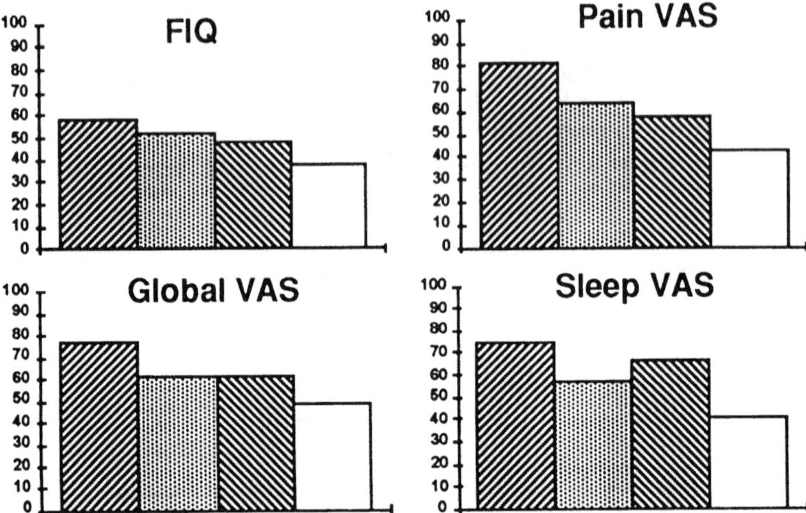

FIGURE 1.—Mean outcomes (statistically significant changes) in the groups treated with placebo (*upward-hatched bars*), amitriptyline (*dotted bars*), fluoxetine (*downward-hatched bars*), or a combination of amitriptyline and fluoxetine (*open bar*), as measured by the Fibromyalgia Impact Questionnaire (*FIQ*) and the visual analogue scales (*VAS*) for pain, global well-being, and sleep. (Courtesy of Goldenberg D, Mayskiy M, Mossey C, et al: A randomized, double-blind crossover trial of fluoxetine and amitriptyline in the treatment of fibromyalgia. *Arthritis Rheum* 39:1852–1859, 1996, copyright American College of Rheumatology.)

Discussion.—In these patients, pain, global well-being, sleep disturbances, and function were improved by fluoxetine and amitriptyline. The combination of fluoxetine and amitriptyline was more effective than either drug alone. Although the visual analogue scores improved for pain, global well-being, and function, the tender-point score did not change significantly. These results are limited by the 6-week treatment period for each drug protocol. Higher doses and longer treatment should be investigated.

► I liked this study but have several problems with it. I suggest caution in its interpretation. Why was benefit from amitriptyline and fluoxetine evident only for the Fibromyalgia Impact Questionnaire and subjective pain, global, and sleep assessments (see Fig 1)? Was this clinically important? Why was the combination not effective for tender-point score, physician global assessment, fatigue, and perception of being refreshed? Given the record of statistically significantly beneficial therapies for fibromyalgia in short-term trials which emerge as unimpressive by 3 or 6 months, why was this not a longer trial? How did patients like this therapy—did they stay on it and would they select it? If this is the best we can do for fibromyalgia, we still have much to accomplish. I applaud the authors' commitment to continue their valuable efforts to help us with the difficult and important problem, and I look forward to their further contributions.

R.S. Panush, M.D.

Psychiatric Diagnoses in Patients With Fibromyalgia Are Related to Health Care–seeking Behavior Rather Than to Illness
Aaron LA, Bradley LA, Alarcón GS, et al (Univ of Alabama, Birmingham)
Arthritis Rheum 39:436–445, 1996 7–13

Introduction.—The relation between psychiatric disorders and health-seeking behavior in patients with fibromyalgia syndrome (FMS) is not known. The frequency of lifetime psychiatric disorders were compared among 64 patients with FMS from a tertiary care setting, 28 community residents with FMS who had not sought medical care for FMS symptoms (FMS nonpatients), and 23 healthy controls.

Methods.—Lifetime psychiatric diagnoses were evaluated using the Computerized Diagnostic Interview Schedule. Current psychological distress was determined by use of the Center for Epidemiological Studies Depression Scale and the Trait Anxiety Inventory.

Results.—The amount of time since onset of symptoms was similar for patients and nonpatients. Patients with FMS differed significantly in number of tender points, pain threshold, pain intensity, and fatigue, compared with nonpatients and controls. Nonpatients had significantly more tender points than controls. Patients with FMS met criteria for a significantly higher number of lifetime psychiatric diagnoses than nonpatients and controls (Fig 1). Patients were significantly more likely to meet criteria for at least 1 psychiatric diagnosis in the anxiety, mood, and body image diagnostic categories, compared with healthy controls (Table 3). There were no between-group differences for nonpatients or controls in the

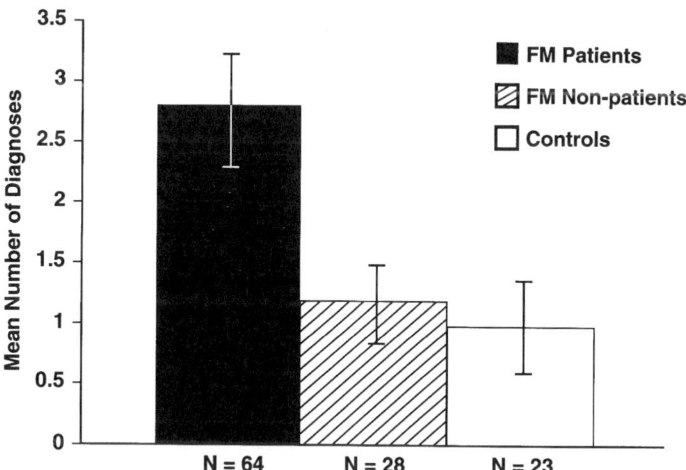

FIGURE 1.—Mean ± SEM number of lifetime psychiatric diagnoses for patients with fibromyalgia (*FM*), FM nonpatients, and healthy controls. Patients with FM met criteria for a significantly greater number of lifetime psychiatric diagnoses than nonpatients and controls ($P = 0.002$). However, there was no significant difference between nonpatients and controls in the number of psychiatric diagnoses. (Courtesy of Aaron LA, Bradley LA, Alarcón GS: Psychiatric diagnoses with fibromyalgia are related to health care–seeking behavior rather than to illness. *Arthritis Rheum* 39:436–445, 1996, copyright American College of Rheumatology.)

TABLE 3.—Percentage of Individuals with Psychiatric Diagnoses by Subject Group

Diagnosis	FMS patients (n = 64)	FMS nonpatients (n = 28)	Controls (n = 23)	P
Anxiety	60	36	26	0.008*
Simple phobia	38	18	4	0.001
Panic disorder with agoraphobia	11	0	0	0.050†
Mood	52	18	22	0.002*
Major depressive episode	39	11	9	0.001
Major depression—recurrent episode	25	7	4	0.014†
Dysthymic disorder	22	7	0	0.004
Bipolar disorder	13	4	0	0.043†
Body image	34	14	4	0.002*
Somatization disorder	23	10	0	0.004
Behavior/character	27	14	13	0.23

*Probability of meeting criteria for at least 1 diagnosis in this category: $P < 0.01$, fibromyalgia syndrome (*FMS*) patients vs. controls; *P* not significant, FMS nonpatients vs. controls.

†Group differences did not reach the stringent significance level of $P < 0.01$ established by the Bonferroni correction procedure.

(Courtesy of Aaron LA, Bradley LA, Alarcón GS: Psychiatric diagnoses with fibromyalgia are related to health care–seeking behavior rather than to illness. *Arthritis Rheum* 39:436–445, 1996, copyright American College of Rheumatology.)

frequency of psychiatric diagnoses within any category. Compared with nonpatients, patients had higher psychological distress levels. Nonpatients had higher distress than controls. After controlling for pain threshold and fatigue, there were no differences in psychological distress between patients and nonpatients.

Conclusions.—Patients with FMS had significantly greater numbers of lifetime psychiatric diagnoses, compared with nonpatients and healthy controls. Patients with FMS may benefit from consultation with health professionals skilled in the use of psychotropic medications and behavioral treatments for chronic pain syndrome and related psychiatric problems.

▶ I have argued for decades that fibromyalgia and its sister labels (chronic fatigue syndrome, irritable bowel syndrome, etc.) are used for individuals who have no primary organ system dysfunction, including no primary psychiatric disease, but whose need for reassurance regarding healthfulness elicits a response from Western medicine that is certain to be iatrogenic. These are individuals living their lives in a process that demands somatizing. And the process is a consequence of the challenge to prove they are ill in a climate that insinuates it is "in their mind." I have set out these arguments in a recent article.

The article abstracted here offers data that support my synthesis. What distinguishes those individuals with aches and pains who cope, somehow, without seeking medical care from those who have arrived at the station of the fibromyalgia label is a lifetime of episodes of the inability to cope. It would follow that palliation that addresses the aches and pains is off the mark. The issue for these dreadfully ill yet nondiseased individuals that needs redress relates to compromised coping.

N.M. Hadler, M.D.

Reference

1. Hadler NM: If you have to prove you are ill, you can't get well: The object lesson of fibromyalgia. *Spine* 21:2397–2400, 1996.

Miscellaneous Disorders

Lead Article

My pick for this year is...no selection. For a simple reason—nothing emerged from those articles I reviewed that was of "landmark" quality, a finding that will importantly affect the way I think or act in rheumatology. This was probably because those articles which I reviewed were generally the ones that none of the other editors were interested in: fibromyalgia, pain, soft tissue rheumatism, crystals, infections, and other topics that have never captured the spotlight or excited the imagination of rheumatologists.

Still, there were several articles that merit brief mention, contributions that will influence my practice, reading, and teaching. I liked the paper by Smith, Triantafillou, Parker, et al. (Abstract 6–4); if inflammatory processes indeed play an important role in early osteoarthritis (OA), or even in some circumstances in OA, then our current approach to treating of OA is wrong.

I also liked the paper by Aker, Gross, Goldsmith, et al. (Abstract 7–2). My 1996 pick of the year[1] told us we really don't know how to manage back pain; it's no surprise that we don't know how to manage neck pain either.

I also found the paper by Kennedy and Felson to be interesting (A prospective long-term study of fibromyalgia syndrome. *Arthritis Rheum* 39:482–485, 1996). These authors told us that, after 15 years of follow-up, patients with fibromyalgia had largely unchanged findings, but nonetheless felt better despite whatever physicians offered, suggesting the importance of developing adequate coping mechanisms. Therein, I think, lies a valuable insight in caring for these patients (however one thinks about fibromyalgia).

And, I liked the paper by Walsh, Wong, Pringle, et al. (Abstract 6–11). This article reminds us of how little attention, still, is given to osteoporosis, and suggests opportunities for rheumatologists in education and patient care.

I offer now my "near picks"—articles not selected for inclusion in the YEAR BOOK but which piqued my interest, and I hope the interest of other readers, for the reasons related.

First is one I've been waiting for—a report of a woman with RA who developed lipoid pneumonia from cod-liver oil capsules![2]

The next is from Beer Sheva, Israel, and is titled "QuestionnaireImpact FibromyalgiatheofVersionHebrewaofValidation: FibromyalgiawithWomenofStatusHealthandDisabilityFunctionalAssessing."[3] (Hebrew reads from right to left.) I know and like these authors, having spent a month last year as their guest visiting professor, but why shouldn't a valid instrument remain valid in good translation? My experience at the medical school in Beer Sheva was delightful. The city is in the (Negev) desert and serves, in part, a large Bedouin community. I marveled at the juxtaposition of past and present illustrated by Bedouins coming to clinic atop their camels while conversing on cellular telephones!

The story by David Pisetsky tells of an elderly academician infuriated by the vicissitudes of managed care who is ultimately pushed over the edge. It is timely, poignant, and provocative, the accompanying commentaries are thoughtful, also.

The editorial "point/counterpoint" of Sanford Roth and Richard Glazier is lively.[5, 6] Should rheumatology try and evolve to large multispecialty arthritis centers managing all aspects of musculoskeletal diseases, as proposed by Roth? Or, should rheumatology provide expert management of complex problems and educate others to care for much of the less complicated, more common musculoskeletal problems, as advocated by Glazier? My own view is that, despite the appeal of Sandy Roth's vision, the notion of Richard Glazier is more consistent with today's realities. I think we'll see some of Sandy's centers, but most of rheumatology will probably be devoted to development of new knowledge, to education of others, and to care of difficult patients.

I came across an interesting piece in *Science News* about MQ—"mensch quotient."[7] Mensch is a wonderful Yiddish term that has no good English counterpart. A mensch is a gentleman; a man of integrity and honor; one who treats others with dignity, respect, empathy, and compassion. Psychologists at the University of California, Berkeley devised a questionnaire to measure MQ. They found that MQs did not necessarily correlate with IQs and that people with high MQs "live much easier in the world" and negotiate life's exigencies well, as would be expected.

Asclepios, the Greek god of medicine, was the son of Apollo, god of art, music, and literature, exemplifying a relationship of medicine to the humanities and arts. What cultural interests do today's physicians pursue? A survey in *The Lancet*[8] offered interesting data. Norwegian physicians, despite working 25% more hours than other university graduates, devoted similar amounts of time to cultural activities. However during the past year, only 43% of doctors (and 33% of university graduates) read a nonmedical book, 38% went to the opera or ballet, 64% to concerts, 75% to the theater, and 78% to the movies. I wonder what the others did? Perhaps I'm simple, but nearly one fourth of physicians not going to the movies and over one half not reading a book in the past year is distressing. I've always thought that the compleat physician should have broad education and interests.

And then there are some great titles: "Why man is such a sweaty and thirsty naked animal: A speculative review,"[9] "My organ is bigger than your organ,"[10] "My organ is more important than your organ,"[11] and the provocative "Milk allergy: An autoallergic disease of cattle."[12] These are for the reader interested in some rather unusual offerings.

Richard S. Panush, M.D.

References

1. Malmivaara A, Häkkinen U, Aro T, et al: The treatment of acute low back pain: Bed rest, exercises, or ordinary activity? *N Engl J Med* 332:351–355, 1995. (1996 YEAR BOOK OF RHEUMATOLOGY, pp 2–4.)
2. Dawson JK, Abernathy VE, Graham DR, et al: A woman who took cod-liver and smoked. *Lancet* 347:1804, 1996.
3. Buskila D, Neumann L: Assessing functional disability and health status of women with fibromyalgia: Validation of a Hebrew version of the Fibromyalgia Impact Questionnaire. *J Rheumatol* 23:903–906, 1996.
4. Pisetsky DS: Final act. *Arthritis Care and Research* 9:248–250, 1996.
5. Roth SH: The future of rheumatology: new directions? *J Rheumatol* 23:1492–1494, 1996.
6. Glazier R: The future of rheumatology: Paradigm shift or turf war? *J Rheumatol* 23:1494–1496, 1996.
7. *Science News,* 15 April 1995, p 233.
8. Nyelenna M, Aasland OG, Falkum E: Survey of Norwegian doctor's cultural activities. *Lancet* 348:1693–1695, 1996.
9. Newman RW: Why man is such a sweaty and thirsty naked animal: A speculative review. *Hum Biol* 42:12–27, 1990.
10. Goldsmith LA: My organ is bigger than your organ. *Arch Dermatol* 126:301–302, 1990.
11. Bernhard JD: My organ is more important than your organ (letter). *Arch Dermatol* 126:827, 1990.
12. Campbell SG: Milk allergy: An autoallergic disease of cattle. *Cornell Vet* 60:684–721, 1970.

Ultrasound Therapy in Musculoskeletal Disorders: A Meta-analysis

Gam AN, Johannsen F (Bispebjerg Hosp, Copenhagen)
Pain 67:85–91, 1995 7–14

Objective.—Many papers have reported the beneficial results of ultrasound in the treatment of musculoskeletal disorders. A meta-analysis of the effectiveness of therapeutic ultrasound in the treatment of pain in musculoskeletal disorders was done.

Methods.—A total of 293 papers on therapeutic ultrasound located using Index Medicus and Medline were reviewed, and 22 were selected that compared ultrasound treatment with sham-ultrasound treatment, nonultrasound treatment, and untreated groups. Two standardized effect sizes ($d_{d/r}$ and $d_{d/s}$) were applied to each study to permit the evaluation of the effect of ultrasound treatment on pain.

Results.—Some studies lacked information about dropouts, randomization methods, and ultrasound and sham-ultrasound instrumentation and methods used. Of the 16 studies that compared ultrasound and sham-ultrasound treatment, it was possible to pool the data from 13. Using the 2 standardized effect sizes, no treatment effect of ultrasound was found.

The d/s test established a significant effect from the degree of blinding, whereas the d/r test showed a trend. It was not possible to analyze the effect of randomization because of insufficient data description.

Conclusion.—The effectiveness of ultrasound treatment for pain is not established by the published studies.

▶ I am keeping a list of lost illusions in rheumatology, to which I now add the presumption of efficacy of ultrasound for musculoskeletal disorders. Others on my list (from previous YEAR BOOKS) include: that changes in weather affect RA symptoms, that traction helps back pain, that the duration of morning stiffness reflects disease actively, that whiplash is a real syndrome, that injections really get into joints, that external application of heat cools and cold warms joints, that walk times help in assessing rheumatologic functional status, that joint abuse causes osteoarthritis, and that effective therapies exist for fibromyalgia syndrome.[1]

R.S. Panush, M.D.

Reference

1. 1996 YEAR BOOK OF RHEUMATOLOGY, pp 44–45.

All-*Trans*-Retinoic Acid in POEMS Syndrome: Therapeutic Effect Associated With Decreased Circulating Levels of Proinflammatory Cytokines

Authier F-J, Belec L, Levy Y, et al (Université Paris XII; Hôpital Henri Mondor, Créteil, France)

Arthritis Rheum 39:1423–1426, 1996 7–15

Objective.—Increased levels of proinflammatory cytokines have been associated with POEMS (plasma cell dyscrasia with polyneuropathy, organomegaly, endocrinopathy, monoclonal [M] protein, skin changes). Because tretinoin possibly can inhibit the production of these cytokines, the effect of administration of tretinoin, with and without concurrent radiotherapy, was evaluated in a patient with POEMS syndrome and atherosclerotic myeloma.

> *Case Report.*—Patient, 58, with POEMS syndrome, thrombocytosis, and 2 monoclonal gammopathies, had multiple osteosclerotic lesions with dystrophic plasmacytosis and IgAλ. The patient received 90 mg/day of all-*trans*-retinoic acid for 50 days, no treatment for 70 days because of lymphopenia, and 75 mg/day of all-*trans*-retinoic acid for 180 days. A 40-gray pelvic irradiation was performed from day 26 to day 50. Neuropathy was evaluated, and platelet count, C-reactive protein, IgGκ, IgAλ, and cytokine levels were determined.

Results.—Levels of interleukin (IL)-1β, IL-6, and tumor necrosis factor-α increased initially, normalized in 5–7 days, increased during radiotherapy, normalized against 13 days into radiotherapy, increased again when tretinoin was discontinued, and normalized again after reintroduction of the drug. Platelet counts, serum C-reactive protein, and monoclonal IgAλ levels paralleled cytokine levels. Monoclonal IgGκ levels began to increase after the first withdrawal of tretinoin and remained unchanged thereafter.

Conclusion.—All-*trans*-retinoic acid appears to downregulate the production of proinflammatory cytokines associated with POEMS.

▶ This is one of those types of papers I usually skim briefly. No, let's be honest here. It's one of those I don't read. But this afternoon, mindful of my frequent exhortations to my residents regarding the educational opportunities inherent in any clinical experience, I asked what I could learn from this paper. The POEMS syndrome is a diagnosis I have never made, and not an entity I have thought about much. But the findings of Authier et al. are provocative. This patient had elevated plasma levels of IL-1β, IL-6, and tumor necrosis factor-α; all became completely normal within 7 days of receiving tretinoin therapy. The graphic illustration of this in Figure 2 of the original article is vivid. There was associated clinical improvement in certain features. How did tretinoin normalize these cytokines? How was this linked to clinical features of POEMS syndrome? Can this observation be exploited and extrapolated for other inflammatory disorders?

R.S. Panush, M.D.

Measurement of Pain: The Psychometric Properties of the Pain-O-Meter, a Simple, Inexpensive Pain Assessment Tool That Could Change Health Care Practices

Gaston-Johansson F (Johns Hopkins Univ, Baltimore, Md)

J Pain Symptom Manage 12:172–181, 1996 7–16

Background.—The literature documents that clinical assessment of patient pain by physicians and nurses has been inadequate. Because adequate assessment is necessary for adequate management, valid and reliable tools for pain assessment are needed; none of the available tools seem well suited for use in clinical practice. The best qualities of several existing tools have been combined into 1 pain assessment tool, the Pain-O-Meter (POM). The validity of this tool was examined.

Product Description.—The POM is composed of hard plastic and measures 8 × 2 × 1 inch. Patients rate their pain with the tool in 2 ways. First, the tool includes a 10-cm long visual analogue scale (VAS) with a moveable marker (Fig 1). Second, the tool lists word descriptors (WDs), of which 15 are sensory and 11 affective. An intensity value (1–5) is assigned to each WDs, and a pain intensity score is provided for the sensory and

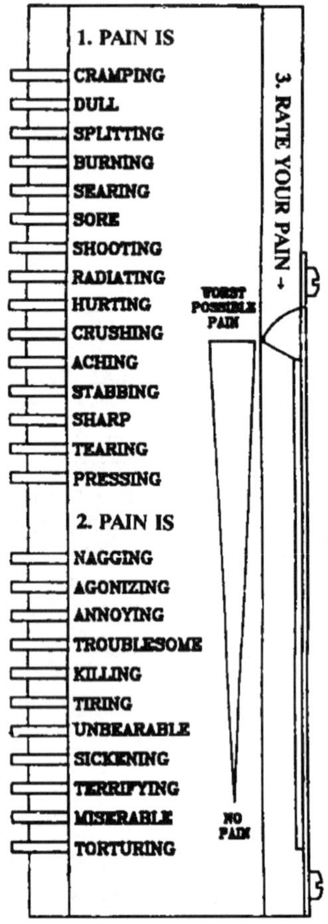

FIGURE 1.—Side 1 of the Gaston-Johansson Pain-O-Meter (U.S. patent 5,018,256, May 28, 1991). (Reprinted by permission of Elsevier Science, Inc. from Measurement of pain: The psychometric properties of the Pain-O-Meter, a simple, inexpensive pain assessment tool that could change health care practices, by Gaston-Johansson F. *J Pain Symptom Manage* 12:172–181. Copyright 1996 by the U.S. Cancer Pain Relief Committee.)

affective categories. Information about pain duration and location can be recorded on the back side of the POM (Fig 2).

Methods.—The test–retest reliability and concurrent and construct validity of the POM-VAS and POM-WDs for 279 patients with acute or chronic pain were examined in a pyschometric study using correlational and comparative designs.

Results.—Test–retest reliability was high for both measures of pain intensity. The concurrent validity of the POM-WDs was supported by

Gaston-Johansson Pain-O-Meter

SIDE II

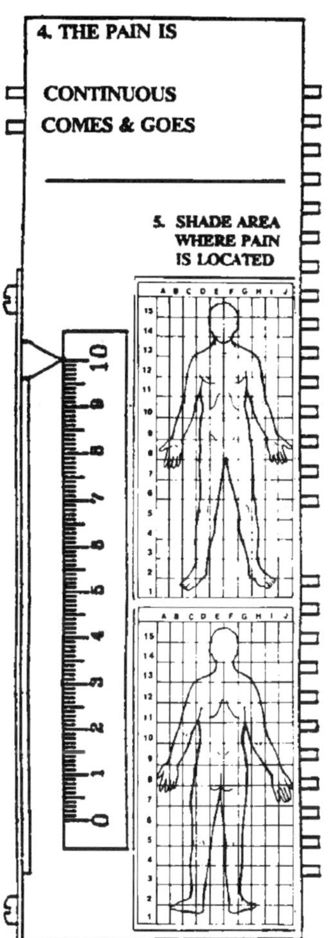

FIGURE 2.—Side 2 of the Gaston-Johansson Pain-O-Meter (U.S. patent 5,018,256, May 28, 1991). (Reprinted by permission of Elsevier Science, Inc. from Measurement of pain: The psychometric properties of the Pain-O-Meter, a simple, inexpensive pain assessment tool that could change health care practices, by Gaston-Johansson F. *J Pain Symptom Manage,* 12:172–181. Copyright 1996 by the U.S. Cancer Pain Relief Committee.)

correlations between the POM-WDs, the McGill Pain Questionnaire, and the POM-VAS. Significant decreases in both pain scores occurring after treatment with pain medication supported construct validity.

Conclusions.—Through better documentation of pain and evaluation of pain relief measures, tools such as the Pain-O-Meter may improve communication between patients and health care providers, thus improving the quality of care provided for pain.

▶ Why didn't I think of this?

R.S. Panush, M.D.

Treatment of 100 Patients With Primary Amyloidosis: A Randomized Trial of Melphalan, Prednisone, and Colchicine Versus Colchicine Only

Skinner M, Anderson JJ, Simms R, et al (Boston Univ)

Am J Med 100:290–298, 1996 7–17

Objective.—Primary amyloidosis (AL) results in an overproduction of a monoclonal immunoglobulin protein. Although there is no treatment for AL, colchicine has been found to be beneficial in treating inflammation. Because some patients have benefitted from treatment with immunosuppressive drugs, a study was initiated to test whether melphalan, prednisone, and colchicine (MPC) is better than colchicine (C) alone for treating patients with AL.

Methods.—One hundred patients with AL who had been admitted between 1987 and 1992 were randomly allocated to receive either 0.6 mg of colchicine twice daily (group A; $n = 50$) or 0.15–0.25 mg of melphalan per kg body weight per day, 1.5 mg of prednisone per kg per day for 4 days, and 0.6 mg of colchicine twice daily on the days on which melphalan was not received every 6 weeks (group B; $n = 50$) for 1 year. Patients were followed for at least 18 months. The outcome measure was survival.

Results.—Survival was 6.7 months in group A and 12.2 months in group B. Overall survival was 8.4 months. Survival of patients with organ system involvement was 4.4 months for cardiac involvement, 18.7 months for renal improvement, 5.9 months for neurologic involvement, and 11.8 months for other organ involvement. The treatment effect for MPC was significant only for patients with neurologic or other organ system involvement. Improvement and survival measures were significantly better in patients who did not have cardiac or gastrointestinal involvement. The only adverse effects observed in patients taking colchicine was diarrhea. Two melphalan-treated patients experienced decreased blood counts. Infection developed in 2 other melphalan-treated patients: 1 with *Klebsiella* pneumonia and the other with coccidiomycosis. Both survived.

Conclusion.—Patients with AL and no renal or cardiac involvement who were treated with MPC improved and had increased survival.

▶ Nice work on a tough and, fortunately, uncommon problem. The survival data were still pretty grim, even if quantitatively better with MPC.

R.S. Panush, M.D.

Delayed Diagnosis of Acute Rheumatic Fever in Adults: A Forgotten Cause of Febrile Polyarthritis

Chan AW, Webb G, Vellend H, et al (Univ of Toronto)
J Rheumatol 23:1999–2001, 1996 7–18

Objective.—Difficulties and delays may arise in the diagnosis of acute rheumatic fever (ARF). The diagnosis and management of 3 cases of ARF were described.

Case 1.—Oriental man, 30, with aortic insufficiency, polyarthritis for 4 days, and fever for 3 weeks had had ARF at age 13 years and had received monthly injections for 6 years. He had elevated blood pressure, a diastolic and pansystolic murmur, an erythrocyte sedimentation rate of 61 mm/hr, and a new first-degree heart block. A migratory pattern of polyarthritis developed. His antistreptolysin O titer was elevated. His polyarthritis resolved with aspirin therapy. Three years after discharge, he receives penicillin V, 250 mg orally twice daily.

Case 2.—Italian man, 39, with fever, sore throat, and polyarthralgia for 2 weeks and a remote history of ARF had a throat culture positive for β-hemolytic group A streptococci. Migrating arthralgia developed despite antibiotic treatment. His hemoglobin level, leukocyte count, erythrocyte sedimentation rate, antistreptolysin titer, and C-reactive protein level were elevated. He had first-degree heart block and received a diagnosis of acute myocarditis. When polyarthralgia did not improve, he was treated with penicillin and aspirin, which was later changed to prednisone. He continues to receive penicillin prophylaxis.

Case 3.—Canadian man, 63, with vomiting and weakness for 2 days, had had ARF at age 20 years and underwent aortic valve replacement at age 55 years. He had chronic atrial fibrillation. When hospitalized, he had mild biventricular failure, aortic stenosis, aortic insufficiency, and mitral regurgitation. Arthralgias developed 1 day after admission, and he received a diagnosis of infective endocarditis. On day 6 ARF was diagnosed, and the patient was treated with penicillin, aspirin, and misoprostol. An upper gastrointestinal hemorrhage occurred on day 25 with hypotension and cardiac arrest. He died, and necropsy showed pericardial adhesions, cardiomegaly, and dilatation. Aschoff's nodules and Anitchkov's myocytes were present in the myocardium.

Discussion.—The risk for recurrence of ARF varies with the individual patient but is correlated with the presence and number of episodes of rheumatic heart disease. Although the use of prophylactic antistreptococcal drugs is debated, premature termination of prophylactic treatment in patients with valve disease increases the risk for recurring ARF.

► I hope I (and my colleagues) don't overlook this. We made this diagnosis several months ago, using confirmation by our nonagenerian Chairman Emeritus (who ran a rheumatic fever service half a century ago) as our definite diagnostic "test."

R.S. Panush, M.D.

The Successful Treatment of Autoimmune Hepatitis With 6-Mercaptopurine After Failure With Azathioprine

Pratt DS, Flavin DP, Kaplan MM (New England Med Ctr, Boston; Tufts Univ, Boston)

Gastroenterology 110:271–274, 1996 7–19

Background.—Glucocorticoids are the treatment of choice for autoimmune hepatitis, but their adverse effects make long-term use unacceptable. Thus other immunosuppressive agents, such as azathioprine, have been used to replace glucocorticosteroids in the long term. Azathioprine is a purine analogue derived from 6-mercaptopurine. Although these 2 agents are often used interchangeably, they have different toxicity profiles and may have clinical differences relevant to immunosuppressive activity in individual patients. Three patients with autoimmune hepatitis who were intolerant of or unresponsive to azathioprine responded well to 6-mercaptopurine.

Case 1.—Girl 13 years of age, who had jaundice at initial assessment was given azathioprine as an adjunct to glucocorticoids to induce remission and lower the glucocorticoid dose. However, neither laboratory tests nor liver biopsy showed improvement in the autoimmune hepatitis, despite prolonged treatment. Treatment with glucocorticoids and 6-mercaptopurine subsequently induced complete remission, which was sustained with 6-mercaptopurine alone.

Case 2.—Boy, 17 years of age, who had jaundice at initial assessment experienced incapacitating gastrointestinal side effects with azathioprine. However, he had no problems with 6-mercaptopurine.

Case 3.—Man, 35 years of age, who had jaundice at initial assessment had fevers and arthralgias develop that were temporally related to azathioprine. Because these adverse effects are so rare, the patient was rechallenged. The identical symptoms recurred. Treatment with 6-mercaptopurine, however, was effective and well tolerated.

Conclusions.—Patients with autoimmune hepatitis who are unresponsive to or intolerant of azathioprine treatment should be given a trial of 6-mercaptopurine as a glucocorticoid-sparing agent. The difference between azathioprine and 6-mercaptopurine in efficacy and toxicity may be related to individual differences in metabolism.

▶ There are several reasons for treatment failures with azathioprine, and among the most common are gastrointestinal intolerance, fever, and inefficacy. This paper describes 3 patients with autoimmune hepatitis who were either intolerant of or unresponsive to azathioprine who responded to its metabolite 6-mercaptopurine. One can imagine many ways to explain this phenomenon, but the major take-home lesson is that when azathioprine fails in the treatment of chronic active hepatitis, 6-mercaptopurine may be effective. This is certainly something that may also be useful in the care of patients with systemic lupus erythematosus and RA.

M. Reichlin, M.D.

Growth of Acid Fast L Forms From the Blood of Patients With Sarcoidosis

Almenoff PL, Johnson A, Lesser M, et al (Veterans Affairs Med Ctr, Hampton, Va; Veterans Affairs Med Ctr, Bronx, NY; Mount Sinai School of Medicine, NY; et al)

Thorax 51:530–533, 1996 7–20

Introduction.—Although the pathogenesis of sarcoidosis is still uncertain, the available evidence suggests that mycobacteria are involved. Acid-fast cell wall deficient forms (CWDF) of bacilli have been isolated from many different sources in patients with sarcoidosis, including blood, bronchial washings, and ocular anterior chamber fluid. However, there is no proof that these bacilli are of mycobacterial origin. A monoclonal antibody against *Mycobacterium tuberculosis* H_{37} RV whole cell antigen was used to further characterize CWDF isolated from the blood of patients with sarcoidosis.

Methods.—Blood cultures were prepared from 20 patients with active sarcoidosis and 20 healthy controls. The blood cultures were analyzed for mycobacterial L forms using a mouse monoclonal antibody against *M. tuberculosis* and indirect fluorescent antibody analysis.

Results.—All but 1 of the blood cultures from patients with sarcoidosis grew CWDF. The bacilli showed positive staining with the mouse monoclonal antibody as well as with a modified Kinyoun stain. None of the 20 control blood samples grew any CWDF.

Conclusion.—Acid-fast CWDF can be isolated from the blood of nearly all patients with sarcoidosis. These organisms are mycobacterial in origin, as shown by both indirect fluorescent antibody analysis and modified Kinyoun stain. Specific DNA sequencing studies will probably be needed to determine whether the isolated bacilli are CWDF of *M. tuberculosis*, a related organism, or a new species.

▶ We draw closer to an understanding of sarcoidosis with the isolation of mycobacterial L forms (CWDF or spheroblasts) from the blood of 19 of 20 patients with active sarcoidosis (vs. 0 of 20 controls). Such deficient microbes are notoriously difficult to eradicate, so we are not there yet.

E.C. LeRoy, M.D.

Tumour Necrosis Factor-α Gene Expression by Alveolar Macrophages in Human Lung Allograft Recipient With Recurrence of Sarcoidosis

Martel S, and the Toulouse Lung Transplantation Group (CHU Rangueil, Toulouse, France)

Eur Respir J 9:1087–1089, 1996 7–21

Objective.—Tumor necrosis factor-α (TNF-α) is suspected of being involved in the development of sarcoid granulomas in the lung. Alveolar macrophages from patients with sarcoidosis have enhanced TNF-α gene expression. A case of recurrence of sarcoidosis in an allograft 2 years after lung transplantation without an increase in TNF-α gene expression by alveolar macrophages at recurrence but a later increase when granulomas were associated with acute rejection was studied.

Case Report.—Man, 25, who underwent a single lung transplant for end-stage lung fibrosis as a result of stage IV sarcoidosis, experienced a rejection episode at 14 months posttransplant and was treated with prednisone. Two months later, a febrile bronchitis developed as a result of *Myxovirus influenzae* infection. At 22 months after transplantation, a second rejection episode was treated with prednisone. A biopsy specimen 2 months later confirmed recurrent sarcoidosis, and the patient's prednisone dose was increased. One month later, the granulomas were no longer observable and the prednisone dose was reduced. One month later, prominent granulomas consistent with grade-1 rejection were observed and continued despite a steroid pulse treatment. The patient's forced expiratory volume in 1 sec dropped to 1.45 L. His respiratory function stabilized for 2 months and then dropped again. After biopsy, bronchiolitis obliterans syndrome was suspected. Respiratory function again stabilized after steroid treatment, and the patient is still alive 54 months after transplantation. Whereas no increased expression of TNF-α gene was detected in alveolar macrophages when his sarcoidosis first recurred, significantly increased expression was seen with the grade-1 rejection episode. When steroid dosage was increased and granulomas disappeared, gene expression returned to normal, but it peaked again when bronchiolitis obliterans syndrome was diagnosed and was as high as that found during the grade-1 rejection episode.

Conclusion.—The behavior of alveolar macrophages in patients with lung transplantation is an indicator of disease progression. Whereas TNF-α is not implicated in early stages of granuloma formation, it appears to stimulate a recurrence of the fibroproliferative process.

► In at least 6 of 8 human lung allograft recipients who receive transplants for pulmonary sarcoidosis, there has been a recurrence of the granulomatous sarcoid lesion and, at least in the case reported in this study, the concomitant occurrence of BOS; thus, the stimulus for recurrence must be blood-borne. Perhaps adoptive transfer of human material from sarcoid patients in SCID mice could be instructive. The etiopathogenesis of sarcoid remains elusive.

E.C. LeRoy, M.D.

Ultrasound-guided Fine-needle Aspiration Cytology of Non-palpable Supraclavicular Lymph Nodes in Sarcoidosis

Lohela P, Tikkakoski T, Strengell L, et al (Kiljava Hosp, Finland; Oulu Univ, Finland; Hyvinkas Hosp, Finland)

Acta Radiol 37:896–899, 1996 7–22

Introduction.—The diagnosis of sarcoidosis has historically been based on surgical histologic biopsy, transbronchial biopsy, or biopsy via mediastinoscopy. Only a few trials have evaluated the accuracy of palpation-guided fine-needle aspiration biopsy (FNAB) in the diagnosis of sarcoidosis. A prospective investigation was conducted to determine the incidence of enlarged supraclavicular lymph nodes by US and the diagnostic yield of US-guided FNAB in the diagnosis of sarcoidosis.

Methods.—All consecutive patients with suspected sarcoidosis underwent supraclavicular US during a 54-month period. Chest radiographs revealed hilar or mediastinal adenopathy (17 patients), interstitial parenchymal changes (5 patients), hilar adenopathy (4 patients), and apical infiltrates (1 patient). Ultrasound-guided FNAB of the lymph node was performed in all patients with enlarged supraclavicular lymph nodes.

Results.—Twenty-seven (10.8%) of 250 patients evaluated by US had enlarged nonpalpable supraclavicular lymph nodes. Twenty and 7 patients, respectively, had unilateral or bilateral supraclavicular lymphadenopathy. All enlarged lymph nodes were focal lesions that were noncompressible and hypoechoic (Figure). Twenty-five cytologic specimens were quantitatively sufficient. The cytologic diagnosis was granulomatous inflammation suggestive of sarcoidosis in 22 specimens. Of 5 aspirates, 3 yielded reactive hyperplasia and 2 specimens were insufficient. Diagnoses were confirmed by positive bronchial mucosal and renal cutting needle biopsies and clinical follow-up.

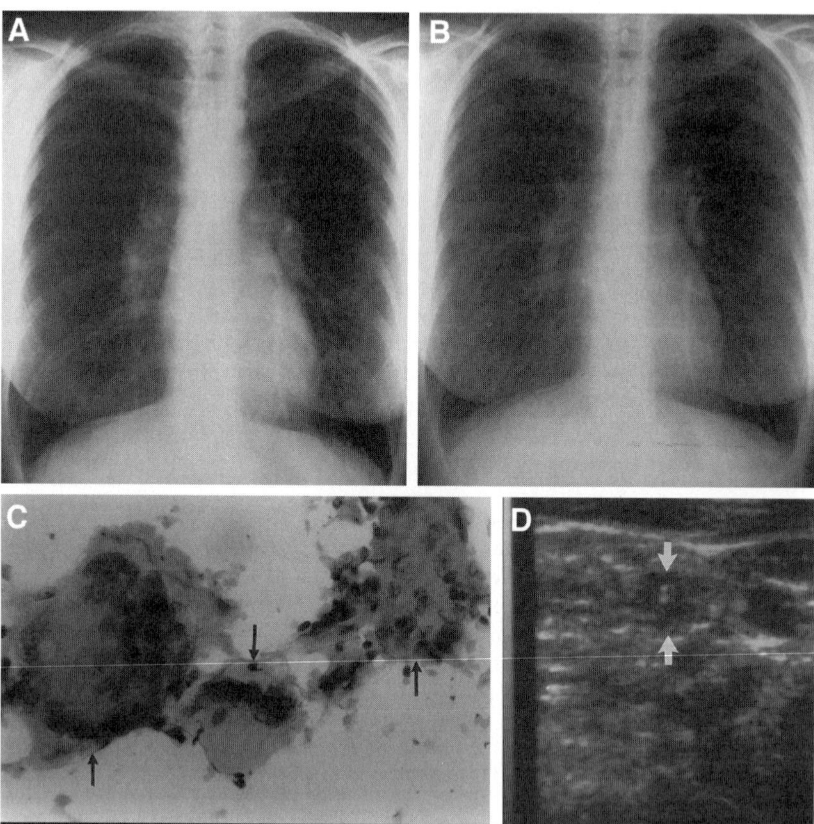

FIGURE.—Imaging of a 45-year-old woman with erythema nodosum and arthralgia. **A,** chest radiograph shows bilateral hilar adenopathy but no changes in the lung parenchyma. **B,** after 18 months' follow-up, the chest radiograph showed normal results, and the patient was asymptomatic. **C,** cytologic aspirate shows 3 small epitheloid cell granulomas with 3 multinucleated giant cells (*arrows*) consistent with sarcoidosis. Five-needle aspiration biopsy (FNAB) smear; toluidine-blue; original magnification, ×200. **D,** ultrasonogram of an enlarged supraclavicular lymph node (*arrows*) during the FNAB. The needle tip echo is easily seen. (Courtesy of Lohela P, Tikkakoski T, Strengell L, et al: Ultrasound-guided fine-needle aspiration cytology of non-palpable supraclavicular lymph nodes in sarcoidosis. *Acta Radiol* 37:896–899, 1996.)

Conclusion.—Supraclavicular US was able to detect nonpalpable enlarged lymph nodes in 10.8% of patients with sarcoidosis. For this patient subset, more invasive diagnostic methods can be avoided by using US combined with aspiration cytology to provide cytologic evidence of granulomatous disease similar to sarcoidosis.

► A histologic diagnosis of sarcoidosis remains the "gold standard" for diagnosis. This prospective study demonstrates—in 250 Finnish patients in whom the diagnosis of sarcoidosis was entertained—that US could detect nonpalpable supraclavicular lymphadenopathy in 11% and that 93% of these could be reliably diagnosed by FNAB, thus avoiding more invasive techniques such as surgical transbronchial or mediastinoscopic biopsy. This approach should reduce both cost and suffering. Both US and FNAB can be done at 1 sitting.

E.C. LeRoy, M.D.

An Exon Skipping Mutation of a Type V Collagen Gene (COL5A1) in Ehlers-Danlos Syndrome

Nicholls AC, Oliver JE, McCarron S, et al (Clinical Research Centre, Harrow, England; Strangeways Research Lab, Cambridge, England; Univ of Wisconsin, Madison)

J Med Genet 33:940–946, 1996 7–23

Background.—The Ehlers-Danlos syndrome (EDS), a heterogeneous group of inherited connective tissue disorders, is characterized by skin hyperextensibility, joint hypermobility, easy bruising, and cutaneous fragility. The EDS has 9 discrete clinical subtypes. The biochemical and molecular features of a type V collagen defect in 1 patient with atypical EDS II were presented.

Case Report.—Woman, 24, had generalized skin fragility with extensive scarring of the forehead, shins, and knees. She also had scattered bruising on the arms and legs. Marked generalized joint laxity was present with severe premature bilateral hallux valgus. She had diamond-shaped feet, short stature, mild thoracic kyphoscoliosis, pectus excavatum, and audible mitral valve prolapse. Clinically, the patient's cutaneous fragility and other features suggested type I or II EDS. Her short stature and scoliosis initially suggested EDS VII.

Electron microscopic examination of skin tissue showed abnormal collagen fibrillogenesis with longitudinal sections showing a marked disruption of fibril packing, resulting in very irregular outlines in transverse sections. The collagens produced by cultured fibroblasts were analyzed, and the type V collagen was found to have a population of α1(V) chains shorter than normal. Peptide mapping showed a possible deletion in the triple helical domain. A 54 bp deletion was shown by RT-PCR amplification of messenger RNA (mRNA) covering the whole of this COL5A1 domain. Six Gly-X-Y triplets were lost, but the essential triplet amino acid sequence and C-propeptide structure were maintained, which allowed mutant protein chains to be incorporated into triple helices. In a genomic DNA analysis, a de novo G^{+3} T transversion in a 5' splice site of one COL5A1 allele was identified. This mutation is analogous to mutations causing exon skipping in the major collagen genes COL1A1, COL1A2, and COL3A1, as seen in patients with osteogenesis imperfecta and EDS type IV.

Conclusion.—This patient produced both normal and shortened α1(V) chains, some carrying a deletion in the triple helical domain as a result of skipping a 54 bp exon in the mRNA transcripts because of a point mutation in 1 COL5A1 allele. This report gives the first characterization of a naturally occurring structural mutation in a human type V collagen gene.

▶ Collagens are characterized by repeating Gly-X-Y sequences, permitting a very tight α helix tertiary structure because Gly has no side chain, which would, if present, require an expanded helix; these triplets are often arranged in 54 (3 × 18) bp exons of which type V collagen has 66 compared with 52 for type I collagen. These fibrillar collagens (types I, III, and V) have many more exons than other proteins.

Skin fragility, papyraceous scar formation, and hyperelastic skin are relatively common and are associated with skeletal/joint abnormalities in the now nearly a dozen subtypes of the EDS, which are steadily being defined on a molecular basis by such reports as the excellent one presented here. Clinically, the patient could be classified as EDS I/II or, with kyphoscoliosis, EDS VII. Careful molecular analysis eliminated the possibility that the defect was that of EDS VII (a failure of an enzyme that converts procollagen to collagen) and identified a point mutation in the splice site causing the transcriptional apparatus to skip the 49th exon (counting from the 5' end of the molecule). This powerful experiment of nature also, by showing abnormal collagen fiber formation, demonstrates that collagen type V is critical to the formation of the major collagen fibril, composed largely of type I collagen.

This is a striking example of the power of molecular techniques (in expert hands) to define the lesion in the inherited disorders of connective tissue. The next major breakthrough will be replacement of the defective mutation by gene therapy.

E.C. LeRoy, M.D.

The Clinical Spectrum of Remitting Seronegative Symmetrical Synovitis with Pitting Edema

Olivé A, and The Catalán Group for the Study of RS_3PE (Hosp Universitari Germans Trias I Pujol, Badalona, Spain)

J Rheumatol 24:333–336, 1997 7–24

Introduction.—Previously, there have been reports of patients with symmetric synovitis that involved the wrists and flexor digitorum tendon sheaths and that was associated with marked pitting edema of the dorsum of the hands. The patients, mostly older men who were negative for rheumatoid factor, responded to low-dose corticosteroids and to hydroxychloroquine. Since then, more cases have been reported and the syndrome of remitting seronegative symmetric synovitis with pitting edema remains controversial. Clinical manifestations, laboratory features, and evolution of disease were studied in several patients with this disorder.

Patients.—Twenty-seven patients with remitting seronegative symmetric synovitis with pitting edema participated in this retrospective multicenter study. They were all older than 50 years, had bilateral pitting edema of both hands, were seronegative for rheumatoid factor, and had sudden onset of polyarthritis. The patients, 9 women (33.3%) and 18 men (66.6%), ranged in age from 58 to 92 years (mean age, 71.7 years).

Results.—Polymyalgia rheumatica was found in 2 patients. Edema of both hands and polyarthritis were the main clinical features. Polyarthritis involved ankles in 7 patients (25.9%), knees in 9 (33.3%), elbows in 3 (11.1%), shoulders in 13 (48%), wrists in 15 (55.5%), proximal interphalangeal joints in 19 (70.4%), and metacarpophalangeal joints in 22 patients (81.5%). In 8 patients, antinuclear antibodies were positive at low titer. One patient had erosions. T lymphoma was seen in 2 patients, and myelodysplastic syndrome was seen in 1 patient.

Conclusion.—Remitting seronegative symmetric synovitis with pitting edema may not be a distinct clinical entity because it is a heterogeneous syndrome that is evidenced by the presence of erosions, clinical history, and evolution to hematologic disease. These patients require meticulous follow-up.

▶ It is now more than 10 St. Patrick's Days ago that Dan McCarty published a report[1] of 10 patients with symmetric synovitis of wrists and hands associated with impressive hand edema. Patients were characteristically older men who were rheumatoid factor negative. In the ensuing decade, more than 35 additional cases have been reported, and the overlapping features with polymyalgia rheumatica and seronegative RA have led several experienced clinicians to question the distinctiveness of RS_3PE (remitting seronegative symmetric synovitis with pitting edema). A Catalan (Barcelona) group for the study of RS_3PE now analyzes 27 additional patients who demonstrate clinical heterogeneity, leading the Catalans to conclude that RS_3PE may not be a distinct clinical entity. What will be the Irish rejoiner?

E.C. LeRoy, M.D.

Reference

1. McCarty DJ, O'Duffy D, Pearson L, et al: Remitting seronegative symmetrical synovitis with pitting edema: RS_3PE syndrome. *JAMA* 254:2763–2767, 1985.

Yttrium-90 Radiochemical Synovectomy in Chronic Knee Synovitis: A One Year Retrospective Review of 133 Treatment Interventions

Asavatanabodee P, Sholter D, Davis P (Univ of Alberta, Edmonton)

J Rheumatol 24:639–642, 1997 7–25

Introduction.—The radioisotope yttrium-90 (Y-90) has been used, primarily in Europe and Australia, for 25 years to treat chronic synovitis. The effectiveness of Y-90 was retrospectively studied in 85 patients (118 knees)

TABLE 6.—The Relation Between General Disease Activity and Clinical Response to Yttrium-90 at 9 Months

Disease Activity (Total of 91 Joints)	Excellent and Good Response (N = 50) (%)	Fair and Poor Response (N = 41) (%)
Active (N = 27)	8/27 (30)*	19/27 (70)
Inactive (remission) or local synovitis (N = 64)	42/64 (66)	22/64 (34)

*$P < 0.001$ compared with benefit in patients in remission or with local synovitis.

(Courtesy of Asavatanabodee P, Sholter D, Davis P: Yttrium-90 radiochemical synovectomy in chronic knee synovitis: A one year retrospective review of 133 treatment interventions. *J Rheumatol* 24:639–642, 1997.)

and prospectively studied in 13 patients (15 knees) with chronic knee synovitis refractory to other medical therapies.

Methods.—The mean patient age was 48 years and the duration of joint involvement was an average of 9 years. Seventy-one patients were in remission from generalized disease or had isolated knee synovitis and 27 patients had active generalized disease. Results of injection with Y-90 were rated, at 3, 6, 9, and 12 months, as excellent, good, fair, or poor. Assessment variables included presence of joint effusion, joint tenderness, joint range of motion, and pain scores rated by a Visual Analogue Scale.

Results.—Treatment benefit was able to be assessed in 81%, 82%, 80%, and 75% of knees at 3, 6, 9, and 12 months, respectively. When successful treatment was considered to be excellent and good response, 49%, 48%, 57%, and 46% of knees were considered to be treated successfully at 3, 6, 9, and 12 months. Twenty-six knees in 16 patients were re-injected with Y-90 because of poor response. Of 15 joints available for 9-month evaluation, 8 (53%) were given an upgraded response, 8 had no change, and 1 was downgraded from poor to fair. Radiographic examination showed excellent or good response in 78% of patients with stage 1 and 54% with stage 4 radiographs, respectively. Patients with inactive generalized disease or only localized synovitis were significantly more likely to have excellent or good responses, compared with patients with active generalized disease (66% vs. 30%) (Table 6). Patients with excellent or good responses were more likely than patients with poor or fair responses to have shorter duration of involvement and shorter duration of generalized disease.

Conclusions.—Successful response to Y-90 was observed in many patients with chronic knee synovitis refractory to other medical interventions. Minimal radiologic change, localized joint disease, and shorter duration of disease were predictive of treatment success. Relapses and primary treatment failures may be successfully treated with re-injection.

▶ Radiosynovectomy of the knee in patients with RA using colloidal Y-90 has been with us for more than 2 decades, and the results continue to be favorable. About half get good results, and about half of those who do not have a good result respond well to a second injection. In selected patients, this seems to be a reasonable therapeutic choice. As expected, those with a structurally intact joint, shorter duration, and fewer systemic signs of disease do better. There is no information regarding cost comparisons.

E.C. LeRoy, M.D.

Subject Index*

A

Abdomen
scintigraphy, three-phase, in lupus vasculitis of gastrointestinal tract, *97:* 177
Abuse
physical, in women with fibromyalgia syndrome, *96:* 225
sexual
in women with fibromyalgia, *96:* 225
in women with fibromyalgia syndrome, *97:* 227
Acid
-fast L forms from blood in sarcoidosis, growth of, *98:* 271
α_1-Acid glycoprotein
as marker for articular destruction in rheumatoid arthritis, *98:* 33
Acquired immunodeficiency syndrome (*See also* HIV)
arthritis in, inflammatory, hydroxychloroquine in, *97:* 43
Acral
skin, silicone granuloma in, in patient with silicone-gel breast implants and scleroderma, *97:* 379
ACTH
secretion, intact, in active rheumatoid arthritis, *98:* 51
for synovitis, acute crystal-induced, *96:* 297
Acute phase response
in early rheumatoid arthritis, individual relationship between progression of radiological damage and, *98:* 34
Adenocarcinoma
ovarian, Raynaud's phenomenon as presenting sign of, *97:* 248
Adenosine
mediation of antiinflammatory effects of adenosine kinase inhibitor (in mice), *97:* 75
receptor stimulation inhibiting synoviocyte collagenase gene expression, *98:* 145
Adhesion
molecule 1, intercellular
expression on scleroderma fibroblasts and endothelial cells in early disease stage, up-regulation by interferon-gamma and tumor necrosis factor-α, *98:* 143
monoclonal antibody to, in refractory rheumatoid arthritis, *96:* 87
in scleroderma fibroblasts, *96:* 158
molecule, soluble, in peripheral blood in scleroderma, *96:* 160
Adrenal
insufficiency, secondary, perioperative steroid requirements in, *98:* 52
α_2-Adrenergic antagonist
blockade of vasospastic attacks in idiopathic Raynaud's disease by, *97:* 243
Adrenocorticotropic
hormone
secretion, intact, in acute rheumatoid arthritis, *98:* 51
for synovitis, acute crystal-induced, *96:* 297
African-Americans
rheumatoid arthritis in, lack of rheumatoid antigenic determinant in, *97:* 34
Age
disability development with, and running, *96:* 191
musculoskeletal pain related to running and, *98:* 215
-related reduction in gastric mucosal prostaglandin levels increasing susceptibility to aspirin-induced injury (in rat), *96:* 69
-specific incidence rates of myocardial infarction and angina in women with systemic lupus erythematosus, *98:* 116
Aged (*see* Elderly)
AIDS
(*See also* HIV)
arthritis in, inflammatory, hydroxychloroquine in, *97:* 43
Alcoholism
gout and, *98:* 222
Alendronate
effect on fracture risk in women with existing vertebral fractures, *98:* 229
esophageal ulceration due to, *98:* 232
esophagitis due to, *98:* 231
in osteoporosis
discussion of, *98:* 226
postmenopausal, effect of 3 years of treatment, *98:* 228

* *All entries refer to the year and page number(s) for data appearing in this and previous editions of the* Year Book.

postmenopausal, effect on bone mass of spine, hip, and total body over 3 years, *98:* 226
postmenopausal, in prevention of nonvertebral fractures, *98:* 227
protocol for, *98:* 231
stimulation of nocturnal parathyroid hormone secretion, *98:* 230
Allopurinol
mouthwashes in methotrexate-induced stomatitis, *96:* 61
Alpha-1 antitrypsin
PiZ allele link with Wegener's granulomatosis, *96:* 241
PiZ gene of, in outcome of PR3-ANCA positive vasculitis, *97:* 312
Alveolar
macrophages express tumor necrosis factor-α gene in lung transplant recipient with recurrence of sarcoidosis, *98:* 272
Alveolitis
fibrosing
lone, interleukin-8 expression in, *97:* 222
in scleroderma, *96:* 172
in scleroderma, memory T cells increase in lung interstitium in, *97:* 246
American College of Rheumatology
definition of improvement in rheumatoid arthritis, preliminary, *97:* 48
recommendations for liver biopsy after methotrexate for rheumatoid arthritis, *97:* 79
Amitriptyline
/fluoxetine in fibromyalgia, *98:* 257
Amoxicillin
vs. azithromycin in erythema migrans, *98:* 239
Amyloid
deposits, turnover and regression in vivo, evidence for, *96:* 308
Amyloidosis, *96:* 307
AA, of familial Mediterranean fever, colchicine for, *96:* 307
primary, treatment of, *98:* 268
systemic, presenting as giant cell arteritis and polymyalgia rheumatica, *96:* 256
Anal
function in systemic sclerosis, *98:* 179
Analgesia
epidural, cervical, for pain of digital vasculitis secondary to rheumatoid arthritis, *98:* 198
Anemia
hemolytic, autoimmune, in child with MHC class II deficiency, *96:* 130
in rheumatoid arthritis
erythropoietin for, *96:* 64
iron deficiency diagnosis in, algorithm for, *97:* 52
Anesthetic
intraarticular, effect on pain in osteoarthritis of knee, *98:* 218
Aneurysm
aortic, thoracic, in giant cell arteritis, *96:* 257
Angiitis
primary, of CNS, limitations of invasive modalities in diagnosis, *97:* 329
Angina
in women with systemic lupus erythematosus, age-specific incidence rates of, *98:* 116
Angiography
in CNS disease in Sjögren's syndrome, correlation with anti-Ro/SS-A autoantibodies, *96:* 116
Angioplasty
intracranial, for vascular stenosis due to atherosclerosis and vasculitis, results, *97:* 326
Angiotropic
large cell lymphoma with mononeuritis multiplex mimicking systemic vasculitis, *97:* 320
Ankle
problems in rheumatoid arthritis, *96:* 49
surgery in psoriasis, *96:* 272
Ankylosing
spondylitis (*see* Spondylitis, ankylosing)
Annexin V
antibody to, antiphospholipid and lupus anticoagulant properties of, *97:* 143
Anorexia
in Lyme borreliosis, early, with erythema migrans, *98:* 237
Antibiotics
plus corticosteroids in *Staphylococcus aureus* arthritis, experimental, *98:* 232
use in rheumatoid arthritis patients treated with methotrexate, *96:* 60
Antibody(ies)
to annexin V, antiphospholipid and lupus anticoagulant properties of, *97:* 143
anti-β_2 glycoprotein I, in monozygotic twin sisters, *96:* 139
anticardiolipin

clinical consequences of "low titers", *98:* 112
family study of, and associated conditions, *97:* 144
in hepatitis C, chronic, *97:* 153
IgG, monoclonal, in antiphospholipid syndrome, thrombogenic properties of (in mice), *98:* 111
in polymyalgia rheumatica and giant cell arteritis, *97:* 323
anticentromere, and HLA class II genes, in scleroderma, *97:* 212
anti-chromo, in connective tissue disease, *96:* 148
anticytoplasmic, perinuclear, in minocycline-induced arthritis, *98:* 196
anti-DNA
anti-idiotypic, in systemic lupus erythematosus, *97:* 164
DNA mimics self-protein as target for, in systemic lupus erythematosus, *96:* 107
double-strand, cross-reactive, induction by immunization with bacterial DNA (in mice), *96:* 112
topoisomerase I, coexisting with anti-Sm antibodies, report of 3 cases, *98:* 102
anti-dorsal root ganglion neuron, in dorsal root ganglionitis with Sjögren's syndrome, *97:* 199
anti-endothelial cell, in vasculitis, pathogenic role of (in mice), *98:* 192
anti-F(ab')$_2$, IgG, cross-reactivity with DNA and other nuclear antigens, *98:* 104
antigen system, anti-Sa, for rheumatoid arthritis, *96:* 35
antihistone, in scleroderma, and lung fibrosis, *96:* 169
anti-La/SS-B, detected by ELISA, utility for diagnosis of systemic lupus erythematosus, *98:* 99
antimyeloperoxidase
in arthritis, minocycline-induced, *98:* 196
in neutrophil activation, *97:* 309
antimyenteric neuronal, in scleroderma, *96:* 149
antineutrophil cytoplasmic
assay to distinguish between vasculitic disease activity and complications of cytotoxic therapy, *96:* 240
in Wegener's granulomatosis, *97:* 314
in Wegener's granulomatosis, and cyclophosphamide response, *96:* 238
antinuclear
determination in routine laboratory, *98:* 97
enzyme immunoassay for, *98:* 98
interferon-gamma–inducible protein p16 as target of, in systemic lupus erythematosus, *96:* 110
positive test, in children without autoimmune disease, *97:* 178
antiphosphatidylethanolamine, as the only antiphospholipid antibodies, *98:* 107
antiphospholipid, *97:* 141
antiphosphatidylethanolamine antibodies as the only, *98:* 107
in children with idiopathic cerebral ischemia, *96:* 142
with CNS disease in systemic lupus erythematosus, *97:* 145
directed against epitopes of oxidized phospholipids, *98:* 109
epilepsy in systemic lupus erythematosus and, *96:* 144
miscarriage associated with, recurrent, aspirin and heparin in pregnant women with, *98:* 115
during pregnancy, and refractory HELLP syndrome, *96:* 141
specificity and cofactor dependence in, from patients with parvovirus B19 infection and systemic lupus erythematosus, *98:* 110
syndrome (*see* Antiphospholipid, syndrome)
thrombosis and, natural history and risk factors, *98:* 113
in twin sisters, monozygotic, *96:* 139
antiribosomal P protein, and lupus erythematosus, neuropsychiatric systemic, *98:* 118
antiribosomal PO protein, in CNS disease in systemic lupus erythematosus, *97:* 162
anti-RNP, detected by ELISA, utility for diagnosis of systemic lupus erythematosus, *98:* 99
anti-Ro/SS-A, detected by ELISA, utility for diagnosis of systemic lupus erythematosus, *98:* 99
anti-Scl-70, and natural killer cells and γδ T cells in scleroderma, *97:* 227
anti-Sm
coexisting with anti-DNA topoisomerase I antibodies, report of 3 cases, *98:* 102

detected by ELISA, utility for diagnosis of systemic lupus erythematosus, *98:* 99
anti-topoisomerase I, severe scleroderma with, and HLA-DRw11 allele, *96:* 151
anti-U1 nuclear ribonucleoprotein, and major histocompatibility complex class II gene, *96:* 97
anti-U3RNP, serum, and pulmonary hypertension in diffuse scleroderma, *98:* 169
autoantibody (*see* Autoantibody)
to C1q, changes predicting kidney relapses in systemic lupus erythematosus, *97:* 159
DNA, double-stranded, circulating titer reduction after LJP 394, *98:* 126
to histone DNA complexes, more sensitive and specific for scleroderma than lupus, *96:* 153
to HIV-1 gp41 and HLA class II antigen-derived peptides in systemic lupus erythematosus, *97:* 158
monoclonal
CAMPATH-1H, for refractory rheumatoid arthritis, *97:* 99
CD4, for early rheumatoid arthritis, *97:* 102
chimeric, anti-CD4, in rheumatoid arthritis with methotrexate, *97:* 103
chimeric, to tumor necrosis factor-α, in rheumatoid arthritis, *96:* 85
to intercellular adhesion molecule 1 in refractory rheumatoid arthritis, *96:* 87
recognize cardiolipin bound to epitopes of oxidized low-density lipoprotein, *98:* 109
nucleosome-restricted, in kidney in lupus with proteinuria (in mice), *96:* 113
Anticardiolipin
antibodies (*see* Antibodies, anticardiolipin)
-positive patients with malignancy, increased thromboembolic incidence in, *97:* 151
Anti-CD4
chimeric monoclonal antibody in rheumatoid arthritis with methotrexate, *97:* 103
synergy with anti-tumor necrosis factor in amelioration of collagen-induced arthritis, *96:* 91
Anti-CD5
ricin A chain immunoconjugate in systemic lupus erythematosus, *96:* 134
Anti-CENP-B
response of uranium miners exposed to quartz dust, and scleroderma, *97:* 217
Anticentromere
antibody and HLA class II genes in scleroderma, *97:* 212
Anti-chromo
antibodies in connective tissue disease, *96:* 148
Anticoagulant
lupus, properties, annexin V antibody with, *97:* 143
protein I in placenta in antiphospholipid antibody syndrome, *96:* 145
Anticytoplasmic
antibodies, perinuclear, in minocycline-induced arthritis, *98:* 196
Anti-DNA
antibodies
anti-idiotypic, in systemic lupus erythematosus, *97:* 164
DNA mimics a self-protein as target for, in systemic lupus erythematosus, *96:* 107
double-strand, cross-reactive, induction by immunization with bacterial DNA (in mice), *96:* 112
autoantibodies, lupus, repertoire cloning of, *98:* 85
topoisomerase I antibodies coexisting with anti-Sm antibodies, report of 3 cases, *98:* 102
Anti-dorsal root
ganglion neuron antibody in dorsal root ganglionitis with Sjögren's syndrome, *97:* 199
Anti-double strand DNA autoantibody
mechanisms of cellular penetration and nuclear localization of, *98:* 82
Anti-endothelial cell
antibodies in vasculitis, pathogenic role of (in mice), *98:* 192
Anti-F(ab')$_2$
antibody, IgG, cross-reactivity with DNA and other nuclear antigens, *98:* 104
system depletion and active systemic lupus erythematosus, *97:* 165
Antigen(s)
-antibody system specific for rheumatoid arthritis, SA, *96:* 35
autoantigen

α-fodrin as, in primary Sjögren's syndrome, *98:* 131
-specific T cell proliferation induced by ribosomal P2 protein in systemic lupus erythematosus, *96:* 109
-based heteropolymers for binding and clearing autoantibodies via erythrocyte complement receptor 1, *96:* 94
-derived peptides, HLA class II, antibodies to, in systemic lupus erythematosus, *97:* 158
DNA, cross-reactivity with IgG anti-F(ab')$_2$ antibody, *98:* 104
HLA class II, and neuropsychiatric systemic lupus erythematosus, *98:* 96
lymphocyte function-associated antigen 3 in scleroderma fibroblasts, *96:* 158
neutrophil cytoplasmic, autoantibodies to, in predicting relapse in systemic vasculitis, *97:* 310
nuclear, cross-reactivity with IgG anti-F(ab')$_2$ antibody, *98:* 104

Antigenic
determinant, rheumatoid, most African-Americans with rheumatoid arthritis do not have, *97:* 34

Antihistone antibodies
in scleroderma, and lung fibrosis, *96:* 169

Antiidiotypes
to anti-double stranded DNA, some autoantibodies to Ro/SS-A and La/SS-B are, *98:* 100

Anti-idiotypic anti-DNA antibodies
in lupus erythematosus, systemic, *97:* 164

Antiinflammatory
drugs, in knee osteoarthritis progression, *97:* 258
drugs, nonsteroidal
alendronate combined with, and esophageal lesions, *98:* 231
in bursitis, trochanteric, *98:* 248
cognitive decline in elderly and, *97:* 125
cost savings with stepped-care prescribing protocol, *97:* 5
effects on glomerular filtration rate in elderly, acute and chronic, *97:* 113
effects on renal function in hypertension, *97:* 121
gastroduodenal injury due to, in children, *97:* 117
hospitalization for acute renal failure and, *97:* 124
in rheumatoid arthritis, cost of misoprostol prophylaxis in, *96:* 65
in rheumatoid arthritis, stopping of, high dose fish oil after, *97:* 129
small intestine inflammation and blood loss due to, sulfasalazine and other disease-modifying antirheumatic drugs in, *96:* 71
ulcer due to, duodenal, prevention of, famotidine in, *98:* 40
ulcer due to, duodenal, prevention of, misoprostol dosage in, *97:* 116
ulcer due to, gastric (*see* Ulcer, gastric, NSAID-induced)
ulcer due to, peptic, bleeding, risk of, *96:* 68
ulcer due to, peptic, *Helicobacter pylori* infection increasing risk of, *97:* 126
use by Medicaid patients, prior authorization requirements for, *97:* 7
effects of adenosine kinase inhibitor mediated by adenosine (in mice), *97:* 75
effects of interleukin-13 on synovial fluid macrophages in rheumatoid arthritis, *98:* 23

Anti-interleukin 12
treatment of Lyme borreliosis (in mice), *98:* 240

Anti-La/SS-B
antibodies detected by ELISA, utility for diagnosis of systemic lupus erythematosus, *98:* 99

Antimyeloperoxidase
antibodies
in arthritis, minocycline-induced, *98:* 196
in neutrophil activation, *97:* 309
solid phase assays of autoantibodies to lactoferrin and histone in systemic vasculitis, *96:* 249

Antimyenteric neuronal antibodies
in scleroderma, *96:* 149

Antineutrophil
cytoplasmic antibodies (*see* Antibody, antineutrophil cytoplasmic)
cytoplasmic autoantibodies
in kidney failure in scleroderma, *96:* 244
with perinuclear staining pattern, and respiratory tract lesions, *96:* 246

Antinuclear
antibody (*see* Antibody, antinuclear)

Antiperinuclear factor
rheumatoid arthritis heterogeneity and, *96:* 37

Antiphosphatidylethanolamine
antibodies as the only antiphospholipid antibodies, *98:* 107
Antiphospholipid
antibodies (*see* Antibody, antiphospholipid)
autoantibodies bind to apoptotic thymocytes in a β_2-glycoprotein-I dependent manner, *98:* 108
properties of annexin V antibody, *97:* 143
syndrome, *96:* 139
anticardiolipin antibodies in, monoclonal IgG, thrombogenic properties of (in mice), *98:* 111
hepatitis C virus causing, *97:* 153
in lupus erythematosus, systemic, associated with anti-β_2-glycoprotein-I, *97:* 147
ocular vaso-occlusive disease in, *97:* 148
ovarian cancer and, *96:* 140
placenta in, β2 glycoprotein I and anticoagulant protein I in, *96:* 145
thrombosis in, induction by immunoglobulin G, M and A (in mice), *97:* 141
thrombosis in, management, *97:* 150
Anti-proteinase 3
neutrophil activation by, *97:* 309
Antirheumatic drugs
death due to, in rheumatoid arthritis, *97:* 111
disease-modifying, for NSAID-induced small intestinal inflammation and blood loss, *96:* 71
second-line, effects on progression or regression of rheumatoid nodules, *97:* 77
Antiribosomal
P protein antibodies and neuropsychiatric systemic lupus erythematosus, *98:* 118
PO protein antibodies, in CNS disease in systemic lupus erythematosus, *97:* 162
Anti-RNP
antibodies detected by ELISA, utility for diagnosis of systemic lupus erythematosus, *98:* 99
Anti-Ro/SS-A
antibodies detected by ELISA, utility for diagnosis of systemic lupus erythematosus, *98:* 99
autoantibodies in Sjögren's syndrome
in CNS disease, *96:* 116
heart block in adult with, complete, *98:* 139
Anti-Sa system
for rheumatoid arthritis, *96:* 35
Anti-Scl-70
antibodies, and natural killer cells and γδ T cells in scleroderma, *97:* 227
Anti-Sm
antibodies
coexisting with anti-DNA topoisomerase I antibodies, report of 3 cases, *98:* 102
detected by ELISA, utility for diagnosis of systemic lupus erythematosus, *98:* 99
Anti-topoisomerase I
antibodies
coexisting with anti-Sm antibodies, report of 3 cases, *98:* 102
in scleroderma, severe, and HLA-DRw11 allele, *96:* 151
α1-Antitrypsin
PiZ allele link with Wegener's granulomatosis, *96:* 241
PiZ gene of, in outcome of PR3-ANCA positive vasculitis, *97:* 312
Anti-tumor
necrosis factor synergy with anti-CD4 in amelioration of collagen-induced arthritis, *96:* 91
Anti-U1
nuclear ribonucleoprotein antibody, and major histocompatibility complex class II gene, *96:* 97
Anti-U3RNP
antibody, serum, and pulmonary hypertension in diffuse scleroderma, *98:* 169
Aorta
thoracic, aneurysm and rupture in giant cell arteritis, *96:* 257
Apoptosis
acceleration of lymphocytes in systemic lupus erythematosus, *96:* 106
endothelial cell, in scleroderma, *98:* 160
of Fas^{high} synovial T cells by *Borrelia*-reactive Fas $\text{ligand}^{\text{high}}$ γδ T cells in Lyme arthritis, *98:* 241
in rheumatoid arthritis, *98:* 25
Apoptotic
thymocytes, antiphospholipid autoantibodies binding to, and β_2-glycoprotein-I, *98:* 108
Arteritis
giant cell
amyloidosis presenting as, systemic, *96:* 256
anticardiolipin antibody in, *97:* 323
aorta in, thoracic, aneurysm and rupture, *96:* 257

disease patterns and tissue cytokine profiles in, *98:* 188
polymyalgia rheumatica with, methotrexate in, *98:* 201
steroid-related complications and mortality in, *96:* 212
survival, long-term, *97:* 327
Takayasu's, *96:* 259
renovascular hypertension due to, *97:* 325
temporal *(see* Arteritis, giant cell *above)*
Artery(ies)
digital, occlusion, due to interferon, *98:* 182
lesions in Behçet's disease, *97:* 359
temporal, biopsy, in suspected giant cell arteritis, prediction of results, *96:* 16
Arthralgia
in Lyme borreliosis, early, with erythema migrans, *98:* 237
Arthritis
acute, in hospital, rheumatologic *vs.* nonrheumatologic care of, *96:* 18
bacterial cell wall-induced, retrovirus-mediated gene transfer to synovium in (in rat), *97:* 105
collagen-induced
anti-CD4 synergy with anti-tumor necrosis factor in amelioration of, *96:* 91
collagen peptide modulating, oral immunodominant, *97:* 38
progression of, interleukin-10 inhibition of (in mice), *98:* 66
progression of, leukotriene B_4 in, *96:* 34
taxol in, *96:* 88
type II, interleukin-10 expression and chemokine regulation during evolution of (in mice), *97:* 226
degenerative, major orthopedic surgery for, gender differences in, *96:* 187
gonococcal, *96:* 309
gouty
acute, ketorolac in, *96:* 298
acute, ketorolac *vs.* indomethacin in, *97:* 367
in osteoarthritis, nodal, *98:* 221
recurrent, nontophaceous, urate lowering drugs for, cost effectiveness of, *97:* 365
infectious, *98:* 232
inflammation in, somatostatin-induced modulation of (in rabbit), *97:* 39
inflammatory
active, in AIDS, hydroxychloroquine in, *97:* 43
chronic, early onset, team managed outpatient care of, *97:* 24
chronic, soft tissue lesions around heel in, ultrasound-guided injection of, *96:* 273
genetic typing in, outcome prediction in, *96:* 31
juvenile, *96:* 274
chronic, markers of disease activity in, serum p55 and p75 tumor necrosis factor receptors as, *98:* 70
chronic, systemic-onset, methotrexate response in, *96:* 276
knee, local heat and cold treatment for, *96:* 72
Lyme
Borrelia burgdorferi detected by DNA amplification in synovial tissue in, *98:* 236
in children, clinical spectrum and outcome, *96:* 292
T cells in, *Borrelia*-reactive Fas ligand^{high} $\gamma\delta$, apoptosis of Fas^{high} CD4+ synovial T cells by, *98:* 241
treatment, *96:* 294
minocycline-induced, with fever, livedo reticularis, and pANCA, *98:* 196
neutrophil activating peptide-78 in, epithelial, *96:* 33
parvovirus B19 causing, variable clinical picture of, *97:* 388
patients, direct medical costs unique to, *98:* 7
pristane-induced, as new model for rheumatoid arthritis (in rat), *98:* 69
protection against, activation of T cells recognizing self 60-kD heat shock protein for (in rat), *96:* 89
psoriatic
fibroblast function in, *96:* 269
gut inflammation in, ileocolonoscopy of, *97:* 338
immunohistochemical markers for, *96:* 270
methotrexate in, long-term, outcome, *96:* 271
progression, clinical indicators of, *97:* 340
sulfasalazine for, *97:* 340
reactive, post-*Salmonella,* clinicopathology, *97:* 335
rheumatoid (*see* Rheumatoid arthritis)
Staphylococcus aureus, experimental, corticosteroids plus antibiotics in, *98:* 232
tuberculous, and gout, *98:* 222

vaccinia virus expressing heat shock protein 60-kD for (in rat), *96:* 90

Arthrodesis
- radiolunate, for rheumatoid wrist, radiological evolution of wrist after, *97:* 56

Arthropathy
- crystal-related, *98:* 220
- dialysis, outcome after kidney transplant, *97:* 387
- idiopathic destructive, clinical, light, and electron microscopic studies, *98:* 223

Arthroplasty
- hip, total
  - for osteoarthritis, cost effectiveness of, *97:* 271
  - for rheumatoid arthritis, predicting length of stay after, *98:* 13
- joint, total, corticosteroid injection in rheumatoid arthritis does not increase rate of, *98:* 53
- knee, total
  - for rheumatoid arthritis, predicting length of stay after, *98:* 13
  - variation in rheumatologists' and family physicians' perceptions of indications for and outcomes of, *98:* 11

Arthroscopy
- knee
  - articular cartilage, *vs.* plain radiography and MRI, *96:* 189
  - office-based, complications of, *97:* 265
  - osteoarthritis, study results, *97:* 266
- needle, disclosing articular cartilage abnormalities, physical exam of knee predicting, *97:* 251
- office-based, evolution of procedure, *97:* 264

Articular
- cartilage, knee
  - abnormalities, compartment-directed physical examination predicting, *97:* 251
  - arthroscopy *vs.* plain radiography and MRI of, *96:* 189
- destruction in rheumatoid arthritis, prediction of, *98:* 33

Aspiration
- cytology, ultrasound-guided fine-needle, of non-palpable supraclavicular lymph nodes in sarcoidosis, *98:* 273

Aspirin
- gastric adaptation to, role of gastric blood flow, neutrophil infiltration and mucosal cell proliferation in (in rat), *96:* 68
- -induced injury to gastric mucosa, age-related reductions in gastric mucosal prostaglandin levels increasing susceptibility to (in rat), *96:* 69
- low-dose prophylactic, and gout, *98:* 222
- in pregnant women with recurrent miscarriage associated with antiphospholipid antibodies, *98:* 115

Atherosclerosis
- vascular stenosis due to, intracranial angioplasty for, results, *97:* 326

Athletes
- female ex-athletes, risk of osteoarthritis of hips and knees in, *98:* 214

Audiovestibular
- involvement in scleroderma, *96:* 168

Auranofin
- in rheumatoid arthritis
  - *vs.* phenytoin and chloroquine, *97:* 61
  - *vs.* sulfasalazine, efficacy and toxicity of, *98:* 43

Autoantibody(ies)
- anti-DNA, lupus, repertoire cloning of, *98:* 85
- antiendothelial cell immunoglobulin G, from scleroderma, inducing leukocyte adhesion to vascular endothelial cells, *97:* 205
- antineutrophil cytoplasmic
  - in kidney failure in scleroderma, *96:* 244
  - with perinuclear staining pattern, and respiratory tract lesions, *96:* 246
- antiphospholipid, bind to apoptotic thymocytes in a β_2-glycoprotein I-dependent manner, *98:* 108
- anti-Ro/SS-A, in Sjögren's syndrome
  - in CNS disease, *96:* 116
  - heart block in adult with, complete, *98:* 139
- -associated congenital heart block, outcome, *96:* 117
- binding and clearing, via erythrocyte CR1, antigen-based heteropolymers as potential therapy for, *96:* 94
- DNA, anti-double strand, mechanisms of cellular penetration and nuclear localization of, *98:* 82

expression lack in children born to mothers with silicone breast implants, *97:* 381
Fcγ receptor specific, circulating, in scleroderma, *97:* 213
to fibrillarin in scleroderma, *98:* 159
to histone in systemic vasculitis, *96:* 249
to lactoferrin in systemic vasculitis, *96:* 249
lupus, to DNA cross-react with SnRNP A and D polypeptides, *96:* 108
in lupus erythematosus, systemic, *97:* 161
against muscle-cell membrane proteins in myositis, *98:* 208
in myositis, relation to MHC class II alleles in four ethnic groups, *98:* 207
to neutrophil cytoplasmic antigen predicting relapse in systemic vasculitis, *97:* 310
against nucleolus organizer region, clinical relevance and HLA association of, *96:* 147
production, pathogenic, in systemic lupus erythematosus, role of CD40 ligand hyperexpression in, *98:* 88
to ribosomal P, lupus hepatitis with, *97:* 179
to Ro/SS-A and La/SS-B, some are antiidiotypes to anti-double stranded DNA, *98:* 100
to topoisomerase I in scleroderma, *96:* 152
in vasculitis, urticarial, *97:* 161
Autoantigen
α-fodrin as, in primary Sjögren's syndrome, *98:* 131
-specific T cell proliferation induced by ribosomal P2 protein in systemic lupus erythematosus, *96:* 109
Autoimmune
anemia, hemolytic, in child with MHC class II deficiency, *96:* 130
disease
cyclosporine in, and grapefruit juice, *98:* 124
silica exposure and, *97:* 370
Goodpasture syndrome, α3 chain of type IV collagen inducing, *96:* 262
hearing loss, methotrexate for, *96:* 310
hepatitis
6-mercaptopurine after azathioprine failure in, *98:* 270
minocycline-induced, *97:* 170
response, trichloroethene-induced (in mice), *97:* 171
sialoadenitis induced by immunization with carbonic anhydrase II (in mice), *97:* 202
Autoimmunity
SLE-related, to double-stranded DNA and histones, viral DNA binding protein generating, *97:* 139
Autonomic
dysfunction in diffuse scleroderma *vs.* CREST, *96:* 173
neuropathy in systemic lupus erythematosus and scleroderma, *97:* 236
Autoreactivity
to heat shock protein 60 predicts disease remission in oligoarticular juvenile rheumatoid arthritis, *98:* 73
Avian
scleroderma, endothelial cell apoptosis in, *98:* 160
Azathioprine
failure in autoimmune hepatitis, 6-mercaptopurine after, *98:* 270
in rheumatoid arthritis, with methotrexate, *97:* 69
Azithromycin
vs. amoxicillin in erythema migrans, *98:* 239

B

B cell(s)
CD40 ligand hyperexpression by, in systemic lupus erythematosus, *98.* 88
hyperactivity in systemic lupus erythematosus, and interleukin-10, *96:* 101
Babesiosis
concurrent Lyme disease and, *98:* 238
Back
pain, low
acute, bed rest, exercises or ordinary activity in, *96:* 2
acute, outcomes and costs of care by primary care practitioners, chiropractors and orthopedic surgeons, *97:* 294
chronic, sacroiliac joint in, *96:* 5
chronic, spa therapy in, effectiveness of, *97:* 295
diagnostic testing for, physician variation in, *96:* 4
management of, chiropractic *vs.* hospital outpatient, *97:* 293
non-specific, traction efficacy for, *97:* 292

Bacterial
cell wall-induced arthritis, retrovirus-mediated gene transfer to synovium in (in rat), *97:* 105
Balneotherapy
for rheumatoid arthritis, *97:* 96
Bed
rest for acute low back pain, *96:* 2
Behçet's disease
arterial lesions in, *97:* 359
interleukin-10 and IL-12 levels in, systemic, *98:* 204
myelodysplastic syndromes and, *98:* 206
portal vein cavernous transformation as manifestation of, *97:* 356
Behçet's syndrome, *98:* 204
Beraprost
in Raynaud's phenomenon, primary, *98:* 185
Biology
of osteoarthritis, *98:* 217
Biopsy
lip, for early expression of E-selectin, tumor necrosis factor-α, and mast cell infiltration in systemic sclerosis, *98:* 155
liver, after methotrexate in rheumatoid arthritis
American College of Rheumatology recommendations for, *97:* 79
cost effectiveness of, *97:* 80
microscopy in, light and electron, *97:* 82
muscle
abnormalities in systemic lupus erythematosus, *96:* 119
needle, in rheumatology practice, *96:* 286
renal, findings in cyclosporine treated-rheumatoid arthritis, *98:* 49
shoulder tendon, in organ culture producing procollagenase and metalloproteinase tissue inhibitor, *97:* 291
temporal artery, in suspected giant cell arteritis, prediction of results, *96:* 16
Birth
country of, and systemic lupus erythematosus, *97:* 154
Bladder
cancer in Wegener's granulomatosis, *97:* 305
Bleeding
peptic ulcer, risk with NSAIDs, *96:* 68
Bleomycin
-induced pulmonary fibrosis, effects of relaxin on (in mice), *98:* 142
Block
heart (*see* Heart, block)
Blood
cells
red (*see* Erythrocyte)
white (*see* Leukocyte)
count decrease due to melphalan in primary amyloidosis, *98:* 268
flow
cerebral, abnormalities, and low pain thresholds in fibromyalgia in women, *97:* 284
cerebral, measurements in fibromyalgia, *97:* 285
gastric, role in gastric adaptation to aspirin (in rat), *96:* 68
loss, small intestine, NSAID-induced, sulfasalazine and other disease-modifying antirheumatic drugs in, *96:* 71
peripheral
mononuclear cells, collagen-stimulated, augmented interleukin-6 secretion in, in scleroderma, *96:* 162
soluble adhesion molecules in, in scleroderma, *96:* 160
pressure, ambulatory, effects of enalapril and nifedipine in hypertension on, *97:* 121
from sarcoidosis patients, growth of acid-fast L forms in, *98:* 271
tests in systemic lupus erythematosus disease activity assessment, *96:* 118
Body
total body bone mass, effect of alendronate over 3 years in postmenopausal osteoporosis on, *98:* 226
Bone
bipartite, tophi in, *98:* 222
destruction progression in wrists and fingers in rheumatoid arthritis, *96:* 28
erosion in rheumatoid arthritis of wrist, MRI scoring of, *97:* 47
loss
generalized, in early rheumatoid arthritis, *96:* 212
glucocorticoid-induced, in postmenopausal women, etidronate with ergocalciferol in prevention of, *97:* 277
after ovariectomy, exercise protecting against (in rat), *96:* 210

in postmenopausal women, long-term effects of calcium supplementation on, *97:* 275
spinal, due to low-dose corticosteroids in rheumatoid arthritis, calcium and vitamin D_3 supplementation in prevention of, *98:* 56
in spine and femur, etidronate reversing, in corticosteroid-induced osteoporosis, *97:* 278
marrow
mononuclear cells in Paget's disease, measles virus nucleocapsid mRNA in, *97:* 385
transplantation, allogenic, from donor with systemic lupus erythematosus, *98:* 92
mass
in rheumatoid arthritis, effect of hormone replacement therapy on, *96:* 215
in rheumatoid arthritis, effect of pamidronate on, *98:* 60
of spine, hip, and total body in postmenopausal osteoporosis, effect of alendronate over 3 years on, *98:* 226
metabolism in rheumatoid arthritis, *96:* 38
mineral
density, and lifetime milk consumption in older women, *96:* 206
density, decreased axial, in perimenopausal women with rheumatoid arthritis, *96:* 214
density, increase after alendronate for 3 years in postmenopausal osteoporosis, *98:* 228
density, lumbar, low, and major depression, *96:* 207
density, radiographic, in hip osteoarthritis, *97:* 256
density in rheumatoid arthritis, effect of low-dose corticosteroids on, *97:* 133
metabolism in juvenile rheumatoid arthritis, *98:* 76
mineralization in juvenile rheumatoid arthritis, *98:* 76
Paget's disease of, monostotic, bone scintigraphy of, *97:* 384
scintigraphy (*see* Scintigraphy, bone)
tripartite, tophi in, *98:* 222
Borrelia burgdorferi
detection by DNA amplification in synovial tissue in Lyme arthritis, *98:* 236
DNA is undetectable by polymerase chain reaction in skin lesions of morphea, scleroderma, or lichen sclerosus et atrophicus in North American patients, *98:* 242
in fasciitis, diffuse, with peripheral eosinophilia, *96:* 289
-reactive Fas ligand^{high} $\gamma\delta$ T cells in Lyme arthritis, apoptosis of Fas^{high} CD4+ synovial T cells by, *98:* 241
Borreliosis
Lyme (*see* Lyme, disease)
Breast
feeding
Raynaud's phenomenon and, *98:* 180
rheumatoid arthritis and, juvenile, *97:* 342
rheumatoid arthritis and prolactin and, *98:* 39
implant
connective tissue diseases risk after, *96:* 301
HLA typing in, *97:* 382
removal, review of, *97:* 375
silicone, explanted, analysis of, *96:* 304
silicone, gel, and blood silicone elevated levels, *97:* 373
silicone, gel, silicone granuloma in acral skin and scleroderma in patient with, *97:* 379
silicone, lack of autoantibody expression in children born to mothers with, *97:* 381
silicone, microbial presence at surface of, *97:* 377
silicone, risk of systemic lupus erythematosus after, *96:* 303
Bromocriptine
in lupus erythematosus, systemic, *97:* 186
Bronchiolitis
obliterans organizing pneumonia as first manifestation of polymyositis, *98:* 209
Bronchoalveolar
lavage
in fibrosing alveolitis in scleroderma, *96:* 172
fluid, from scleroderma, platelet-derived growth factor and transforming growth factor-β1 in, *97:* 214

Bupivacaine
cervical epidural, for pain of digital vasculitis secondary to rheumatoid arthritis, *98:* 198
injection, intraarticular, for pain in osteoarthritis of knee, *98:* 218
Bursitis
of iliopsoas, pain as only clinical indicator of, *97:* 297
trochanteric, *98:* 248
tuberculous, imaging findings, *98:* 235

C

Calcific
tendinitis in proximal thigh, *96:* 229
Calcinosis
diltiazem for, *97:* 351
Calcitonin
salmon, intermittent nasal, to prevent postmenopausal lumbar spine bone loss, *97:* 276
Calcium
channel blockers
lupus erythematosus due to, subacute cutaneous, *98:* 117
in scleroderma, left ventricular myocardial perfusion and function after, *98:* 176
pyrophosphate dihydrate crystal-induced acute tenosynovitis, *97:* 368
supplementation
in postmenopausal women, long-term effects on bone loss and fractures, *97:* 275
prophylactic, for spinal bone loss secondary to low-dose corticosteroids in rheumatoid arthritis, *98:* 56
CAMPATH-1H
monoclonal antibody for refractory rheumatoid arthritis, *97:* 99
Cancer
anticardiolipin-positive patients with, increased thromboembolic incidence in, *97:* 151
bladder, in Wegener's granulomatosis, *97:* 305
development after cyclophosphamide-treated rheumatoid arthritis, *97:* 110
ovarian, with antiphospholipid antibody syndrome, *96:* 140
polymyositis and dermatomyositis associated with, *96:* 283
risk and rheumatoid arthritis, *98:* 28
Candidiasis
liver, polyarteritis nodosa mimicking, CT of, *96:* 247
Carbonic anhydrase II
immunization with, inducing autoimmune sialoadenitis (in mice), *97:* 202
Carcinoma
(*See also* Cancer)
renal cell, interleukin-2 and lymphokine activated killer cells for, rapid exacerbation of scleroderma after, *96:* 181
Cardiac (*see* Heart)
Cardiolipin
recognition by monoclonal antibodies to epitopes of oxidized low-density lipoprotein, *98:* 109
Cardiorespiratory
responses to incremental exercise in systemic sclerosis, *98:* 171
Cardiovascular
fitness and health in end-stage osteoarthritis, *97:* 254
Care
of back pain, acute low, outcomes and costs with primary care practitioners, chiropractors and orthopedic surgeons, *97:* 294
continuity of, increasing HMO patients' satisfaction with physician performance, *97:* 15
health (*see* Health, care)
managed, effects on specialty practice at university medical center, *97:* 12
primary (*see* Primary care)
rheumatologic *vs.* nonrheumatologic, of acute arthritis in hospital, *96:* 18
rheumatology specialist, *97:* 19
team managed outpatient, for inflammatory arthritis, early onset chronic, *97:* 24
Carpal
tunnel syndrome surgery, prognostic value of hand symptom diagram in, *98:* 249
Carpometacarpal
joint osteoarthritis and obesity, in women, *98:* 214
Cartilage
articular
abnormalities, needle arthroscopy for, *97:* 251
knee, arthroscopy *vs.* plain radiography and MRI of, *96:* 189
defects, deep, in knee, chondrocyte transplant for, *96:* 197

human, synovial fibroblasts in rheumatoid arthritis attach and invade, when engrafted into SCID mice, *98:* 68
metabolism in rheumatoid arthritis, *96:* 38

Cauda
equina compression by epidural lipomatosis in obesity, *97:* 299

Caudate
nucleus, cerebral blood flow abnormalities in, and low pain thresholds in fibromyalgia in women, *97:* 284

CD4
monoclonal antibody in early rheumatoid arthritis, *97:* 102

CD4+
synovial T cells, Fas^{high}, apoptosis by *Borrelia*-reactive Fas ligand^{high} γδ T cells in Lyme arthritis, *98:* 241

CD40
ligand hyperexpression by B and T cells in systemic lupus erythematosus, *98:* 88

CD56+ cells
T and non-T, impaired recovery and cytolytic function in systemic lupus erythematosus, *98:* 90

CDR
molecular localization of anti-idiotypic anti-DNA antibodies in systemic lupus erythematosus, *97:* 164

Cell(s)
B
CD40 ligand hyperexpression by, in systemic lupus erythematosus, *98:* 88
hyperactivity in systemic lupus erythematosus, and interleukin-10, *96:* 101
blood
red (*see* Erythrocyte)
white (*see* Leukocyte)
endothelial (*see* Endothelium, cells)
gastric mucosal, proliferation, role in gastric adaptation to aspirin (in rat), *96:* 68
giant cell arteritis (*see* Arteritis, giant cell)
killer
lymphokine activated, for renal cell carcinoma, rapid exacerbation of scleroderma after, *96:* 181
natural, in scleroderma, and anti-scl-70 antibodies, *97:* 227
mast, infiltration in salivary glands in early systemic sclerosis, *98:* 155
mononuclear
infiltration in scleroderma, animal model of, *97:* 209
marrow, in Paget's disease, measles virus nucleocapsid mRNA in, *97:* 385
peripheral blood, collagen-stimulated, augmented interleukin-6 secretion in, in scleroderma, *96:* 162
muscle-cell membrane proteins, autoantibodies against, in myositis, *98:* 208
NIH-3T3, α1 (I) procollagen gene expression in, stimulation by HTLV-1 Tax gene, *98:* 147
T (*see* T cell)

Cellular
penetration mechanisms of anti-double strand DNA autoantibody, *98:* 82

Central nervous system
angiitis of, primary, limitation of invasive modalities in diagnosis, *97:* 329
disease
in lupus erythematosus, systemic, and antiphospholipid antibodies, *97:* 145
in lupus erythematosus, systemic, antiribosomal PO protein antibodies and PO fusion protein in, *97:* 162
in Sjögren's syndrome, anti-Ro/SSA autoantibodies in, *96:* 116
vasculitis, sensitivities of noninvasive tests for, *96:* 260

Cerebral
blood flow
abnormalities in fibromyalgia in women, and low pain thresholds, *97:* 284
measurements in fibromyalgia, *97:* 285
dysfunction in fibromyalgia, *97:* 285
ischemia, idiopathic, antiphospholipid antibodies in, in children, *96:* 142

Cerebrospinal fluid
analysis for cerebral dysfunction in fibromyalgia, *97:* 285

Cervical
(*See also* Neck)
epidural analgesia for pain of digital vasculitis secondary to rheumatoid arthritis, *98:* 198
spine (*see* Spine, cervical)

Chemokine
regulation in type II collagen-induced arthritis (in mice), *97:* 226

Chest
CT, high-resolution, in systemic lupus erythematosus, *97:* 189
Children
(*See also* Juvenile)
anemia in, autoimmune hemolytic, with MHC class II deficiency, *96:* 130
antinuclear antibody test in, positive, without autoimmune disease, *97:* 178
born to mothers with silicone breast implants, lack of autoantibody expression in, *97:* 381
cerebral ischemia in, idiopathic, antiphospholipid antibodies in, *96:* 142
connective tissue disease in, systemic, incidence of, *96:* 276
dermatomyositis in, mineral metabolism in, *96:* 216
fibromyalgia syndrome in, outcome, *97:* 283
gastroduodenal injury in, NSAID-induced, *97:* 117
heart block in, congenital
autoantibody-associated, outcome, *96:* 117
complete, long-term outcome of mothers of children with, *98:* 105
Lyme arthritis in, clinical spectrum and outcome, *96:* 292
Lyme disease in, pitfalls in diagnosis and treatment, *97:* 386
methotrexate bioavailability in, oral, influence of food on, *97:* 72
scleroderma progression in, linear, to fatal systemic sclerosis, *96:* 164
Chills
in Lyme borreliosis, early, with erythema migrans, *98:* 237
Chiropractic
vs. hospital outpatient management of low back pain, *97:* 293
Chiropractor
care for acute low back pain, outcomes and costs, *97:* 294
Chloroquine
in rheumatoid arthritis
early, *vs.* low-dose cyclosporine, *96:* 80
reducing bioavailability of methotrexate, *96:* 58
vs. phenytoin and auranofin, *97:* 61
Choctaw Indians
in Oklahoma, increased prevalence of systemic sclerosis in, *98:* 163
Chondrocyte
transplant for deep cartilage defects in knee, *96:* 197
Churg-Strauss syndrome
corticosteroids, pulse cyclophosphamide and plasma exchanges in, factors predicting poor prognosis, *97:* 316
with polyarteritis nodosa, outcome, *96:* 248
Cigarette
smoking and rheumatoid arthritis lung disease, *98:* 26
Cloning
repertoire, of lupus anti-DNA autoantibodies, *98:* 85
Cloxacillin
/dexamethasone in experimental *Staphylococcus aureus* arthritis, *98:* 233
cM-T412
methotrexate and, in rheumatoid arthritis, *97:* 103
CNS (*see* Central nervous system)
Coccidioidomycosis
after melphalan in primary amyloidosis, *98:* 268
Cod-liver oil
capsules, lipoid pneumonia, and rheumatoid arthritis, *98:* 261
Cognitive
decline in elderly, and nonsteroidal antiinflammatory drugs, *97:* 125
COL5A1
exon skipping mutation of, in Ehlers-Danlos syndrome, *98:* 275
Colchicine
in amyloidosis
AA, of familial Mediterranean fever, *96:* 307
primary, *98:* 268
Cold
sensitivity, cooling in, digital vascular responses to, *98:* 183
treatment, local, effects on temperature of arthritic knees, *96:* 72
Collagen
degradation products, cross-linked, in urine in scleroderma, *97:* 224
disease, heart involvement in, *96:* 165
gene expression during postnatal skin development and fibrosis (in mice), *97:* 230
-induced arthritis (*see* Arthritis, collagen-induced)
peptide, oral immunodominant human, modulating collagen-induced arthritis, *97:* 38

-stimulated peripheral blood mononuclear cells in scleroderma, augmented interleukin-6 secretion in, *96:* 162
synthesis, heterogeneity in normal and systemic sclerosis skin fibroblasts, *98:* 148
type I
binding region for *Yersinia enterocolitica* adhesion YadA on, *97:* 337
gene expression in fascial fibroblasts in diffuse fasciitis with eosinophilia, *98:* 203
type II, binding region for *Yersinia enterocolitica* adhesion YadA on, *97:* 337
type III gene expression in fascial fibroblasts in diffuse fasciitis with eosinophilia, *98:* 203
type IV, α3 chain of, inducing autoimmune Goodpasture syndrome, *96:* 262
type V gene mutation, exon skipping, in Ehlers-Danlos syndrome, *98:* 275
type VI gene expression in fascial fibroblasts in diffuse fasciitis with eosinophilia, *98:* 203
type VII in skin in scleroderma, transforming growth factor-β regulating, *96:* 163
vascular disease, histopathologic spectrum of palisaded neutrophilic and granulomatous dermatitis in, *96:* 120
Collagenase
gene expression, synoviocyte, inhibition by adenosine receptor stimulation, *98:* 145
levels and joint involvement in osteoarthritis, *96:* 204
Complement
C1q deficiency, hereditary, in systemic lupus erythematosus, *96:* 126
receptor 1, erythrocyte, antigen-based heteropolymers for binding and clearing autoantibodies via, *96:* 94
serum, determinations in quiescent systemic lupus erythematosus, *98:* 120
Compression
cauda equina, by epidural lipomatosis in obesity, *97:* 299
Computed tomography
in alveolitis, fibrosing, in scleroderma, *96:* 172
in bursitis, tuberculous, *98:* 235
chest, high-resolution, in systemic lupus erythematosus, *97:* 189
of lung involvement, discrete, in systemic lupus erythematosus, *97:* 175
postcontrast, of polyarteritis nodosa mimicking liver candidiasis, *96:* 247
in tenosynovitis, tuberculous, *98:* 235
of tophi in knee, intraarticular, *98:* 222
in vasculitis, CNS, *96:* 260
Computerized
databases for diagnosis of rheumatoid arthritis, sensitivity and specificity of, *96:* 13
heart rate variability of autonomic dysfunction in diffuse scleroderma *vs.* CREST, *96:* 173
Connective tissue
disease
anti-chromo antibodies in, *96:* 148
mixed, differentiation, HLA type as predictor of, *96:* 104
mixed, pulmonary hypertension in, diltiazem and oxygen for, *96:* 180
pulmonary hypertension in, long-term iloprost infusion in, *96:* 177
risk after breast implant, *96:* 301
systemic, incidence in children, *96:* 276
undifferentiated, methotrexate in, *98:* 123
growth factor gene expression in systemic sclerosis, *97:* 216
Cooling
digital pressure responses to, in scleroderma *vs.* Raynaud's phenomenon, *96:* 175
digital vascular responses to, in subjects with cold sensitivity, primary Raynaud's phenomenon, or scleroderma spectrum disorders, *98:* 183
Corticosteroid(s)
(*See also* Steroids)
-induced bone loss in postmenopausal women, etidronate with ergocalciferol in prevention of, *97:* 277
-induced osteoporosis (*see* Osteoporosis, corticosteroid-induced)
injection
local, for trochanteric bursitis, *98:* 248
in rheumatoid arthritis does not increase rate of total joint arthroplasty, *98:* 53

single, cortisol level reduction after, *97:* 132
in joint destruction in rheumatoid arthritis, *97:* 134
low-dose, in rheumatoid arthritis
effect on bone mineral density, *97:* 133
effectiveness of, moderate-term, *98:* 54
long-term, serious adverse events in, *96:* 78
spinal bone loss secondary to, calcium and vitamin D_3 supplementation in prevention of, *98:* 56
oral, and prevention of secondary osteoporosis, *98:* 225
plus antibiotics in *Staphylococcus aureus* arthritis, experimental, *98:* 232
in polyarteritis nodosa and Churg-Strauss syndrome, factors predicting poor prognosis, *97:* 316
regenerative repair of epithelium in gastric ulcers reduced by (in rat), *97:* 130
Cortisol
level reduction after single steroid injection, *97:* 132
response, impaired, in active rheumatoid arthritis, *98:* 51
Cost(s)
of back pain care, low, by primary care practitioners, chiropractors and orthopedic surgeons, *97:* 294
direct, of fibromyalgia treatment, *97:* 280
of drug therapy for rheumatoid arthritis, total, *96:* 7
effectiveness
of hip arthroplasty, total, for hip osteoarthritis, *97:* 271
of liver biopsy in rheumatoid arthritis with methotrexate, *97:* 80
of MRI in polymyositis, *97:* 352
of urate lowering drugs in recurrent gouty arthritis, *97:* 365
indirect and nonmedical, in rheumatoid arthritis and osteoarthritis, *98:* 6
medical, direct, unique to arthritis patients, *98:* 7
of misoprostol prophylaxis for rheumatoid arthritis with nonsteroidal antiinflammatory drugs, *96:* 65
savings with nonsteroidal anti-inflammatory drugs, stepped-care prescribing protocol, *97:* 5
Cough
after methotrexate, approach to, *97:* 86
C1q
antibodies to, changes predicting kidney relapses in systemic lupus erythematosus, *97:* 159
C-reactive protein (*see* Protein, C-reactive)
CREST
autonomic dysfunction in, *96:* 173
Cryoglobulinemia
with hepatitis C virus, interferon alfa-2a in, *96:* 254
mixed
monoclonal, cross-reactive idiotypes, as predictive factor for development of lymphoma in primary Sjögren's syndrome, *98:* 136
type II, interferon-α and 6-methylprednisolone in, *96:* 251
Crystal
calcium pyrophosphate dihydrate crystal-induced tenosynovitis, acute, *97:* 368
-induced diseases, *97:* 365; *96:* 297
-induced synovitis, acute, ACTH for, *96:* 297
-related arthropathies, *98:* 220
submicroscopic, in osteoarthritic synovial fluids, *96:* 300
urate in tophaceous tissue samples, formalin dissolving, *96:* 299
CT (*see* Computed tomography)
CTLA41g
for lupus erythematosus, systemic (in mice), *96:* 138
Culture(s)
-confirmed erythema migrans and early Lyme borreliosis, clinical spectrum of, *98:* 237
scleroderma fibroblast
dermatan sulfate proteoglycan synthesis altered in, *98:* 158
interleukin-4 expression in, *98:* 152
Cutaneous
(*See also* Skin)
fibrosis in scleroderma, animal model of, *97:* 209
lupus erythematosus
chronic, and HLA class II alleles, *96:* 98
subacute, due to calcium channel blockers, *98:* 117

sclerosis, and connective tissue growth factor gene expression, in scleroderma, *97:* 216
Cyclophosphamide
-induced cystitis in Wegener's granulomatosis, *97:* 305
IV, in lupus nephritis, economic impact of treatment, *96:* 10
oral bolus, outpatient monthly, in systemic lupus erythematosus, *97:* 184
pulse
in lupus erythematosus, systemic (in mice), *98:* 127
with plasmapheresis, in systemic lupus erythematosus remission, *96:* 133
in polyarteritis nodosa and Churg-Strauss syndrome, *97:* 316
in Wegener's granulomatosis, response to, and antineutrophil cytoplasmic antibodies, *96:* 238
in rheumatoid arthritis, effects on development of malignancy and long-term survival, *97:* 110
in scleroderma, lung function improvement after, *96:* 179
Cyclosporine
in autoimmune diseases, and grapefruit juice, *98:* 124
in rheumatoid arthritis
benefit/risk ratio with, *96:* 84
early, *vs.* chloroquine, *96:* 80
low-dose, *96:* 82
low-dose long-term, effect on kidney function, *97:* 108
renal biopsy findings and follow-up of renal function and, *98:* 49
severe, *vs.* methotrexate, *97:* 106
Cyst
synovial, bicipital, in juvenile rheumatoid arthritis, *97:* 344
Cysteine
extra, in FBN1 polypeptide in novel variant of Marfan's syndrome, *96:* 306
Cystitis
cyclophosphamide-induced, in Wegener's granulomatosis, *97:* 305
Cytokine
chemotactic novel, for neutrophils in arthritis, *96:* 33
endothelium-derived, involvement in scleroderma, immunoglobulin G antiendothelial cell autoantibodies inducing, *97:* 205
production
in osteoarthritis, early, and synovial membrane inflammation, *98:* 217
in POEMS syndrome, effect of all-*trans*-retinoic acid on, *98:* 264
in psoriatic arthritis, *96:* 269
profiles, tissue, in giant cell arteritis, *98:* 188
Cytology
aspiration, ultrasound-guided fine-needle, of non-palpable supraclavicular lymph nodes in sarcoidosis, *98:* 273
Cytolytic
function of CD56+ T and non-T cells in systemic lupus erythematosus, *98:* 90
Cytotoxic
products, transformation of lupus-inducing drugs to, by activated neutrophils, *96:* 131
therapy complications distinguished from vasculitic disease activity by antineutrophil cytoplasmic antibody assay, *96:* 240
Cytoxan (*see* Cyclophosphamide)

D

Database
computerized, for diagnosis of rheumatoid arthritis, sensitivity and specificity of, *96:* 13
online biomedical, in rheumatology, performance of, *96:* 11
Death
antirheumatic drugs causing, in rheumatoid arthritis, *97:* 111
in temporal arteritis, *96:* 212
Dehydroepiandrosterone
in lupus erythematosus, systemic, trial results, *97:* 194
Deoxyribonucleic acid (*see* DNA)
Depression
major, and low lumbar bone mineral density, *96:* 207
Dermatan
sulfate proteoglycan synthesis alteration in fibroblast skin cultures in systemic sclerosis, *98:* 158
Dermatitis
neutrophilic and granulomatous, palisaded, in collagen vascular disease, histopathologic spectrum of, *96:* 120
Dermatomyositis
amyopathic and myopathic, muscle dysfunction in, *96:* 279
cancer associated with, *96:* 283

cutaneous lesions of, microvascular injury in pathogenesis of, *97:* 353
management, MRI and magnetic resonance spectroscopy in, *96:* 281
mineral metabolism in, *96:* 216
Dexamethasone
/cloxacillin in experimental *Staphylococcus aureus* arthritis, *98:* 233
Dialysis
arthropathy, outcome after kidney transplant, *97:* 387
Diarrhea
after colchicine in primary amyloidosis, *98:* 268
after zolpidem in fibromyalgia, *98:* 256
Diclofenac
in rheumatoid arthritis, salsalate as efficacious as, *97:* 118
Dietary
intake related to progression of osteoarthritis of knee, *98:* 219
Digital
artery occlusion due to interferon, *98:* 182
pressure responses to cooling in scleroderma *vs.* Raynaud's phenomenon, *96:* 175
ulcers, ischemic, in systemic sclerosis, IV iloprost for, *98:* 184
vascular responses to cooling in subjects with cold sensitivity, primary Raynaud's phenomenon, or scleroderma spectrum disorders, *98:* 183
vasculitis secondary to rheumatoid arthritis, cervical epidural analgesia for pain of, *98:* 198
Diltiazem
for calcinosis, *97:* 351
lupus erythematosus due to, subacute cutaneous, *98:* 118
with oxygen in pulmonary hypertension of mixed connective tissue disease, *96:* 180
in scleroderma, left ventricular myocardial perfusion and function after, *98:* 176
Diphtheria
fusion protein, interleukin-2, for refractory rheumatoid arthritis, *97:* 100
Disability
development with age, and running, *96:* 191
fibromyalgia syndrome and, *98:* 254
functional, in rheumatoid arthritis, changes in, and rheumatology visit frequency, *98:* 8
in rheumatoid arthritis, long-term, reduction with antirheumatic drug-based treatment strategies, *97:* 2
work, predictors in rheumatoid arthritis, follow-up, *97:* 58
Diuretics
gout and, *98:* 222
DNA
amplification detecting *Borrelia burgdorferi* in synovial tissue in Lyme arthritis, *98:* 236
antibodies
double-stranded, circulating titer reduction after LJP 394, *98:* 126
to histone DNA complexes, more sensitive and specific for scleroderma than lupus, *96:* 153
anti-DNA autoantibodies
double strand, mechanisms of cellular penetration and nuclear localization of, *98:* 82
lupus, repertoire cloning of, *98:* 85
anti-double stranded, antiidiotypes to, some autoantibodies to Ro/SS-A and La/SS-B are, *98:* 100
antigen, cross-reactivity with IgG anti-F(ab')$_2$ antibody, *98:* 104
bacterial, immunization with, induction of cross-reactive anti-dsDNA antibodies by (in mice), *96:* 112
binding protein, viral, generating SLE-related autoimmunity to double-stranded DNA and histones, *97:* 139
Borrelia burgdorferi, undetectable by polymerase chain reaction in skin lesions of morphea, scleroderma, or lichen sclerosus et atrophicus in North American patients, *98:* 242
mimics self-protein as target for anti-DNA antibodies in systemic lupus erythematosus, *96:* 107
polymorphisms, HLA and T cell receptor β-chain, in pauciarticular-onset juvenile rheumatoid arthritis, *96:* 275
topoisomerase I, T cell proliferative response due to, in scleroderma, *97:* 219
Doppler
echocardiography
for cardiac involvement in limited systemic sclerosis, *98:* 173

for pulmonary hypertension in limited and diffuse scleroderma, *98:* 168
ultrasound, color-flow, for renal vascular damage in systemic sclerosis, *98:* 177
Dorsal
root ganglionitis with Sjögren's syndrome, anti-dorsal root ganglion neuron antibody in, *97:* 199
Doxycycline
activation of neutrophil procollagenase in presence of, enzyme fragmentation and activity loss after, *97:* 259
Dreaming
abnormal, after zolpidem in fibromyalgia, *98:* 256
Drug(s)
antiinflammatory (*see* Antiinflammatory, drugs)
antirheumatic (*see* Antirheumatic drugs)
lupus-inducing, transformation to cytotoxic products by activated neutrophils, *96:* 131
studies published in symposium proceedings, quality of, *97:* 136
therapy in rheumatoid arthritis (*see* Rheumatoid arthritis, drug therapy in)
Duodenal
ulcer, NSAID-induced, prevention of
famotidine for, *98:* 40
misoprostol dosage for, *97:* 116
Dust
quartz, uranium miners exposed to, anti-CENP-B response of, and scleroderma, *97:* 217
Dystrophy
reflex sympathetic, bone scintigraphy in diagnosis, *97:* 290

E

Echocardiography
Doppler
for cardiac involvement in limited systemic sclerosis, *98:* 173
for pulmonary hypertension in limited and diffuse scleroderma, *98:* 168
transesophageal and transthoracic, in cardiac sarcoidosis masquerading as metastatic tumor, *97:* 355
Echography
in myositis, idiopathic orbital, *96:* 288
Economic
burden of musculoskeletal disorders, in Canada, *96:* 15
impact of lupus nephritis treatment with prednisone and IV cyclophosphamide, *96:* 10
Economics, *98:* 6; *97:* 4; *96:* 4
Edema
pitting, synovitis with, remitting seronegative symmetrical, clinical spectrum of, *98:* 276
Education
in fibromyalgia in women, *96:* 228
medical, continuing, in rheumatic diseases for primary care physicians, *97:* 21
rheumatology, in general practice, trainee study, *97:* 22
Ehlers-Danlos syndrome
exon skipping mutation of type V collagen gene in, *98:* 275
Elastin
degradation products, cross-linked, in urine in scleroderma, *97:* 224
Elderly
arthropathies in, idiopathic destructive, *98:* 223
cognitive decline in, and nonsteroidal antiinflammatory drugs, *97:* 125
glomerular filtration rate in, acute and chronic effects of nonsteroidal antiinflammatory drugs on, *97:* 113
joint symptoms with exercise in, *97:* 274
ketorolac in, intramuscular, gastrointestinal complications of, *97:* 119
kidney dysfunction in, indomethacin-induced, misoprostol protective effect on, *97:* 123
musculoskeletal pain related to running in, *98:* 215
osteoporosis in, in women (*see* Osteoporosis, postmenopausal)
rheumatoid arthritis in
protein metabolism and, *98:* 38
self-reported, validity of, in women, *98:* 32
walking velocity in, determinants of, *96:* 43
Electrical stimulation
pulsed, for knee osteoarthritis, *97:* 261
Electromagnetic
fields, pulsed, for osteoarthritis of knee and cervical spine, *96:* 201
Electron
microscopy
of arthropathies, idiopathic destructive, *98:* 223

in liver biopsy after methotrexate for rheumatoid arthritis, *97:* 82
ELISA
anti-Sm, anti-RNP, anti-Ro/SS-A, and anti-La/SS-B antibodies detected by, utility for diagnosis of systemic lupus erythematosus, *98:* 99
for interleukin-2 receptors, soluble serum, in systemic sclerosis, *98:* 151
for quantification of antiribosomal PO protein antibodies in CNS disease in systemic lupus erythematosus, *97:* 162
Employment
status, initial, of physicians completing training in 1994, *97:* 14
Enalapril
in hypertension, *97:* 121
Endothelin-1
levels, circulating, in scleroderma subsets, *96:* 157
localization and binding sites in scleroderma skin, *96:* 154
production in fibroblasts from scleroderma, *96:* 156
Endothelium
activated, in vascular injury in systemic lupus erythematosus, *97:* 168
cell(s)
anti-endothelial cell antibodies in vasculitis, pathogenic role of (in mice), *98:* 192
apoptosis in scleroderma, *98:* 160
scleroderma, class II MHC and ICAM-1 expression on, up-regulation by interferon-gamma and tumor necrosis factor-α, in early disease stage, *98:* 143
vascular, leukocyte adhesion to, immunoglobulin G antiendothelial cell autoantibodies from scleroderma inducing, *97:* 205
Enzyme
fragmentation and activity loss after activation of neutrophil procollagenase in presence of doxycycline, *97:* 259
immunoassay for antinuclear antibodies, *98:* 98
-linked immunosorbent assay (*see* ELISA)
Eosinophil
major basic protein, elevated levels in scleroderma, *97:* 228
Eosinophilia
peripheral, with diffuse fasciitis, *Borrelia burgdorferi* in, *96:* 289
Eosinophilic
fasciitis
diffuse, increased expression of transforming growth factor-β1, fibronectin, and collagen genes in fascial fibroblasts in, *98:* 203
idiopathic, with renal involvement, methotrexate in, *97:* 249
Epidemiology, *98:* 1
Epidermal
growth factor-like motifs of FBN1 polypeptide, extra cysteine in, in novel variant of Marfan's syndrome, *96:* 306
Epidural
analgesia, cervical, for pain of digital vasculitis secondary to rheumatoid arthritis, *98:* 198
lipomatosis, cauda equina compression by, in obesity, *97:* 299
Epilepsy
antiphospholipid antibodies and, in systemic lupus erythematosus, *96:* 144
Epithelium
neutrophil activating peptide-78, in arthritis, *96:* 33
regenerative repair in gastric ulcer, corticosteroids reducing (in rat), *97:* 130
Epitopes
of oxidized phospholipids, antiphospholipid antibodies directed against, *98:* 109
Epstein-Barr virus
clonality in lymphomas in rheumatoid arthritis, *98:* 30
infection in methotrexate-related B lymphoproliferative disease in rheumatoid arthritis, *97:* 88
Ergocalciferol
with etidronate to prevent glucocorticoid-induced bone loss in postmenopausal women, *97:* 277
Erythema
migrans
azithromycin *vs.* amoxicillin in, *98:* 239
culture-confirmed, with early Lyme borreliosis, clinical spectrum of, *98:* 237
Erythrocyte
complement receptor 1, antigen-based heteropolymers for binding and clearing autoantibodies via, *96:* 94

/leukocyte casts appearance, urinary, and onset of renal relapse in systemic lupus erythematosus, *97:* 174
sedimentation rate
as marker for articular destruction in rheumatoid arthritis, *98:* 33
normal, polymyalgia rheumatica with, *97:* 322
Erythropoietin
for anemia in rheumatoid arthritis, *96:* 64
Escherichia coli
dnaJ heat shock protein, immune responses to, in juvenile rheumatoid arthritis, *96:* 278
E-selectin
expression in salivary glands in early systemic sclerosis, *98:* 155
Esophagitis
alendronate causing, *98:* 231
Esophagus
ulceration due to alendronate, *98:* 232
Estrogen
exogenous, safety of use by women with systemic lupus erythematosus, *97:* 188
scleroderma fibroblasts and, *96:* 158
Ethnicity
in lupus erythematosus, systemic, *97:* 154
myositis and relation of MHC class II alleles and autoantibodies in, *98:* 207
Etidronate
cyclical
with ergocalciferol to prevent glucocorticoid-induced bone loss in postmenopausal women, *97:* 277
intermittent, in postmenopausal osteoporosis, *96:* 217
in osteoporosis, corticosteroid-induced, for prevention, *98:* 6
in osteoporosis, corticosteroid-induced, reversing bone loss of spine and femur, *97:* 278
Exercise
for back pain, acute low, *96:* 2
incremental, in systemic sclerosis, cardiorespiratory responses to, *98:* 171
joint symptoms with, in elderly, *97:* 274
muscle oxygen uptake reduction during, in systemic lupus erythematosus, *97:* 155
after ovariectomy (in rat), *96:* 210
Exon
skipping mutation of type V collagen gene in Ehlers-Danlos syndrome, *98:* 275
Extracellular
matrix-degrading phenotype in lung fibroblasts, relaxin-induced, *98:* 142

F

Family
history and gout, *98:* 222
physicians' *vs.* rheumatologists' perceptions of indications for and outcomes of knee replacement, *98:* 11
Famotidine
in prevention of ulcers, NSAID-induced gastric and duodenal, *98:* 40
Fas
expression in salivary glands in primary Sjögren's syndrome, *98:* 133
ligand
expression in salivary glands in primary Sjögren's syndrome, *98:* 133
mutation in systemic lupus erythematosus and lymphoproliferative disease, *98:* 89
ligand^{high} $\gamma\delta$ T cells, *Borrelia*-reactive, in Lyme arthritis, apoptosis of Fas^{high} CD4+ synovial T cells by, *98:* 241
soluble, accumulation in inflamed joints in rheumatoid arthritis, *98:* 24
Fas^{high}
CD4+ synovial cell apoptosis by *Borrelia*-reactive Fas ligand^{high} $\gamma\delta$ T cells in Lyme arthritis, *98:* 241
Fascial
fibroblasts in diffuse fasciitis with eosinophilia, expression of transforming growth factor-β1, fibronectin, and collagen genes in, *98:* 203
Fasciitis
diffuse, *Borrelia burgdorferi* in, *96:* 289
eosinophilic, *98:* 203
diffuse, increased expression of transforming growth factor-β1, fibronectin, and collagen genes in fascial fibroblasts in, *98:* 203
idiopathic, with renal involvement, methotrexate in, *97:* 249
Fatigue
in Lyme borreliosis, early, with erythema migrans, *98:* 237

Fatty acid
supplement, omega-3, in active rheumatoid arthritis, *96:* 77
FBN1 polypeptide
extra cysteine in, in novel variant of Marfan's syndrome, *96:* 306
Fcγ receptor
II-mediated signal transduction, effect of tumor necrosis factor-induced integrin activation on, *97:* 309
-specific autoantibodies, circulating, in scleroderma, *97:* 213
Febrile
polyarthritis due to acute rheumatic fever in adults, *98:* 269
Feeding
breast (*see* Breast, feeding)
Fellowship
in musculoskeletal medicine, extended, opinions of recent and current rheumatology fellows about, *96:* 12
Femur
bone loss in corticosteroid-induced osteoporosis, etidronate reversing, *97:* 278
neck mechanical strength decrease after ovariectomy, exercise protecting against (in rat), *96:* 210
Fever
in arthritis, minocycline-induced, *98:* 196
in Lyme borreliosis, early, with erythema migrans, *98:* 237
Mediterranean, familial, AA amyloidosis of, colchicine for, *96:* 307
after methotrexate, approach to, *97:* 86
rheumatic
acute, in adults, delayed diagnosis of, *98:* 269
Jones criteria for diagnosis, guideline maintenance and revision, *97:* 9
Fibrillarin
autoantibodies to, in scleroderma, *98:* 159
Fibrinolysis
markers in Raynaud's phenomenon and scleroderma, *97:* 208
Fibroblast(s)
fascial, in diffuse fasciitis with eosinophilia, expression of transforming growth factor-β1, fibronectin, and collagen genes in, *98:* 203
function in psoriatic arthritis, *96:* 269
lung, effects of relaxin on, *98:* 142
scleroderma
cultures, interleukin-4 expression in, *98:* 152
endothelin-1 production increase in, *96:* 156
ICAM-1 and class II MHC expression on, up-regulation by interferon-gamma and tumor necrosis factor-α, in early disease stage, *98:* 143
ICAM-1 and lymphocyte function-associated antigen 3 in, *96:* 158
skin, cultures, altered dermatan sulfate proteoglycan synthesis in, *98:* 158
skin, heterogeneity of collagen synthesis in, *98:* 148
skin, heterogeneity of collagen synthesis in, *98:* 148
synovial, in rheumatoid arthritis attach and invade human cartilage when engrafted into SCID mice, *98:* 68
Fibromyalgia, *98:* 250; *97:* 280; *96:* 219
cerebral blood flow abnormalities and low pain thresholds in, in women, *97:* 284
cerebral dysfunction in, *97:* 285
education and physical training for women with, *96:* 228
fluoxetine/amitriptyline in, *98:* 257
orthostatic sympathetic derangement in, *98:* 252
patients, psychiatric diagnoses in, related to health care-seeking behavior rather than to illness, *98:* 259
pressure pain sensibility increase in, *97:* 288
prevalence and characteristics in general population, *96:* 223
rate increase after cervical spine injury, *98:* 250
in rheumatology practice, in Canada, *97:* 281
sexual abuse in women with, prevalence, *96:* 227
skeletal muscle of, increased incidence of a resonance in phosphodiester region of ^{31}P nuclear magnetic resonance spectra in, *96:* 220
with spinal pain, prevalence and treatment outcome, *97:* 282
syndrome
in children, outcome, *97:* 283
disability and, consensus report, *98:* 254
not associated with muscle energy metabolism abnormalities, *96:* 219

primary, ondansetron in, *98:* 256
sexual and physical abuse in women with, *96:* 225
study of, prospective long-term, *98:* 253
substance P CSF level elevation in, *96:* 220
tender point counts as evidence of, *96:* 222
tender point scores assessed by manual palpation in, reliability of, *97:* 287
treatment
cost of, direct, *97:* 280
group, *98:* 255
zolpidem in, *98:* 255
Fibronectin
expression in fascial fibroblasts in diffuse fasciitis with eosinophilia, *98:* 203
Fibrosing
alveolitis (*see* Alveolitis, fibrosing)
Fibrosis
cutaneous, in scleroderma, animal model of, *97:* 209
pulmonary
antihistone antibodies in scleroderma and, *96:* 169
bleomycin-induced, effects of relaxin on (in mice), *98:* 142
fatal, complicating low-dose methotrexate therapy in rheumatoid arthritis, *97:* 83
in sclerosis, systemic, and elevated serum tumor necrosis factor-α levels, *98:* 156
in scleroderma, and interleukin-4 expression, *98:* 152
skin, postnatal development, transforming growth growth factor-β1 and collagen gene expression during (in mice), *97:* 230
Finger
bone destruction progression in, in rheumatoid arthritis, *96:* 28
joints, gouty arthritis and nodal osteoarthritis in, *98:* 221
Fish oil
high-dose, in rheumatoid arthritis after stopping nonsteroidal antiinflammatory drugs, *97:* 129
Flulike
symptoms after zolpidem in fibromyalgia, *98:* 256
Fluoxetine
/amitriptyline in fibromyalgia, *98:* 257
Flushing
after iloprost in systemic sclerosis, *98:* 184
α-Fodrin
as autoantigen in primary Sjögren's syndrome, *98:* 131
Folic acid
supplement during methotrexate therapy in rheumatoid arthritis, *96:* 57
Food
influence on oral methotrexate bioavailability in children, *97:* 72
Foot
problems in rheumatoid arthritis, *96:* 49
surgery in psoriasis, *96:* 272
Formalin
dissolving urate crystals in tophaceous tissue samples, *96:* 299
Fracture
nonvertebral, prevention with alendronate in postmenopausal osteoporosis, *98:* 227
in postmenopausal women, long-term effects of calcium supplementation on, *97:* 275
risk
in osteoporosis, and high-intensity strength training, *96:* 208
in spondylitis, ankylosing, *96:* 266
in women with existing vertebral fractures, effect of alendronate on, *98:* 229
Free radical
-mediated injury in scleroderma, *98:* 161

G

Gamma-linoleic acid
in rheumatoid arthritis, *98:* 63
Ganglionitis
dorsal root, with Sjögren's syndrome, anti-dorsal root ganglion neuron antibody in, *97:* 199
Gangrene
prevention with IV iloprost in systemic sclerosis, *98:* 184
Gastric
(*See also* Gastrointestinal)
adaptation to aspirin, role of gastric blood flow, neutrophil infiltration and mucosal cell proliferation in (in rat), *96:* 68
blood flow, role in gastric adaptation to aspirin (in rat), *96:* 68
mucosa

cell proliferation, role in gastric adaptation to aspirin (in rat), *96:* 68
prostaglandin levels, age-related reductions in, increasing susceptibility to aspirin-induced injury (in rat), *96:* 69
ulcer (*see* Ulcer, gastric)
Gastroduodenal
injury, NSAID-induced, in children, *97:* 117
Gastrointestinal
(*See also* Gastric; Intestine)
complications
of ketorolac, in elderly, *97:* 119
in rheumatoid arthritis with nonsteroidal antiinflammatory drugs, misoprostol reducing, *97:* 114
tract, lupus vasculitis of, three-phase abdominal scintigraphy in, *97:* 177
Gender
differences in major orthopedic surgery for degenerative arthritis, *96:* 187
Gene(s)
collagen
expression during postnatal skin development and fibrosis (in mice), *97:* 230
type V, exon skipping mutation, in Ehlers-Danlos syndrome, *98:* 275
types I, III, and VI, expression in fascial fibroblasts in diffuse fasciitis with eosinophilia, *98:* 203
collagenase, synoviocyte, expression inhibited by adenosine receptor stimulation, *98:* 145
connective tissue growth factor, expression in scleroderma, *97:* 216
HLA
class II, and anticentromere antibody in scleroderma, *97:* 212
-DRB1, and disease severity in rheumatoid arthritis, *98:* 21
-DRB and -DQB, and outcome in rheumatoid arthritis, *97:* 35
MHC class II, and anti-U1 small nuclear ribonucleoprotein antibody, *96:* 97
PiZ, of alpha-1 antitrypsin, in outcome of PR3-ANCA positive vasculitis, *97:* 312
procollagen, α1 (I), expression in NIH-3T3 cells stimulated by HTLV-1 Tax gene, *98:* 147
Tax, HTLV-1, stimulation of α1 (I) procollagen gene expression in NIH-3T3 cells by, *98:* 147
transfer to synovium, retrovirus-mediated, in bacterial cell wall-induced arthritis (in rat), *97:* 105
tumor necrosis factor-α, expression by alveolar macrophages in lung transplant recipient with recurrence of sarcoidosis, *98:* 272
Genetic
anticipation in familial rheumatoid arthritis, *96:* 30
further evidence for, *98:* 20
association of juvenile rheumatoid arthritis and interleukin-1α polymorphism, *96:* 274
associations with rheumatoid arthritis, and prolactin, *98:* 39
epidemiology of rheumatoid arthritis, *97:* 37
typing in inflammatory arthritis, outcome prediction in, *96:* 31
Genetics
in rheumatoid arthritis, *97:* 33; *96:* 28
Giant cell arteritis (*see* Arteritis, giant cell)
Glomerular
deposits in lupus nephritis, nucleosomes and histones in, *98:* 93
filtration rate, in elderly, acute and chronic effects of nonsteroidal antiinflammatory drugs on, *97:* 113
Glomerulonephritis
in chronic granulomatous disease and systemic lupus erythematosus, *97:* 156
Glucocorticoids (*see* Corticosteroids)
Glycoprotein
α_1-acid, as marker for articular destruction in rheumatoid arthritis, *98:* 33
-I
β_2-, and antiphospholipid autoantibody binding to apoptotic thymocytes, *98:* 108
β_2-, in placenta in antiphospholipid antibody syndrome, *96:* 145
anti-β_2-, and antiphospholipid syndrome in systemic lupus erythematosus, *97:* 147
anti-β_2-, antibodies, in monozygotic twin sisters, *96:* 139
Gold
in rheumatoid arthritis
early, *97:* 63
second course of, *97:* 62
Gonococcal
arthritis, *96:* 309

Goodpasture syndrome
autoimmune, α3 chain of type IV collagen inducing, *96:* 262
Gout
of spine, *97:* 369
tuberculous arthritis and, *98:* 222
Gouty arthritis (*see* Arthritis, gouty)
Granuloma
silicone, in acral skin, in patient with silicone gel breast implants and scleroderma, *97:* 379
Granulomatosis
Wegener's (*see* Wegener's granulomatosis)
Granulomatous
dermatitis in collagen vascular disease, histopathologic spectrum of, *96:* 120
disease, chronic, and glomerulonephritis, *97:* 156
Grapefruit
juice, and cyclosporine in autoimmune diseases, *98:* 124
Group
treatment of fibromyalgia, *98:* 255
Growth
factor
connective tissue, gene expression in scleroderma, *97:* 216
epidermal growth factor-like motifs of FBN1 polypeptide, extra cysteine in, in novel variant of Marfan's syndrome, *96:* 306
insulin-like, in Werner syndrome with osteoporosis, *96:* 209
platelet-derived, β, receptors, expression increase in psoriatic arthritis, *96:* 269
platelet-derived, in bronchoalveolar lavage fluid from scleroderma, *97:* 214
production increase in psoriatic arthritis, *96:* 269
transforming (*see* Transforming growth factor)
Guidelines, *98:* 2
for monitoring drug therapy in rheumatoid arthritis, *98:* 2
Gut
inflammation in psoriatic arthritis, ileocolonoscopy of, *97:* 338

H

Hand
osteoarthritis
obesity and, in women, *98:* 213
yoga-based regimen for, *96:* 200
rheumatoid arthritis, radiography of, *97:* 46
symptom diagram in surgery for carpal tunnel syndrome, prognostic value of, *98:* 249
Headache
after iloprost in systemic sclerosis, *98:* 184
in Lyme borreliosis, early, with erythema migrans, *98:* 237
after zolpidem in fibromyalgia, *98:* 256
Health
care, *98:* 15
-seeking behavior, psychiatric diagnoses in fibromyalgia patients related to, *98:* 259
system, evolving, role of rheumatologist in, *96:* 19
outcomes of telephone interventions in rheumatoid arthritis or osteoarthritis, *98:* 10
sciences, *98:* 1
Hearing
loss, autoimmune, methotrexate for, *96:* 310
Heart
block
complete, congenital, long-term outcome of mothers of children with, *98:* 105
complete, in adult with Sjögren's syndrome and anti-Ro/SS-A autoantibodies, *98:* 139
congenital, autoantibody-associated, outcome, *96:* 117
dysfunction, subsequent, in systemic sclerosis, thallium perfusion defects predict, *98:* 175
involvement
in collagen diseases, *96:* 165
in sclerosis, limited systemic, comprehensive noninvasive assessment of, *98:* 173
rate
resting, in systemic lupus erythematosus disease activity assessment, *96:* 118
variability, computerized, in autonomic dysfunction in diffuse scleroderma *vs.* CREST, *96:* 173
sarcoidosis masquerading as metastatic tumor, echocardiography in, *97:* 355
Heat
shock protein
Escherichia coli, dnaJ, immune responses to, in juvenile rheumatoid arthritis, *96:* 278

60, autoreactivity to, predicts disease remission in oligoarticular juvenile rheumatoid arthritis, *98:* 73
60-kD, self, T cells recognizing, activation of T cells can protect against arthritis (in rat), *96:* 89
60-kD, vaccinia virus expressing, therapeutic effect in arthritis (in rat), *96:* 90
treatment, local, effects on temperature of arthritic knees, *96:* 72

Heel
pain in Reiter's disease, bone scintigraphy of, *97:* 334
soft tissue lesions in chronic inflammatory arthritis, ultrasound-guided injection of, *96:* 273

Helicobacter pylori
infection increasing risk of peptic ulcer with chronic use of nonsteroidal antiinflammatory drugs, *97:* 126

HELLP syndrome
refractory, and antiphospholipid antibodies during pregnancy, *96:* 141

Hemolytic
anemia, autoimmune, in child with MHC class II deficiency, *96:* 130

Hemorrhagic
rupture of shoulder, *96:* 205

Heparin
/aspirin in pregnant women with recurrent miscarriage associated with antiphospholipid antibodies, *98:* 115

Hepatitis
autoimmune
6-mercaptopurine after azathioprine failure in, *98:* 270
minocycline-induced, *97:* 170
C
chronic, anticardiolipin antibodies in, *97:* 153
extrahepatic manifestations of, *97:* 315
virus, causing antiphospholipid syndrome, *97:* 153
virus, with cryoglobulinemia, interferon alfa-2a in, *96:* 254
virus infection in primary Sjögren's syndrome, *98:* 135
lupus, with autoantibodies to ribosomal P, *97:* 179

Hepatotoxicity
of methotrexate in rheumatoid arthritis, *96:* 58
monitoring guidelines, *96:* 55

Heteropolymers
antigen-based, for binding and clearing autoantibodies via erythrocyte complement receptor 1, *96:* 94

Hip
arthroplasty, total
for osteoarthritis, cost effectiveness of, *97:* 271
for rheumatoid arthritis, predicting length of stay after, *98:* 13
bone mass in, effect of alendronate over 3 years in postmenopausal osteoporosis on, *98:* 226
osteoarthritis (*see* Osteoarthritis, hip)

Histocompatibility
complex, major (*see* Major histocompatibility complex)

Histone(s)
autoantibodies to, in systemic vasculitis, *96:* 249
autoimmunity to, SLE-related, viral DNA binding protein generating, *97:* 139
in glomerular deposits in lupus nephritis, *98:* 93

History
family, and gout, *98:* 222

HIV
infection
lupus erythematosus and, systemic, *96:* 128
polyarteritis nodosa-like vasculitis in, *96:* 250
joint destruction in, progressive, with rheumatoid arthritis, *97:* 41
type 1 gp41, antibodies to, detection in systemic lupus erythematosus, *97:* 158

HLA
association of autoantibodies against nucleolus organizer region, *96:* 147
class II
alleles, and chronic cutaneous lupus erythematosus, *96:* 98
antigen-derived peptides, antibodies to, detection in systemic lupus erythematosus, *97:* 158
antigens and neuropsychiatric systemic lupus erythematosus, *98:* 96
genes and anticentromere antibody in scleroderma, *97:* 212
DNA polymorphisms in pauciarticular-onset juvenile rheumatoid arthritis, *96:* 275
-DR polymorphism in polymyalgia rheumatica, molecular analysis of, *98:* 199

-DR4
career prospects in rheumatology and, *97:* 40
molecules, peptide binding specificity of, *97:* 33
-DRB and -DQB genes, outcome in rheumatoid arthritis, *97:* 35
-DRB1
alleles, rheumatoid susceptible, as genetically recessive, *96:* 28
genes and disease severity in rheumatoid arthritis, *98:* 21
DRw11 allele in severe scleroderma with anti-topoisomerase I antibodies, *96:* 151
markers and prediction of clinical course and outcome in rheumatoid arthritis, *98:* 22
type as predictor of mixed connective tissue disease differentiation, *96:* 104
typing in women with breast implants, *97:* 382
HMO
patients' satisfaction with physician performance, increasing with continuity of care, *97:* 15
Hodgkin's disease
risk in rheumatoid arthritis, *98:* 29
spontaneous regression in patients treated with methotrexate for rheumatoid arthritis and other rheumatic diseases, *98:* 46
Hormone
adrenocorticotropic
secretion, intact, in active rheumatoid arthritis, *98:* 51
for synovitis, acute crystal-induced, *96:* 297
parathyroid, nocturnal secretion, alendronate stimulation of, *98:* 230
replacement therapy, effect on bone mass in rheumatoid arthritis, *96:* 215
supplement for cyclical rashes in systemic lupus erythematosus, *97:* 191
Hospital
arthritis in, acute, rheumatologic *vs.* nonrheumatologic care of, *96:* 18
length of stay after hip or knee replacement for rheumatoid arthritis, predicting, *98:* 13
utilization, effect of physician-payment mechanisms on, in Canada, *98:* 15
vs. chiropractic outpatient management of low back pain, *97:* 293
Hospitalization
for kidney failure, acute, and NSAIDs, *97:* 124
HTLV-1
Tax gene stimulation of α1 (I) procollagen gene expression in NIH-3T3 cells, *98:* 147
Human immunodeficiency virus (*see* HIV)
Hydroxychloroquine
in arthritis, inflammatory, in AIDS, *97:* 43
ocular toxicity monitoring practices with, *96:* 14
in osteoarthritis, erosive, *97:* 262
in pregnant women with systemic lupus erythematosus, *98:* 122
in rheumatoid arthritis
early, *96:* 54
with methotrexate and sulfasalazine, *97:* 1
vs. tenidap and piroxicam, *97:* 127
5-Hydroxytryptamine
type 3 receptor antagonist ondansetron in primary fibromyalgia syndrome, *98:* 256
L-5 Hydroxytryptophan
exposure, eosinophilia-myalgia syndrome after, *96:* 182
Hypergammaglobulinemia
immunoglobulin M, with idiopathic eosinophilic fasciitis, methotrexate in, *97:* 249
Hyperprolactinemia
longstanding, in systemic lupus erythematosus, *96:* 125
Hypersensitivity
delayed, silicone gel repeated exposure inducing, *97:* 371
to molybdenum as trigger of antinuclear antibody-negative systemic lupus erythematosus, *96:* 132
Hypertension
enalapril and nifedipine in, *97:* 121
gout and, *98:* 222
kidney function in, effect of NSAIDs on, *97:* 121
pulmonary
in connective tissue disease, long-term iloprost infusion in, *96:* 177
in connective tissue disease, mixed, diltiazem and oxygen for, *96:* 180
in scleroderma, diffuse, and serum anti-U3RNP antibody, *98:* 169
in scleroderma, limited and diffuse, *98:* 168
renovascular, due to Takayasu's arteritis, *97:* 325

Hypertrophy
synovial membrane, in rheumatoid arthritis of wrist, MRI scoring of, *97:* 47
Hyperuricemia
oxipurinol in, *98:* 224
Hypothenar
hammer syndrome, accelerated progressive scleroderma in, *97:* 234

I

ICAM-1 (*see* Adhesion, molecule 1, intercellular)
Ileocolonoscopy
of gut inflammation in psoriatic arthritis, *97:* 338
Iliopsoas
bursitis, pain as only clinical indicator of, *97:* 297
Iloprost
infusion, long-term, in pulmonary hypertension in connective tissue diseases, *96:* 177
IV, in systemic sclerosis for treatment of ischemic digital ulcers and prevention of gangrene, *98:* 184
Imaging
findings in tuberculous tenosynovitis and bursitis, *98:* 235
magnetic resonance (*see* Magnetic resonance imaging)
neuroimaging of CNS disease in Sjögren's syndrome, correlation with anti-Ro/SS-A antibodies, *96:* 116
Immune
response to *Escherichia coli*, dnaJ heat shock protein in juvenile rheumatoid arthritis, *96:* 278
Immunization
with bacterial DNA, induction of cross-reactive anti-dsDNA antibodies by (in mice), *96:* 112
with carbonic anhydrase II inducing autoimmune sialoadenitis (in mice), *97:* 202
with leukocytes, mononuclear, in rheumatoid arthritis, *97:* 104
Immunoassay
enzyme, for antinuclear antibodies, *98:* 98
Immunoblot
analysis, protein, for α-fodrin as autoantigen in primary Sjögren's syndrome, *98:* 131
Immunodeficiency
disease, severe combined, engraftment of rheumatoid synovial tissue and normal human cartilage in (in mice), *96:* 30
syndrome, acquired
(*See also* HIV)
arthritis in, inflammatory, hydroxychloroquine in, *97:* 43
virus, human (*see* HIV)
Immunofluorescence
technique, indirect, for antinuclear antibodies, in routine laboratory, *98:* 97
Immunogenetic
follow-up of HLA type predicting mixed connective tissue disease differentiation, *96:* 104
susceptibility to neuropsychiatric systemic lupus erythematosus, *98:* 96
Immunogenetics
of rheumatoid arthritis, *98:* 20
of scleroderma, *98:* 143
Immunogenicity
of protein A Lyme vaccine, *96:* 293
Immunoglobulin
A inducing thrombosis in antiphospholipid syndrome (in mice), *97:* 141
G
antiendothelial cell autoantibodies from scleroderma inducing leukocyte adhesion to vascular endothelial cells, *97:* 205
anti-F(ab')$_2$ antibody, cross-reactivity with DNA and other nuclear antigens, *98:* 104
thrombosis in antiphospholipid syndrome induced by (in mice), *97:* 141
IV
high-dose, in systemic lupus erythematosus, *97:* 185
low-dose, failure in refractory rheumatoid arthritis, *98:* 61
in rheumatoid arthritis, juvenile, polyarticular, *98:* 79
in rheumatoid arthritis, juvenile, systemic onset, follow-up, *98:* 77
M
hypergammaglobulinemia with idiopathic eosinophilic fasciitis, methotrexate in, *97:* 249
thrombosis in antiphospholipid syndrome induced by (in mice), *97:* 141

Immunologic
  activity, ongoing, after short courses of pulse cyclophosphamide in systemic lupus erythematosus (in mice), *98:* 127
Immunosorbent assay
  enzyme-linked (*see* ELISA)
Immunosuppressive
  agents for early treatment in lupus nephritis, *96:* 136
Implant
  breast (*see* Breast, implant)
  silicone, *97:* 370
Indians
  Choctaw, in Oklahoma, increased prevalence of systemic sclerosis in, *98:* 163
Indomethacin
  intestinal ulcer due to, oxygen radical scavengers protecting against (in rat), *97:* 122
  kidney dysfunction due to, in elderly, misoprostol protective effect in, *97:* 123
  oral, *vs.* ketorolac for acute gouty arthritis, *97:* 367
Infarction
  myocardial, in women with systemic lupus erythematosus, age-specific incidence rates of, *98:* 116
Infection
  after methotrexate
    in lupus erythematosus, systemic, and in undifferentiated connective tissue disease, *98:* 123
    in rheumatoid arthritis, *96:* 60
Infectious
  arthritis, *98:* 232
Infertility
  rheumatoid arthritis and prolactin, *98:* 39
Inflammation
  in arthritis, somatostatin-induced modulation of (in rabbit), *97:* 39
  intestine, small, NSAID-induced, sulfasalazine and other disease-modifying antirheumatic drugs in, *96:* 71
  monosodium urate monohydrate crystal-induced acute, transforming growth factor β1 to inhibit and prevent (in rat), *98:* 220
  synovial membrane, and cytokine production in early osteoarthritis, *98:* 217
Inflammatory
  arthritis (*see* Arthritis, inflammatory)
  diseases, *97:* 331
Injection
  intraarticular and soft tissue, current practice, *97:* 297
Insulin
  -like growth factor in Werner syndrome with osteoporosis, *96:* 209
Integrin
  activation, tumor necrosis factor-induced, effect on Fcγ receptor II-mediated signal transduction, *97:* 309
Interferon
  -alpha, natural, and 6-methylprednisolone in type II mixed cryoglobulinemia, *96:* 251
  -alpha 2a in cryoglobulinemia with hepatitis C virus, *96:* 254
  -gamma
    –inducible protein p16, as target of antinuclear antibodies in systemic lupus erythematosus, *96:* 110
    scleroderma fibroblasts and, *96:* 158
    up-regulation of class II MHC and ICAM-1 expression on scleroderma fibroblasts and endothelial cells by, in early stage disease, *98:* 143
  Raynaud's syndrome and, *98:* 182
Interleukin
  -1 receptor antagonist in active systemic lupus erythematosus, *97:* 166
  -1α
    polymorphism, genetic association with juvenile rheumatoid arthritis, *96:* 274
    production in synovial membranes in early osteoarthritis, *98:* 217
  -1β
    levels after all-*trans*-retinoic acid in POEMS syndrome, *98:* 265
    production in synovial membranes in early osteoarthritis, *98:* 217
  -2
    diphtheria fusion protein for refractory rheumatoid arthritis, *97:* 100
    receptors, soluble serum, in systemic sclerosis, *98:* 150
    in renal cell carcinoma, rapid exacerbation of scleroderma after, *96:* 181
  -4
    expression in scleroderma skin specimens and scleroderma fibroblast cultures, *98:* 152
    levels, elevated serum, in systemic sclerosis, *98:* 154
  -6

levels after all-*trans*-retinoic acid in POEMS syndrome, *98:* 265
secretion augmented in collagen-stimulated peripheral blood mononuclear cells in scleroderma, *96:* 162
-8 expression in fibrosing alveolitis and scleroderma, *97:* 222
-10
in B lymphocyte hyperactivity and autoantibody production in systemic lupus erythematosus, *96:* 101
expression in type II collagen-induced arthritis (in mice), *97:* 226
inhibition of progression of collagen-induced arthritis (in mice), *98:* 66
levels, elevated serum, in systemic sclerosis, *98:* 154
levels, systemic, in Behçet's disease, *98:* 204
production in rheumatoid arthritis, Sjögren's syndrome and systemic lupus erythematosus, *96:* 100
-12 levels, systemic, in Behçet's disease, *98:* 204
-13
levels, elevated serum, in systemic sclerosis, *98:* 154
in rheumatoid synovium and its anti-inflammatory effects on synovial fluid macrophages in rheumatoid arthritis, *98:* 23
Intestine
(*See also* Gastrointestinal)
small
inflammation and blood loss, NSAID-induced, sulfasalazine and other disease-modifying antirheumatic drugs in, *96:* 71
ischemia in scleroderma, *96:* 167
ulcer, indomethacin-induced, oxygen radical scavengers protecting against (in rat), *97:* 122
Intraarticular
anesthetic, effect on pain in osteoarthritis of knee, *98:* 218
injections, current practice survey, *97:* 297
tophi in knee, CT of, *98:* 222
Intracranial
angioplasty for vascular stenosis due to atherosclerosis and vasculitis, *97:* 326
Iron
deficiency in rheumatoid arthritis and anemia, algorithm for diagnosis, *97:* 52
as marker for articular destruction in rheumatoid arthritis, *98:* 33
Ischemia
cerebral, idiopathic, antiphospholipid antibodies in, in children, *96:* 142
intestine, small, in scleroderma, *96:* 167
Ischemic
digital ulcers in systemic sclerosis, IV iloprost for, *98:* 184
Isoprostane
overproduction in scleroderma, *98:* 161

J

Joint
arthroplasty, total, corticosteroid injection in rheumatoid arthritis does not increase rate of, *98:* 53
carpometacarpal, osteoarthritis, and obesity, in women, *98:* 214
destruction in rheumatoid arthritis
glucocorticoids and, *97:* 134
progressive, and HIV, *97:* 41
finger, gouty arthritis and nodal osteoarthritis in, *98:* 221
inflamed, in rheumatoid arthritis, accumulation of soluble Fas in, *98:* 24
involvement in osteoarthritis, collagenase, stromelysin 1 and TIMP 1 in, *96:* 204
movement range utilization, in primates *vs.* humans, osteoarthritis evolutionary frame, *96:* 194
patellofemoral, osteoarthritis, and obesity, in women, *98:* 214
sacroiliac, in chronic low back pain, *96:* 5
small, arthropathy in, idiopathic destructive, *98:* 223
symptoms with exercise in elderly, *97:* 274
tibiofemoral, osteoarthritis of, *96:* 196
obesity and, in women, *98:* 214
twenty-eight–joint count for rheumatoid arthritis activity assessment, validity and reliability of, *96:* 42
Juice
grapefruit, and cyclosporine in autoimmune diseases, *98:* 124
Juvenile
(*See also* Children)
arthritis (*see* Arthritis, juvenile)

arthritis, rheumatoid (*see* Rheumatoid arthritis, juvenile)
myositis, broadened spectrum of, *96:* 284
-onset ankylosing spondylitis, early recognition of, differentiation from juvenile rheumatoid arthritis, *97:* 348
spondyloarthropathy, synovium in, expression of tumor necrosis factor-α and -β and their receptors in, *98:* 71

K

Keratan sulfate
antigenic, levels in osteoarthritis, *96:* 204
Ketorolac
in arthritis, acute gouty, *96:* 298
vs. indomethacin, *97:* 367
gastrointestinal complications of, in elderly, *97:* 119
Kidney
biopsy findings in cyclosporine treated-rheumatoid arthritis, *98:* 49
disease in Sjögren's syndrome, biochemical markers of, *97:* 198
dysfunction, indomethacin-induced, in elderly, misoprostol protective effect on, *97:* 123
eluates of lupus with proteinuria, nucleosome-restricted antibodies in (in mice), *96:* 113
failure
acute, hospitalization for, and NSAIDs, *97:* 124
gout and, *98:* 222
in scleroderma, and antineutrophil cytoplasmic autoantibodies, *96:* 244
function
in hypertension, effect of NSAIDs on, *97:* 121
in rheumatoid arthritis patients treated with cyclosporine, *98:* 49; *97:* 108
involvement
in fasciitis, idiopathic eosinophilic, methotrexate for, *97:* 249
in lupus erythematosus, recent-onset systemic, predictors of, *97:* 172
relapse in systemic lupus erythematosus
changes in antibodies to C1q predicting, *97:* 159
onset, and appearance of urinary erythrocyte/leukocyte casts, *97:* 174
transplant, dialysis arthropathy outcome after, *97:* 387
vascular damage in systemic sclerosis, *98:* 177
Killer cells
lymphokine activated, for renal cell carcinoma, rapid exacerbation of scleroderma after, *96:* 181
natural, in scleroderma, and anti-scl-70 antibodies, *97:* 227
Klebsiella
pneumonia after melphalan in primary amyloidosis, *98:* 268
Klinefelter's syndrome
with lupus erythematosus, systemic, testosterone for, *97:* 193
Knee
arthritis, local heat and cold treatment for, *96:* 72
arthropathy in, idiopathic destructive, *98:* 223
arthroplasty, total
for rheumatoid arthritis, predicting length of stay after, *98:* 13
variation in rheumatologists' and family physicians' perceptions of indications for and outcomes of, *98:* 11
arthroscopy, office-based, complications of, *97:* 265
cartilage
articular, abnormalities, compartment-directed physical examination predicting, *97:* 251
articular, arthroscopy *vs.* plain radiography and MRI of, *96:* 189
defects, deep, chondrocyte transplant for, *96:* 197
osteoarthritis (*see* Osteoarthritis, knee)
synovitis, chronic, yttrium-90 radiochemical synovectomy in, *98:* 277
tophi in, intraarticular, CT of, *98:* 222

L

Laboratory
routine, antinuclear antibody determination in, *98:* 97
Lacrimal
glands
lymphocytic infiltration in, and decreased reflex tearing, *98:* 137
in Sjögren's syndrome, common T cell receptor clonotype in, *98:* 134
Lactoferrin
autoantibodies to, in systemic vasculitis, *96:* 249

La/SS-B
autoantibodies to, some are antiidiotypes to anti-double stranded DNA, *98:* 100
Lavage
bronchoalveolar
in fibrosing alveolitis in scleroderma, *96:* 172
fluid, from scleroderma, platelet-derived growth factor and transforming growth factor-β1 in, *97:* 214
Length of stay
after hip or knee replacement for rheumatoid arthritis, predicting, *98:* 13
Leukemia
after methotrexate in rheumatoid arthritis, temporal association, *97:* 90
myeloid, acute, allogenic bone marrow transplantation from donor with systemic lupus erythematosus in, *98:* 92
virus type 1, human T cell, Tax gene, stimulation of α1 (I) procollagen gene expression in NIH-3T3 cells by, *98:* 147
Leukocyte
adhesion to vascular endothelial cells, immunoglobulin antiendothelial cell autoantibodies from scleroderma inducing, *97:* 205
/erythrocyte casts, urinary, appearance of, and onset of renal relapse in systemic lupus erythematosus, *97:* 174
mononuclear, immunization with, in rheumatoid arthritis, *97:* 104
Leukocytoclastic
vasculitis after staphylococcal protein A column immunoadsorption therapy, *97:* 318
Leukotriene
B_4 in progression of collagen-induced arthritis, *96:* 34
Lichen
sclerosus et atrophicus skin lesions, *Borrelia burgdorferi* DNA is undetectable by polymerase chain reaction in, in North American patients, *98:* 242
Life
expectancy in Marfan's syndrome, *96:* 305
Light
microscopy
of arthropathies, idiopathic destructive, *98:* 223
in liver biopsy after methotrexate for rheumatoid arthritis, *97:* 82
Linoleic acid
gamma-, in rheumatoid arthritis, *98:* 63
Lip
biopsy for early expression of E-selectin, tumor necrosis factor-α, and mast cell infiltration in systemic sclerosis, *98:* 155
Lipoid
pneumonia, rheumatoid arthritis, and cod-liver oil capsules, *98:* 261
Lipomatosis
epidural, cauda equina compression by, in obesity, *97:* 299
Lipoprotein
low-density
oxidation of, increased susceptibility, in scleroderma, *97:* 221
oxidized, recognition of cardiolipin by monoclonal antibodies to epitopes of, *98:* 109
Livedo
reticularis in minocycline-induced arthritis, *98:* 196
Liver
biopsy (*see* Biopsy, liver)
candidiasis, polyarteritis nodosa mimicking, CT of, *96:* 247
function, abnormal, in early Lyme borreliosis with erythema migrans, *98:* 237
toxicity of methotrexate in rheumatoid arthritis, *96:* 58
monitoring guidelines, *96:* 55
LJP 394
reduction in circulating dsDNA antibody titer after, *98:* 126
Low back pain (*see* Back, pain, low)
Lumbar
bone mineral density, low, and major depression, *96:* 207
puncture in CNS vasculitis, *96:* 260
spine
bone loss, postmenopausal, intermittent salmon calcitonin to prevent, *97:* 276
stenosis, degenerative, history and physical exam diagnostic value in, *97:* 253
Lung
(*See also* Pulmonary)
cancer risk in rheumatoid arthritis, *98:* 29
disease

chronic, inflammatory, tryptophan metabolism in, *97:* 210
interstitial, severe, treatment, in scleroderma, *96:* 178
preexisting, and methotrexate pneumonitis in rheumatoid arthritis, *97:* 85
restrictive, severe, in scleroderma, *96:* 170
rheumatoid arthritis, *98:* 26
fibroblasts, effects of relaxin on, *98:* 142
function
after cyclophosphamide in scleroderma, *96:* 179
methotrexate and, long-term low-dose, *98:* 48
interstitium, memory T cell increase in, in fibrosing alveolitis in scleroderma, *97:* 246
involvement
discrete, in systemic lupus erythematosus, CT of, *97:* 175
in scleroderma, *98:* 166
in scleroderma, procollagen III predictive value in diagnosis, *97:* 239
transplant recipient with recurrence of sarcoidosis, tumor necrosis factor-α expression by alveolar macrophages in, *98:* 272

Lupus
antibodies to histone DNA complexes more sensitive and specific for scleroderma than lupus, *96:* 153
anticoagulant properties of annexin V antibody, *97:* 143
autoantibodies
anti-DNA, repertoire cloning of, *98:* 85
to DNA cross-react with SnRNP A and D polypeptides, *96:* 108
erythematosus, cutaneous
chronic, and HLA class II alleles, *96:* 98
subacute, due to calcium channel blockers, *98:* 117
erythematosus, systemic, *98:* 81; *97:* 139; *96:* 93
active, and anti-F(ab')$_2$ system depletion, *97:* 165
active, interleukin-1 receptor antagonist and, *97:* 166
alendronate causing esophageal ulcers in, *98:* 232
antibodies to HIV-1 gp41 and HLA class II antigen-derived peptides in, *97:* 158
anti-CD5 ricin A chain immunoconjugate in, *96:* 134
anti-DNA antibodies in, anti-idiotypic, *97:* 164
anti-DNA antibodies in, DNA mimics self-protein as target for, *96:* 107
antinuclear antibody-negative, molybdenum hypersensitivity as trigger of, *96:* 132
antiphospholipid antibodies and epilepsy in, *96:* 144
antiphospholipid antibodies in, specificity and cofactor dependence of, *98:* 110
antiphospholipid syndrome in, associated with anti-β_2-glycoprotein-I, *97:* 147
apoptosis acceleration of lymphocytes in, *96:* 106
autoantibodies in, *97:* 161
B lymphocyte hyperactivity and autoantibody production in, and interleukin-10, *96:* 101
basic mechanisms, *97:* 154
bone marrow transplantation from donor with, allogenic, *98:* 92
bromocriptine in, *97:* 186
CD40 ligand hyperexpression by B and T cells in, *98:* 88
CD56+ T and non-T cells in, impaired recovery and cytolytic function of, *98:* 90
clinical aspects, *98:* 116
clinical studies, *96:* 116
CNS disease in, and antiphospholipid antibodies, *97:* 145
CNS disease in, antiribosomal PO protein antibodies and PO fusion protein in, *97:* 162
C1q deficiency in, hereditary, *96:* 126
CT in, chest high-resolution, *97:* 189
CTLA41g for (in mice), *96:* 138
cyclophosphamide in, outpatient monthly oral bolus, *97:* 184
cyclophosphamide in, pulse (in mice), *98:* 127
dehydroepiandrosterone for, trial results, *97:* 194
diagnosis, *97:* 172
diagnosis, utility of anti-Sm, anti-RNP, anti-Ro/SS-A, and anti-La/SS-B antibodies detected by ELISA for, *98:* 99
disease activity assessment, resting heart rate and blood tests in, *96:* 118
estrogen use and, exogenous, safety of, *97:* 188

fas ligand mutation in, *98:* 89
glomerulonephritis and, *97:* 156
HIV infection and, *96:* 128
hyperprolactinemia in, longstanding, *96:* 125
immunoglobulins for, IV high-dose, *97:* 185
immunopathogenesis, *96:* 97
incidence and prevalence, ethnicity and birth country in, *97:* 154
interferon-gamma–inducible protein p16 as target of antinuclear antibodies in, *96:* 110
interleukin-10 production in, *96:* 100
kidney relapse onset in, and urinary erythrocyte/leukocyte casts appearance, *97:* 174
kidney relapses in, changes in antibodies to C1q predicting, *97:* 159
with Klinefelter's syndrome, testosterone for, *97:* 193
-like syndrome, minocycline-induced, *97:* 170
lung involvement in, discrete, CT of, *97:* 175
methotrexate in, *96:* 137
muscle biopsy abnormalities in, *96:* 119
muscle oxygen uptake reduction during exercise in, *97:* 155
neuropathy in, autonomic and sensorimotor, *97:* 236
neuropsychiatric, and antiribosomal P protein antibodies, *98:* 118
neuropsychiatric, and quinolinic acid, *98:* 95
neuropsychiatric, diagnostic tests in, *97:* 181
neuropsychiatric, immunogenetic susceptibility to, *98:* 96
nonrenal, methotrexate in, *98:* 123
ovulation induction treatment causing, *96:* 123
poly(ADP-ribose) metabolism alteration in family members in, *96:* 128
pregnancy and, hydroxychloroquine in, *98:* 122
prolactin in, *96:* 124
quiescent, serum complement determinations in, *98:* 120
rashes in, cyclical, hormone supplement for, *97:* 191
recent onset, kidney involvement predictors in, *97:* 172
relapse prevention in, *97:* 182
-related autoimmunity to double-stranded DNA and histones, viral DNA binding protein generating, *97:* 139
-related disorders, *98:* 81
risk after breast silicone implant, *96:* 303
severe, remission after plasmapheresis and cyclophosphamide, *96:* 133
T cell proliferation in, autoantigen-specific, induced by ribosomal P2 protein in, *96:* 109
T lymphocytes, deficient type I protein kinase A isozyme activity in, *96:* 105
therapy, *98:* 120; *96:* 133
thrombomodulin marking disease activity in, *96:* 122
in women, age-specific incidence of myocardial infarction and angina in, *98:* 116
hepatitis with autoantibodies to ribosomal P, *97:* 179
-inducing drugs, transformation to cytotoxic products by activated neutrophils, *96:* 131
-like disease, model, (SWR x SJL)F_1 mice as, *96:* 115
nephritis
glomerular deposits in, nucleosomes and histones in, *98:* 93
severe, economic impact of treatment with prednisone and IV cyclophosphamide, *96:* 10
with proteinuria, nucleosome-restricted antibodies in kidney eluates of (in mice), *96:* 113
therapy, *97:* 182
vasculitis of gastrointestinal tract, three-phase abdominal scintigraphy in, *97:* 177
Lyme
arthritis (*see* Arthritis, Lyme)
disease, *98:* 235; *96:* 289
anti-interleukin 12 treatment of (in mice), *98:* 240
babesiosis concurrent with, *98:* 238
in children, pitfalls in diagnosis and treatment, *97:* 386
early, and culture-confirmed erythema migrans, clinical spectrum of, *98:* 237
as infectious and postinfectious syndrome, *96:* 295
outcomes, long-term, *96:* 290
post Lyme syndrome, clinical and neurocognitive features of, *98:* 237

vaccine, protein A, safety and immunogenicity of, *96:* 293

Lymph
  nodes, non-palpable supraclavicular, in sarcoidosis, ultrasound-guided fine-needle aspiration cytology of, *98:* 273

Lymphadenopathy
  in Lyme borreliosis, early, with erythema migrans, *98:* 237

Lymphocyte
  apoptosis acceleration in systemic lupus erythematosus, *96:* 106
  B
    CD40 ligand expression by, in systemic lupus erythematosus, *98:* 88
    hyperactivity in systemic lupus erythematosus, and interleukin-10, *96:* 101
  function-associated antigen 3 in scleroderma fibroblasts, *96:* 158
  T (*see* T cell)

Lymphocytic
  infiltration in lacrimal glands, and decreased reflex tearing, *98:* 137

Lymphokine
  activated killer cells for renal cell carcinoma, rapid exacerbation of scleroderma after, *96:* 181

Lymphoma
  angiotropic large cell, with mononeuritis multiplex mimicking systemic vasculitis, *97:* 320
  development in primary Sjögren's syndrome, predictive factors for, *98:* 136
  malignant, with Sjögren's syndrome, *97:* 197
  non-Hodgkin's
    risk, and rheumatoid arthritis, *98:* 29
    spontaneous regression in patients treated with methotrexate for rheumatoid arthritis and other rheumatic diseases, *98:* 46
  in rheumatoid arthritis, Epstein-Barr virus clonality in, *98:* 30

Lymphoproliferative
  disease
    fas ligand mutation in, *98:* 89
    methotrexate-related, in rheumatoid arthritis, *97:* 88
  disorders, spontaneous regression of, in patients treated with methotrexate for rheumatoid arthritis and other rheumatic diseases, *98:* 46

M

Macrophages
  alveolar, tumor necrosis factor-α expression by, in lung transplant recipient with recurrence of sarcoidosis, *98:* 272
  synovial fluid, in rheumatoid arthritis, antiinflammatory effects of interleukin-13 on, *98:* 23

Magnetic resonance imaging
  in bursitis, tuberculous, *98:* 235
  in dermatomyositis, *96:* 281
    amyopathic and myopathic, muscle dysfunction in, *96:* 279
  dynamic
    for sacroiliitis in spondyloarthropathy, *96:* 267
    for synovitis in rheumatoid arthritis, *96:* 46
  functional, of cervical spine in rheumatoid arthritis, *96:* 48
  of knee articular cartilage, *vs.* arthroscopy and plain radiography, *96:* 189
  in polymyositis, cost effectiveness of, *97:* 352
  of rotator cuff dysfunction in rheumatoid arthritis, *97:* 54
  scoring of synovial membrane hypertrophy and bone erosions in rheumatoid arthritis of wrist, *97:* 47
  in tenosynovitis, tuberculous, *98:* 235
  in vasculitis, CNS, *96:* 260

Magnetic resonance spectra
  ^{31}P, in skeletal muscle in fibromyalgia, increased incidence of a resonance in phosphodiester region of, *96:* 220

Magnetic resonance spectroscopy
  phosphorus-31, in dermatomyositis
    amyopathic and myopathic, muscle dysfunction in, *96:* 279
    data useful in longitudinal management, *96:* 281

Major histocompatibility complex
  class II
    alleles related to autoantibodies in four ethnic groups with myositis, *98:* 207
    deficiency in autoimmune hemolytic anemia in child, *96:* 130
    expression on scleroderma fibroblasts and endothelial cells in early disease stage, up-regulation by interferon-gamma and tumor necrosis factor-α, *98:* 143

gene and anti-U1 small nuclear ribonucleoprotein antibody, *96:* 97
Managed care
effects on specialty practice at university medical center, *97:* 12
Marfan's syndrome, *96:* 305
life expectancy in, *96:* 305
novel variant of, *96:* 306
Marrow
mononuclear cells in Paget's disease, measles virus nucleocapsid mRNA in, *97:* 385
transplantation, allogenic, from donor with systemic lupus erythematosus, *98:* 92
Mast cell
infiltration in salivary glands in early systemic sclerosis, *98:* 155
Matrix
-degrading phenotype, relaxin-induced extracellular, in lung fibroblasts, *98:* 142
Measles
virus, nucleocapsid mRNA, in marrow mononuclear cells in Paget's disease, *97:* 385
Medicaid
patients, prior authorization requirement for nonsteroidal antiinflammatory drug use by, *97:* 7
Medical
center, university, potential effects of managed care on specialty practice at, *97:* 12
costs, direct, unique to arthritis patients, *98:* 7
education, continuing, in rheumatic diseases for primary care physicians, *97:* 21
Medicare
preserving and strengthening, *97:* 10
Medicine
musculoskeletal, extended fellowship in, opinions of rheumatology fellows about, *96:* 12
Mediterranean fever
familial, AA amyloidosis of, colchicine for, *96:* 307
Melphalan
in amyloidosis, primary, with colchicine and prednisone, *98:* 268
6-Mercaptopurine
in hepatitis, autoimmune, after azathioprine failure, *98:* 270
Metabolism
bone mineral, in juvenile rheumatoid arthritis, *98:* 76
cartilage and bone, in rheumatoid arthritis, *96:* 38
mineral, in dermatomyositis, in children, *96:* 216
protein, in rheumatoid arthritis and aging, *98:* 38
Metalloproteinase
tissue inhibitor, shoulder tendon biopsy samples in organ culture producing, *97:* 291
Metastases
tumor, cardiac sarcoidosis masquerading as, echocardiography in, *97:* 355
Methotrexate
in arthritis
juvenile chronic, systemic-onset, response to, *96:* 276
psoriatic, long-term therapy, outcome of, *96:* 271
rheumatoid *(see* Methotrexate, in rheumatoid arthritis *below)*
in connective tissue disease, undifferentiated, *98:* 123
fever and cough after, approach to, *97:* 86
for hearing loss, autoimmune, *96:* 310
in idiopathic eosinophilic fasciitis, morphea, IgM hypergammaglobulinemia and kidney involvement, *97:* 249
-induced stomatitis, allopurinol mouthwashes in, *96:* 61
in lupus erythematosus, systemic, *96:* 137
nonrenal, *98:* 123
oral, bioavailability in children, influence of food on, *97:* 72
in polychondritis, relapsing, *98:* 210
in polymyalgia rheumatica, *98:* 200
with giant cell arteritis, *98:* 201
results of open, randomized study, *98:* 201
in rheumatic diseases, and spontaneous regression of lymphoproliferative disorders, *98:* 46
in rheumatoid arthritis
antibiotic use and infection rate after, *96:* 60
with azathioprine, *97:* 69
B lymphoproliferative disease related to, *97:* 88
chimeric monoclonal antibody anti-CD4 with, *97:* 103
chloroquine reducing bioavailability of, *96:* 58
discontinuation analyses, *98:* 45
every-other-week, *97:* 73
folic acid supplement during, *96:* 57

leukemia after, temporal association, *97:* 90
liver biopsy after (*see* Biopsy, liver, after methotrexate in rheumatoid arthritis)
low-dose, causing methotrexate osteopathy, *97:* 91
low-dose, fatal pulmonary fibrosis complicating, *97:* 83
lymphoproliferative disorders and, spontaneous regression of, *98:* 46
monitoring liver toxicity guidelines, *96:* 55
oral administration of easily prepared injectable methotrexate diluted in water, *98:* 44
pneumonitis due to, and preexisting lung disease, *97:* 85
with psoriasis, accelerated nodulosis after, *97:* 74
pulmonary function and, *98:* 48
reactions to, underrecognized postdosing, *96:* 59
study, *96:* 26
sulfasalazine and hydroxychloroquine with, *97:* 1
survival and, *98:* 45
in spondylitis, ankylosing, severe, *97:* 331

Methylprednisolone
with interferon-α in type II mixed cryoglobulinemia, *96:* 251
in myelodysplastic syndrome with systemic vasculitis, *98:* 194

MHC (*see* Major histocompatibility complex)

Microbial
presence at silicone breast implant surface, *97:* 377

Microscopy
light and electron
of arthropathies, idiopathic destructive, *98:* 223
in liver biopsy after methotrexate for rheumatoid arthritis, *97:* 82

Microvascular
injury in pathogenesis of cutaneous lesions in dermatomyositis, *97:* 353

Milk
consumption, lifetime, and bone mineral density in older women, *96:* 206

Mineral
bone (*see* Bone, mineral)
metabolism in dermatomyositis, in children, *96:* 216

Mineralization
bone, in juvenile rheumatoid arthritis, *98:* 76

Minocycline
-induced arthritis with fever, livedo reticularis, and pANCA, *98:* 196
-induced autoimmune hepatitis and systemic lupus erythematosus-like syndrome, *97:* 170
in rheumatoid arthritis, *96:* 73
active, *96:* 74

Miscarriage
recurrent, associated with antiphospholipid antibodies, aspirin and heparin in pregnant women with, *98:* 115

Misoprostol
dosage to prevent NSAID-induced gastric and duodenal ulcer, *97:* 116
prophylaxis
against NSAID-induced gastric ulcers, *96:* 66
for rheumatoid arthritis with nonsteroidal antiinflammatory drugs, cost of, *96:* 65
protective effect on indomethacin-induced kidney dysfunction in elderly, *97:* 123
reducing gastrointestinal complications of NSAIDs in rheumatoid arthritis, *97:* 114

Mitral
regurgitation in limited systemic sclerosis, *98:* 173

Model
animal, of scleroderma with cutaneous fibrosis and mononuclear cell infiltration, *97:* 209
of lupus-like disease, (SWR x SJL)F_1 mice as, *96:* 115
rheumatoid arthritis
engraftment of rheumatoid synovial tissue and normal human cartilage in severe combined immunodeficiency disease as (in mice), *96:* 30
new, pristane-induced arthritis as (in rat), *98:* 69
of thrombosis induction by immunoglobulin G, M and A in antiphospholipid syndrome (in mice), *97:* 141
for total costs of drug therapy for rheumatoid arthritis, *96:* 7

Molecular
analysis of HLA-DR polymorphism in polymyalgia rheumatica, *98:* 199

Molybdenum
hypersensitivity as trigger to antinuclear antibody-negative systemic lupus erythematosus, *96:* 132

Monitoring
guidelines
for drug therapy in rheumatoid arthritis, *98:* 2
for liver toxicity of methotrexate in rheumatoid arthritis, *96:* 55
practices for ocular toxicity with hydroxychloroquine, *96:* 14
Monoclonal
antibody (*see* Antibody, monoclonal)
cryoglobulinemia, mixed, cross-reactive idiotypes, as predictive factor for development of lymphoma in primary Sjögren's syndrome, *98:* 136
rheumatoid factor, cross-reactive idiotypes, as predictive factor for development of lymphoma in primary Sjögren's syndrome, *98:* 136
Monocyte
production enhancement and interleukin-1 receptor antagonist in systemic lupus erythematosus, *97:* 166
Mononeuritis
multiplex with angiotropic large cell lymphoma, mimicking systemic vasculitis, *97:* 320
Mononuclear
cell (*see* Cell, mononuclear)
Monosodium urate
monohydrate crystal-induced acute inflammation, transforming growth factor β1 to inhibit and prevent (in rat), *98:* 220
Morning
stiffness after triazolam in rheumatoid arthritis, *97:* 51
Morphea
Borrelia burgdorferi DNA is undetectable by polymerase chain reaction in skin lesions of, in North American patients, *98:* 242
renal disease and idiopathic eosinophilic fasciitis, methotrexate in, *97:* 249
Mothers
of children with congenital heart block
autoantibody-associated, outcome, *96:* 117
complete, long-term outcome of, *98:* 105
Mouthwashes
allopurinol, in methotrexate-induced stomatitis, *96:* 61
MRI (*see* Magnetic resonance imaging)
Mucosa
gastric
cell proliferation, role in gastric adaptation to aspirin (in rat), *96:* 68
prostaglandin levels, age-related reduction in, increasing susceptibility to aspirin-induced injury (in rat), *96:* 69
Muscle
biopsy
abnormalities in systemic lupus erythematosus, *96:* 119
needle, in rheumatology practice, *96:* 286
-cell membrane proteins, autoantibodies against, in myositis, *98:* 208
dysfunction in dermatomyositis, amyopathic and myopathic, *96:* 279
energy metabolism abnormalities, lack of association with fibromyalgia syndrome, *96:* 219
oxygen uptake reduction during exercise in systemic lupus erythematosus, *97:* 155
skeletal, in fibromyalgia, increased incidence of a resonance in phosphodiester region of ^{31}P nuclear magnetic resonance spectra in, *96:* 220
Musculoskeletal
disorders
economic burden of, in Canada, *96:* 15
impact of, *97:* 18
non-articular, *98:* 246
primary care management of, determinants of physician confidence in, *97:* 23
ultrasound therapy in, *98:* 263
medicine, extended fellowship in, opinions of rheumatology fellows about, *96:* 12
pain related to running, with age, *98:* 215
problems in VDU workers, *98:* 246
Myalgia
-eosinophilia syndrome after L-5 hydroxytryptophan exposure, *96:* 182
in Lyme borreliosis, early, with erythema migrans, *98:* 237
Myelodysplastic
syndromes
Behçet's disease and, *98:* 206
polychondritis and, relapsing, *97:* 361
vasculitis and, systemic, *98:* 193

Myeloid
leukemia, acute, allogenic bone marrow transplantation from donor with systemic lupus erythematosus in, *98:* 92
Myocardial
infarction in women with systemic lupus erythematosus, age-specific incidence rates of, *98:* 116
perfusion and function, left ventricular, in systemic sclerosis after diltiazem, *98:* 176
Myopathy, *98:* 207
Myositis, *97:* 351; *96:* 279
autoantibodies in
against muscle-cell membrane proteins, *98:* 208
relation to MHC class II alleles in four ethnic groups, *98:* 207
juvenile, broadened spectrum of, *96:* 284
orbital, idiopathic, clinical and echographic findings in, *96:* 288

N

Nasal
stimulation with Schirmer test for reflex tearing in Sjögren's syndrome, *98:* 137
Native Americans
in Oklahoma, increased prevalence of systemic sclerosis in, *98:* 163
Nausea
after iloprost in systemic sclerosis, *98:* 184
Neck
(*See also* Spine, cervical)
pain, mechanical, conservative management of, *98:* 247
stiff, in early Lyme borreliosis with erythema migrans, *98:* 237
Neisseria gonorrhoeae
in synovial fluid, polymerase chain reaction for, *96:* 309
Nephritis
lupus
glomerular deposits in, nucleosomes and histones in, *98:* 93
severe, economic impact of treatment with prednisone and IV cyclophosphamide, *96:* 10
Nervous
system, central (*see* Central nervous system)
Neurocognitive
features of post Lyme syndrome, *98:* 237
Neuroimaging
of CNS disease in Sjögren's syndrome, correlation with anti-Ro/SS-A autoantibodies, *96:* 116
Neuronal
antibodies, antimyenteric, in scleroderma, *96:* 149
Neuropathy
autonomic and sensorimotor, in systemic lupus erythematosus and scleroderma, *97:* 236
Neuropsychiatric
involvement in systemic lupus erythematosus (*see* Lupus, erythematosus, systemic, neuropsychiatric)
Neutrophil(s)
activated, transformation of lupus-inducing drugs to cytotoxic products by, *96:* 131
activating peptide-78, epithelial, in arthritis, *96:* 33
activation by anti-proteinase 3 or anti-myeloperoxidase antibodies, *97:* 309
cytoplasmic antigen, autoantibodies to, in predicting relapse in systemic vasculitis, *97:* 310
infiltration, role in gastric adaptation to aspirin (in rat), *96:* 68
procollagenase, activation in presence of doxycycline, causing enzyme fragmentation and activity loss, *97:* 259
Neutrophilic
dermatitis, palisaded, in collagen vascular disease, histopathologic spectrum of, *96:* 120
Nifedipine
in hypertension, *97:* 121
lupus erythematosus due to, subacute cutaneous, *98:* 118
NIH-3T3 cells
α1 (I) procollagen gene expression in, stimulation by HTLV-1 Tax gene, *98:* 147
Nipple
–A manifestation of Raynaud's phenomenon, vasospasm of, *98:* 180
Nocturnal
parathyroid hormone secretion, alendronate stimulation of, *98:* 230
Nodal
osteoarthritis, gouty arthritis in, *98:* 221

Nodulosis
accelerated, after methotrexate in rheumatoid arthritis with psoriasis, *97:* 74
NSAIDs (*see* Antiinflammatory, drugs, nonsteroidal)
Nuclear
antigens, cross-reactivity with IgG anti-F(ab')$_2$ antibody, *98:* 104
localization of anti-double strand DNA autoantibody, *98:* 82
Nucleolus
organizer region, autoantibodies against, clinical relevance and HLA association of, *96:* 147
Nucleosome(s)
in glomerular deposits in lupus nephritis, *98:* 93
-restricted antibodies in kidney in lupus with proteinuria (in mice), *96:* 113

O

Obesity
cauda equina compression by epidural lipomatosis in, *97:* 299
osteoarthritis in women and
hand and knee, *98:* 213
knee, unilateral, *96:* 193
Occipito-cervical
fixation in rheumatoid arthritis, surgical risk factors in, *97:* 55
Ocular
toxicity, hydroxychloroquine-related, monitoring practices, *96:* 14
vaso-occlusive disease in antiphospholipid syndrome, *97:* 148
Office
-based arthroscopy
evolution of procedure, *97:* 264
of knee, complications of, *97:* 265
Oligoarticular
juvenile rheumatoid arthritis, autoreactivity to heat shock protein 60 predicts disease remission in, *98:* 73
Omega-3 fatty acid supplement
in rheumatoid arthritis, active, *96:* 77
Ondansetron
in fibromyalgia syndrome, primary, *98:* 256
Online
biomedical databases in rheumatology, performance of, *96:* 11
Orbital
myositis, idiopathic, clinical and echographic findings in, *96:* 288
Orthopedic
surgeons' care of acute low back pain, outcomes and costs, *97:* 294
surgery, major, for degenerative arthritis, gender differences in, *96:* 187
Orthostatic
sympathetic derangement in fibromyalgia, *98:* 252
Osteoarthritis, *98:* 213; *97:* 251; *96:* 187
biology of, *98:* 217
clinical aspects of, *98:* 219
costs in, indirect and nonmedical, *98:* 6
early, synovial membrane inflammation and cytokine production in, *98:* 217
end-stage, cardiovascular fitness and health in, *97:* 254
epidemiology, *98:* 213
erosive, hydroxychloroquine for, *97:* 262
evolutionary frame, and joint movement range utilization in primates *vs.* humans, *96:* 194
hand
obesity and, in women, *98:* 213
yoga-based regimen for, *96:* 200
hip
arthroplasty for, cost-effectiveness of, *97:* 271
medical management guidelines, *97:* 267
radiography of, *97:* 256
risk, and sports, long-term weight-bearing, in women, *98:* 214
joint involvement in, collagenase, stromelysin 1 and TIMP 1 in, *96:* 204
keratan sulfate in, antigenic, *96:* 204
knee
arthroscopy of, trial results, *97:* 266
electrical stimulation for, pulsed, *97:* 261
electromagnetic fields for, pulsed, *96:* 201
in former runners, soccer players, weight lifters and shooters, *97:* 257
medical management guidelines, *97:* 268
obesity and, in women, *98:* 213
pain mechanisms in, *98:* 218
progression, antiinflammatory drugs in, *97:* 258
progression, relation to dietary intake and serum levels of vitamin D, *98:* 219
risk, and sports, long-term weight-bearing, in women, *98:* 214

triamcinolone hexacetonide for, intraarticular, *97:* 263
unilateral, and obesity, in women, *96:* 193
nodal, gouty arthritis in, *98:* 221
running associated with, follow-up study, *96:* 190
spine, cervical, pulsed electromagnetic fields for, *96:* 201
synovial fluid in, submicroscopic crystals in, *96:* 300
telephone interventions and health outcomes in, *98:* 10
thumb base, trapezium excision for, *96:* 203
tibiofemoral joint, *96:* 196
treatment, direct cost of, *vs.* treatment of fibromyalgia, *97:* 280
Osteopathy
methotrexate, after low-dose methotrexate in rheumatoid arthritis and psoriasis, *97:* 91
Osteoporosis, *98:* 225; *97:* 275; *96:* 187, 206
corticosteroid-induced
bone loss of spine and femur in, etidronate reversing, *97:* 278
prevention of, *96:* 211
prevention of, cyclic etidronate in, *98:* 6
fracture in, risk for, and high intensity strength training, *96:* 208
postmenopausal
alendronate in (*see* Alendronate, in osteoporosis, postmenopausal)
etidronate in, intermittent cyclic, *96:* 217
sodium fluoride in, slow-release, *97:* 279
secondary, prevention of, and oral corticosteroids, *98:* 225
severe, in men, *97:* 277
steroid-induced (*see* Osteoporosis, corticosteroid-induced *above*)
with Werner syndrome, insulin-like growth factor in, *96:* 209
Otoneurologic
tests for cerebral dysfunction in fibromyalgia, *97:* 285
Ovariectomy
exercise after (in rat), *96:* 210
Ovary
adenocarcinoma, Raynaud's phenomenon as presenting sign of, *97:* 248
cancer with antiphospholipid antibody syndrome, *96:* 140
Ovulation
induction treatment inducing systemic lupus erythematosus, *96:* 123
Oxidation
increased susceptibility in low-density lipoproteins isolated from scleroderma, *97:* 221
Oxipurinol
in hyperuricemia, *98:* 224
Oxygen
with diltiazem for pulmonary hypertension in mixed connective tissue disease, *96:* 180
radical scavengers protecting against indomethacin-induced intestinal ulcer (in rat), *97:* 122
uptake, muscle, reduction during exercise in systemic lupus erythematosus, *97:* 155

P

p53
overexpression in rheumatoid arthritis synovium, *98:* 25
p55
tumor necrosis factor-α receptor, serum, as marker of disease activity in juvenile chronic arthritis, *98:* 70
p75
tumor necrosis factor-α receptor, serum, as marker of disease activity in juvenile chronic arthritis, *98:* 70
p80
fusion protein, recombinant soluble, in refractory rheumatoid arthritis, *98:* 62
Paget's disease
of bone, monostotic, bone scintigraphy of, *97:* 384
measles virus nucleocapsid mRNA in marrow mononuclear cells in, *97:* 385
Pain
back (*see* Back, pain)
in bursitis, iliopsoas, pain as only clinical indicator, *97:* 297
chronic
syndromes, *97:* 251
weather changes and, *97:* 289
of digital vasculitis secondary to rheumatoid arthritis, cervical epidural analgesia for, *98:* 198
as fibromyalgia evidence, *96:* 222
heel, in Reiter's disease, bone scintigraphy of, *97:* 334
measurement of, *98:* 265

mechanisms in osteoarthritis of knee, *98:* 218
musculoskeletal, relation to running, with age, *98:* 215
neck, mechanical, conservative management of, *98:* 247
-O-Meter, psychometric properties of, *98:* 265
pressure pain sensibility increase in fibromyalgia, *97:* 288
in rheumatoid arthritis, changes in, and rheumatology visit frequency, *98:* 8
of rheumatoid shoulder, ultrasound of, *96:* 47
spine, in fibromyalgia, prevalence and treatment outcome, *97:* 282
syndrome(s)
greater trochanter, *98:* 248
regional, *98:* 246; *97:* 280; *96:* 187
thresholds, low, in fibromyalgia in women, and cerebral blood flow abnormalities, *97:* 284

Pamidronate
in rheumatoid arthritis, bone mass increase with, *98:* 60

pANCA
in minocycline-induced arthritis, *98:* 196

Parathyroid
hormone secretion, nocturnal, alendronate stimulation of, *98:* 230

Parvovirus B19
arthritis due to, variable clinical picture of, *97:* 388
infection
antiphospholipid antibodies in, specificity and cofactor dependence of, *98:* 110
vasculitis and, chronic and systemic necrotizing, *96:* 237

Patella
tophi in, *98:* 222

Patellofemoral
joint osteoarthritis and obesity, in women, *98:* 214

Pathophysiology
of rheumatoid arthritis, *98:* 20
of scleroderma, *98:* 143

Patient
HMO, satisfaction with physician performance, continuity of care increasing, *97:* 15
-with-patient interaction, impact on perceived rheumatoid arthritis overall disease status, *98:* 12

Payment
physician-payment mechanisms, effect on hospital utilization, in Canada, *98:* 15

D-Penicillamine
low-dose, in rheumatoid arthritis, *96:* 62

Penicillin
in rheumatic fever, acute adult, *98:* 269

Penile
Raynaud's phenomenon, *98:* 180

Peptic ulcer
bleeding, risk with NSAIDs, *96:* 68
NSAID-induced, *Helicobacter pylori* infection increasing risk of, *97:* 126

Peptide
binding specificity of HLA-DR4 molecules, *97:* 33

Phenotype
extracellular matrix-degrading, relaxin-induced, in lung fibroblasts, *98:* 142

Phenytoin
in rheumatoid arthritis, *vs.* auranofin and chloroquine, *97:* 61

Phosphodiester
region of ^{31}P nuclear magnetic resonance spectra in skeletal muscle in fibromyalgia, increased incidence of a resonance in, *96:* 220

Phospholipids
oxidized, antiphospholipid antibodies directed against epitopes of, *98:* 109

Phosphorus-31
magnetic resonance spectra in skeletal muscle in fibromyalgia, increased incidence of a resonance in phosphodiester region of, *96:* 220
magnetic resonance spectroscopy in dermatomyositis
amyopathic and myopathic, muscle dysfunction in, *96:* 279
data useful in longitudinal management, *96:* 281

Physical
abuse in women with fibromyalgia syndrome, *96:* 225
therapy for trochanteric bursitis, *98:* 248
training in fibromyalgia in women, *96:* 228

Physician(s)
completing training in 1994, initial employment status of, *97:* 14

confidence in primary care management of musculoskeletal disorders, determinants of, *97:* 23
family, perceptions of indications for and outcomes of knee replacement, *vs.* rheumatologists' perceptions, *98:* 11
-payment mechanisms, effect on hospital utilization, in Canada, *98:* 15
performance, HMO patients' satisfaction with, increasing with continuity of care, *97:* 15
primary care
back pain care by, acute low, outcomes and costs, *97:* 294
continuing medical education in rheumatic diseases, *97:* 21
variation in diagnostic testing for low back pain, *96:* 4

Physiologic
abnormalities in rheumatoid arthritis lung disease, *98:* 26

Piroxicam
in rheumatoid arthritis, *vs.* tenidap and hydroxychloroquine, *97:* 127

PiZ
allele, alpha-1 antitrypsin, link with Wegener's granulomatosis, *96:* 241
gene of alpha-1 antitrypsin in outcome of PR3-ANCA positive vasculitis, *97:* 312

Placenta
in antiphospholipid antibody syndrome, beta 2 glycoprotein I and anticoagulant protein I in, *96:* 145

Plaquenil (*see* Hydroxychloroquine)

Plasma
exchanges in polyarteritis nodosa and Churg-Strauss syndrome, factors predicting poor prognosis, *97:* 316

Plasmapheresis
with cyclophosphamide, systemic lupus erythematosus remission after, *96:* 133

Platelet
-derived growth factor
β, receptors, expression increase in psoriatic arthritis, *96:* 269
in bronchoalveolar lavage fluid from scleroderma, *97:* 214

Pneumocystis carinii
pneumonia in Wegener's granulomatosis, factors associated with, *97:* 308

Pneumonia
bronchiolitis obliterans organizing, as first manifestation of polymyositis, *98:* 209
Klebsiella, after melphalan in primary amyloidosis, *98:* 268
lipoid, and rheumatoid arthritis and cod-liver oil capsules, *98:* 261
Pneumocystis carinii in Wegener's granulomatosis, factors associated with, *97:* 308

Pneumonitis
methotrexate, in rheumatoid arthritis, and preexisting lung disease, *97:* 85

PO fusion protein
in CNS disease in systemic lupus erythematosus, *97:* 162

POEMS syndrome
all-*trans*-retinoic acid in, *98:* 264

Poly(ADP-ribose)
metabolism alteration in family members in systemic lupus erythematosus, *96:* 128

Polyarteritis nodosa
with Churg-Strauss syndrome, outcome, *96:* 248
corticosteroids, pulse cyclophosphamide and plasma exchanges in, factors predicting poor prognosis, *97:* 316
-like vasculitis in HIV infection, *96:* 250
mimicking hepatic candidiasis, CT of, *96:* 247

Polyarthritis
febrile, due to acute rheumatic fever in adults, *98:* 269

Polychondritis
relapsing
methotrexate in, *98:* 210
myelodysplastic syndrome and, *97:* 361

Polymerase chain reaction
Borrelia burgdorferi DNA is undetectable in skin lesions of morphea, scleroderma, or lichen sclerosus et atrophicus by, in North American patients, *98:* 242
for *Neisseria gonorrhoeae* in synovial fluid, *96:* 309

Polymorphism
HLA-DR, in polymyalgia rheumatica, molecular analysis of, *98:* 199

Polymyalgia
rheumatica
amyloidosis presenting as, systemic, *96:* 256
anticardiolipin antibody in, *97:* 323

with giant cell arteritis, methotrexate in, *98:* 201
HLA-DR polymorphism in, molecular analysis of, *98:* 199
methotrexate in, *98:* 200
methotrexate in, results of open, randomized study, *98:* 201
normal erythrocyte sedimentation rate and, *97:* 322

Polymyositis
bronchiolitis obliterans organizing pneumonia as first manifestation of, *98:* 209
cancer associated with, *96:* 283
MRI in, cost effectiveness of, *97:* 352

Portal
vein cavernous transformation as manifestation of Behçet's disease, *97:* 356

Postmenopausal
bone loss
glucocorticoid-induced, etidronate with ergocalciferol in prevention of, *97:* 277
lumbar spine, intermittent salmon calcitonin to prevent, *97:* 276
osteoporosis (*see* Osteoporosis, postmenopausal)
women
alendronate effect on risk of fractures in women with existing vertebral fractures, *98:* 229
calcium supplementation in, long-term effects on bone loss and fractures, *97:* 275

Postnatal
skin development and fibrosis, transforming growth factor-β1 and collagen gene expression during (in mice), *97:* 230

Practice
general, rheumatology education and management skills in, trainee study, *97:* 22
rheumatology
fibromyalgia in, in Canada, *97:* 281
university, needle muscle biopsy in, *96:* 286
specialty, at university medical center, managed care effects on, *97:* 12
university-based, more aggressive drug treatment of rheumatoid arthritis in, *97:* 70

Practitioner (*see* Physician)

Prednisolone
osteoporosis and, secondary, *98:* 225
in rheumatoid arthritis, active, and intact ACTH secretion but impaired cortisol response, *98:* 51

Prednisone
in amyloidosis, primary, with melphalan and colchicine, *98:* 268
low-dose, in rheumatoid arthritis, spinal bone loss secondary to, calcium and vitamin D_3 supplementation in prevention of, *98:* 57
in lupus nephritis, severe, economic impact of treatment, *96:* 10
in myelodysplastic syndrome with systemic vasculitis, *98:* 194
requirements, perioperative, in secondary adrenal insufficiency, *98:* 52
in rheumatoid arthritis, outcome, *96:* 79

Pregnancy
antiphospholipid antibodies during, and refractory HELLP syndrome, *96:* 141
aspirin and heparin in pregnant women with recurrent miscarriage associated with antiphospholipid antibodies, *98:* 115
lupus erythematosus and, systemic, hydroxychloroquine in, *98:* 122

Premenopausal women
lupus erythematosus in, systemic, and myocardial infarction and angina, *98:* 116

Primary care
management of musculoskeletal disorders, physician confidence in, determinants of, *97:* 23
physicians
care of acute low back pain, outcomes and costs of, *97:* 294
continuing medical education in rheumatic diseases, *97:* 21
setting, impact of rheumatology in, *97:* 17

Pristane
-induced arthritis as new model for rheumatoid arthritis (in rat), *98:* 69

Procollagen
gene, α1 (I), expression in NIH-3T3 cells stimulated by HTLV-1 Tax gene, *98:* 147
III, predictive value in lung involvement diagnosis in scleroderma, *97:* 239

Procollagenase
  neutrophil, activation in presence of doxycycline results in enzyme fragmentation and enzyme activity loss, *97:* 259
  shoulder tendon biopsy samples in organ culture producing, *97:* 291
Prolactin
  link to genetic and reproductive associations with rheumatoid arthritis, *98:* 39
  in lupus erythematosus, systemic, *96:* 124
Prostacyclin
  analog, oral, in primary Raynaud's phenomenon, *98:* 185
Prostaglandin
  levels, gastric mucosal, age-related reduction in, increasing susceptibility to aspirin-induced injury (in rat), *96:* 69
Protein(s)
  A
    column immunoadsorption therapy, staphylococcal, leukocytoclastic vasculitis after, *97:* 318
    Lyme vaccine, safety and immunogenicity of, *96:* 293
  antibodies, anti-ribosomal P, and neuropsychiatric systemic lupus erythematosus, *98:* 118
  anticoagulant, I, in placenta in antiphospholipid antibody syndrome, *96:* 145
  antiribosomal PO, antibodies, in CNS disease in systemic lupus erythematosus, *97:* 162
  C-reactive, in rheumatoid arthritis
    early, and functional outcome, *98:* 34
    early, individual relationship between progression of radiological damage and, *98:* 34
    as marker for articular destruction, *98:* 33
  eosinophil major basic, elevated levels in scleroderma, *97:* 228
  heat shock (*see* Heat, shock protein)
  immunoblot analysis for α-fodrin as autoantigen in primary Sjögren's syndrome, *98:* 131
  interleukin-2 diphtheria fusion, for refractory rheumatoid arthritis, *97:* 100
  kinase A isozyme activity, deficient type I, in systemic lupus erythematosus T lymphocytes, *96:* 105
  metabolism in rheumatoid arthritis and aging, *98:* 38
  muscle-cell membrane, autoantibodies against, in myositis, *98:* 208
  p16, interferon-gamma–inducible, as target of antinuclear antibodies in systemic lupus erythematosus, *96:* 110
  p80 fusion, recombinant soluble, in refractory rheumatoid arthritis, *98:* 62
  PO fusion, in CNS disease in systemic lupus erythematosus, *97:* 162
  ribosomal P2, autoantigen-specific T cell proliferation induced by, in systemic lupus erythematosus, *96:* 109
  viral DNA binding, generating SLE-related autoimmunity to double-stranded DNA and histones, *97:* 139
Proteinuria
  in lupus, nucleosome-restricted antibodies in kidney eluates of (in mice), *96:* 113
Proteoglycan
  synthesis, dermatan sulfate, altered in fibroblast skin cultures in systemic sclerosis, *98:* 158
Psoriasis
  arthritis in (*see* Arthritis, psoriatic)
  foot and ankle surgery in, *96:* 272
  methotrexate in, low-dose, causing methotrexate osteopathy, *97:* 91
  rheumatoid arthritis and, methotrexate in, accelerated nodulosis after, *97:* 74
Psychiatric
  diagnoses in fibromyalgia patients related to health care-seeking behavior rather than to illness, *98:* 259
Psychometric
  properties of Pain-O-Meter, *98:* 265
Psychosocial
  findings and long-term outcome after whiplash injury, *97:* 298
Pulmonary
  (*See also* Lung)
  fibrosis (*see* Fibrosis, pulmonary)
  hypertension (*see* Hypertension, pulmonary)
Puncture
  lumbar, in CNS vasculitis, *96:* 260

Q

Quartz dust
uranium miners exposed to, anti-CENP-B response of, and scleroderma, *97:* 217
Quinolinic acid
neuropsychiatric manifestations of systemic lupus erythematosus and, *98:* 95

R

Radiochemical
synovectomy, yttrium-90, in chronic knee synovitis, *98:* 277
Radiography
abnormalities in rheumatoid arthritis lung disease, *98:* 26
in bursitis, tuberculous, *98:* 235
of hand, in rheumatoid arthritis, *97:* 46
of heel pain in Reiter's disease, *vs.* bone scintigraphy, *97:* 334
in osteoarthritis of hip, and bone mineral density, *97:* 256
plain, of knee articular cartilage, *vs.* arthroscopy and MRI, *96:* 189
in tenosynovitis, tuberculous, *98:* 235
Radiolabelled amyloid P component
studies provide evidence for turnover and regression of amyloid deposits in vivo, *96:* 308
Radiologic
damage in early rheumatoid arthritis, progression of, individual relationship between acute phase response and, *98:* 34
evidence of disease modification after cyclosporine in rheumatoid arthritis, *96:* 82
evolution of rheumatoid wrist after radiolunate arthrodesis, *97:* 56
findings and long-term outcome after whiplash injury, *97:* 298
outcome assessment after methotrexate and azathioprine in rheumatoid arthritis, *97:* 69
progression in early rheumatoid arthritis, measurement and prediction of, *96:* 45
Radiolunate arthrodesis
for rheumatoid wrist, radiological evolution of wrist after, *97:* 56
Rash
cyclical, in systemic lupus erythematosus, hormone supplement for, *97:* 191
Raynaud's disease
idiopathic, blockade of vasospastic attacks by α_2-adrenergic antagonists in, *97:* 243
Raynaud's phenomenon, *98:* 180
discussion of, *97:* 242
evolution of, long-term study, *97:* 237
penile, *98:* 180
as presenting sign of ovarian adenocarcinoma, *97:* 248
primary
cooling in, digital pressure responses to, *96:* 175
cooling in, digital vascular responses to, *98:* 183
prostacyclin analog in, oral, *98:* 185
vasospasm of nipple–A manifestation of, *98:* 180
von Willebrand factor, thrombomodulin, thromboxane, beta-thromboglobulin and fibrinolysis markers in, *97:* 208
Raynaud's syndrome
interferon therapy and, *98:* 182
outcome, long-term, *97:* 231
Red blood cell (*see* Erythrocyte)
Reflex
sympathetic dystrophy, bone scintigraphy for diagnosis, *97:* 290
tearing, decreased, and lymphocytic infiltration in lacrimal glands, *98:* 137
Regurgitation
mitral, in limited systemic sclerosis, *98:* 173
Reiter's disease
heel pain in, bone scintigraphy of, *97:* 334
Relaxin
effects on lung fibroblasts and lung fibrosis, *98:* 142
Renal
(*See also* Kidney)
cell carcinoma, interleukin-2 and lymphokine activated killer cells for, rapid exacerbation of scleroderma after, *96:* 181
Renomegaly
sudden onset unilateral, as initial manifestation of primary Sjögren's syndrome, in teenager, *98:* 129
Renovascular
hypertension due to Takayasu's arteritis, *97:* 325
Reproductive
associations with rheumatoid arthritis, and prolactin, *98:* 39

Research
  epidemiologic, self-administered rheumatoid arthritis disease activity index for, *97:* 44
Resistance
  training, progressive, effect in rheumatoid arthritis, *98:* 37
Respiratory
  cardiorespiratory responses to incremental exercise in systemic sclerosis, *98:* 171
  tract lesions associated with antineutrophil cytoplasmic autoantibodies with perinuclear staining pattern, *96:* 246
Rest
  bed, for acute low back pain, *96:* 2
Retinoic acid
  all-*trans*-, in POEMS syndrome, *98:* 264
Retrovirus
  -mediated gene transfer to synovium in bacterial cell wall-induced arthritis (in rat), *97:* 105
Rheumatic
  conditions, reliability of diagnosis at primary health care level, *96:* 52
  disease
    continuing medical education for primary care physicians, *97:* 21
    methotrexate in, spontaneous regression of lymphoproliferative disorders and, *98:* 46
    systemic, *98:* 187
  fever
    acute, in adults, delayed diagnosis of, *98:* 269
    Jones criteria for diagnosis, guideline maintenance and revision, *97:* 9
Rheumatoid
  antigenic determinant, most African-Americans with rheumatoid arthritis do not have, *97:* 34
  arthritis *(see below)*
  factor, monoclonal, cross-reactive idiotypes, as predictive factor for development of lymphoma in primary Sjögren's syndrome, *98:* 136
  nodules, effect of second-line drugs on progression or regression of, *97:* 77
  shoulder, painful, ultrasound of, *96:* 47
  susceptible alleles of HLA-DRB1 as genetically recessive, *96:* 28
  synovial tissue, engraftment in severe combined immunodeficiency disease (in mice), *96:* 30
  synovium
    interleukin-13 in, *98:* 23
    p53 overexpression in, *98:* 25
Rheumatoid arthritis, *98:* 19; *97:* 29; *96:* 25
  active
    ACTH secretion in, intact, *98:* 51
    cortisol response in, impaired, *98:* 51
    minocycline in, *96:* 74
    omega 3 fatty acid supplement in, *96:* 77
    Rome criteria for, *96:* 50
  activity assessment, 28-joint count for, validity and reliability of, *96:* 42
  in African Americans lacking rheumatoid antigenic determinant, *97:* 34
  anemia in
    erythropoietin for, *96:* 64
    iron deficiency diagnosis in, algorithm for, *97:* 52
  ankle problems in, *96:* 49
  antiinflammatory drugs in, nonsteroidal
    cost of misoprostol prophylaxis and, *96:* 65
    gastrointestinal complications of, misoprostol reducing, *97:* 114
  anti-Sa system for, *96:* 35
  apoptosis in, *98:* 25
  articular destruction in, prediction of, *98:* 33
  assessment, *97:* 44; *96:* 42
  auranofin *vs.* sulfasalazine in, efficacy and toxicity of, *98:* 43
  balneotherapy for, *97:* 96
  in Black-Caribbeans, low prevalence compared with whites, *96:* 41
  bone destruction in, progression in wrists and fingers, *96:* 28
  bone mass in, effect of hormone replacement therapy on, *96:* 215
  bone metabolism in, *96:* 38
  bone mineral density in
    decreased axial, in perimenopausal women, *96:* 214
    effect of low-dose corticosteroids on, *97:* 133
  cancer risk and, *98:* 28
  cartilage metabolism in, *96:* 38
  clinical aspects of, *98:* 26
  clinical course, HLA markers and prediction of, *98:* 22
  cod-liver oil capsules and lipoid pneumonia, *98:* 261
  corticosteroids in
    injection of, no effect on rate of total joint arthroplasty, *98:* 53

low-dose, bone loss in spine secondary to, calcium and vitamin D_3 supplementation in prevention of, *98:* 56
low-dose, long-term, serious adverse events, *96:* 78
low-dose, moderate-term effectiveness of, *98:* 54
costs in, indirect and nonmedical, *98:* 6
cyclophosphamide in, effects on development of malignancy and long-term survival, *97:* 110
cyclosporine in
benefit/risk ratio, *96:* 84
low-dose, *96:* 82
low-dose, long-term, effect on kidney function, *97:* 108
renal biopsy findings and follow-up of renal function and, *98:* 49
death in, antirheumatic drugs causing, *97:* 111
diagnosis
computerized databases for, sensitivity and specificity of, *96:* 13
self-reported, validity of, *98:* 31
self-reported, validity of, in elderly women, *98:* 32
disability in
functional, changes in, and rheumatology visit frequency, *98:* 8
long-term, reduction with antirheumatic drug-based treatment strategies, *97:* 2
disease activity index, self-administered, for epidemiologic research, *97:* 44
disease modifying agents, *97:* 59; *96:* 54
disease severity in, and HLA-DRB1 genes, *98:* 21
disease status, perceived overall, impact of patient-with-patient interaction on, *98:* 12
drug therapy in
costs of, total, *96:* 7
monitoring guidelines, *98:* 2
more aggressive, in university-based practice, *97:* 70
second-line, early, benefit from, 5 year follow-up, *97:* 29
second-line, stopping, *97:* 59
second-line, variation among rheumatologists in use of, *97:* 4
early
acute phase and function in, *98:* 34
bone loss in, generalized, *96:* 212
CD4 monoclonal antibody for, *97:* 102
cyclosporine in, low-dose, *vs.* chloroquine, *96:* 80
drugs for, second line, *97:* 65
gold *vs.* sulfasalazine for, *97:* 63
hydroxychloroquine in, *96:* 54
individual relationship between progression of radiological damage and acute phase response in, *98:* 34
radiological progression of, measurement and prediction, *96:* 45
"sawtooth" treatment strategy in, outcome, *98:* 41
economics, *97:* 4
familial, genetic anticipation in, *96:* 30
further evidence for, *98:* 20
Fas accumulation in inflamed joints in, soluble, *98:* 24
fish oil in, high dose, after stopping nonsteroidal antiinflammatory drugs, *97:* 129
foot problems in, *96:* 49
gamma-linoleic acid in, *98:* 63
genetic associations with, and prolactin, *98:* 39
genetic epidemiology of, *97:* 37
genetics, *97:* 33; *96:* 28
gold in, second course of, *97:* 62
hand, radiography of, *97:* 46
heterogeneity, and antiperinuclear factor, *96:* 37
hip or knee replacement for, predicting length of stay after, *98:* 13
immunization in, mononuclear leukocyte, *97:* 104
immunogenetics of, *98:* 20
improvement in, American College of Rheumatology preliminary definition of, *97:* 48
interleukin-13 anti-inflammatory effects on synovial fluid macrophages in, *98:* 23
interleukin-10 production in, *96:* 100
joint destruction in
glucocorticoids and, *97:* 134
progressive, with HIV, *97:* 41
juvenile, *98:* 70; *97:* 342
bone mineralization and bone mineral metabolism in, *98:* 76
breast feeding and, *97:* 342
changing epidemiology in Rochester, Minnesota 1960-1993, *98:* 74
differentiation from juvenile-onset ankylosing spondylitis, *97:* 348
epidemiology, 1975-1992, *97:* 346

Escherichia coli, dnaJ heat shock protein in, immune responses to, *96:* 278
genetic association with interleukin-1α polymorphism, *96:* 274
oligoarticular, autoreactivity to heat shock protein 60 predicts disease remission in, *98:* 73
pauciarticular-onset, DNA polymorphisms in, *96:* 275
polyarticular, IV immunoglobulin in, *98:* 79
sulfasalazine for, *97:* 349
synovial cysts in, bicipital, *97:* 344
synovium in, expression of tumor necrosis factor-α and -β and their receptors in, *98:* 71
systemic onset, IV immunoglobulin in, follow-up, *98:* 77
lung disease, *98:* 26
lymphoma in, Epstein-Barr virus clonality in, *98:* 30
methotrexate in (*see* Methotrexate, in rheumatoid arthritis)
minocycline in, *96:* 73
model
engraftment of rheumatoid synovial tissue and normal human cartilage in severe combined immunodeficiency disease as (in mice), *96:* 30
pristane-induced arthritis as (in rat), *98:* 69
monoclonal antibody to tumor necrosis factor-α in, chimeric, *96:* 85
occipito-cervical fixation in, surgical risk factors in, *97:* 55
outcome
HLA markers and prediction of, *98:* 22
two and five year, associated with HLA-DRB and DQB genes, *97:* 35
pain in, changes in, and rheumatology visit frequency, *98:* 8
pamidronate in, bone mass increase with, *98:* 60
pathophysiology, *98:* 20; *97:* 33; *96:* 28
D-penicillamine in, low-dose, *96:* 62
phenytoin in, *vs.* auranofin and chloroquine, *97:* 61
in Pima Indians, decreasing incidence and prevalence over 25 years, *96:* 39
prednisone in
outcome, *96:* 79
variation of rheumatologists in use of, *97:* 4
protein metabolism in, and aging, *98:* 38
refractory
active, CAMPATH-1H monoclonal antibody for, *97:* 99
failure of low-dose IV immunoglobulin in, *98:* 61
interleukin-2 diphtheria fusion protein for, *97:* 100
monoclonal antibody to intercellular adhesion molecule 1 in, *96:* 87
tumor necrosis factor receptor p80 fusion protein in, recombinant soluble, *98:* 62
reproductive associations with, and prolactin, *98:* 39
resistance training in, progressive, *98:* 37
rotator cuff dysfunction in, MRI of, *97:* 54
salsalate in, as efficacious as diclofenac, *97:* 118
seropositive, combination drugs for, *97:* 67
severe, cyclosporine *vs.* methotrexate in, *97:* 106
spine in, cervical, MRI of, *96:* 48
stress management in, effects on clinical outcomes, *97:* 94
sulfasalazine *vs.* auranofin in, efficacy and toxicity of, *98:* 43
synovial fibroblasts attach and invade human cartilage when engrafted into SCID mice in, *98:* 68
synovitis in, MRI of, *96:* 46
T cell depletion in, oligoclonal T cell populations after, *97:* 97
telephone interventions and health outcomes in, *98:* 10
tenidap for, *vs.* hydroxychloroquine and piroxicam, *97:* 127
treatment, *98:* 40; *97:* 111
cost of, direct, *vs.* fibromyalgia treatment, *97:* 280
triazolam for, sleep, daytime sleepiness and morning stiffness after, *97:* 51
vasculitis development in, factors associated with, *98:* 196
vasculitis secondary to, digital, cervical epidural analgesia for pain of, *98:* 198
well-controlled, training in, high *vs.* low intensity, *98:* 65
work disability predictors in, follow-up, *97:* 58
wrist

arthrodesis in, radiolunate, radiological evolution of wrist after, *97:* 56
synovial membrane hypertrophy and bone erosions in, MRI scoring of, *97:* 47

Rheumatologic
manifestations of tuberculosis, *98:* 235
vs. nonrheumatologic care of acute arthritis in hospital, *96:* 18

Rheumatologists
Canadian, survey on fibromyalgia in rheumatology practice, *97:* 281
role in health care system, evolving, *96:* 19
variation in use of prednisone and second line agents for rheumatoid arthritis, *97:* 4
vs. family physicians' perceptions of indications for and outcomes of knee replacement, *98:* 11

Rheumatology
career prospects in, and HLA-DR4, *97:* 40
in changing environment, *97:* 1; *96:* 1
clinic, pediatric, children with positive antinuclear antibody test but without autoimmune disease in, *97:* 178
databases in, online biomedical, performance of, *96:* 11
education and management skills in general practice, trainee study, *97:* 22
fellows' opinions about extended fellowship in musculoskeletal medicine, *96:* 12
practice
fibromyalgia in, in Canada, *97:* 281
university, needle muscle biopsy in, *96:* 286
in primary care setting, *97:* 17
specialist care, *97:* 19
training, clinical, in an uncertain future, *96:* 12
visit frequency and changes in functional disability and pain in rheumatoid arthritis, *98:* 8

Ribonucleoprotein
antibody, anti-U1 nuclear, and major histocompatibility complex class II gene, *96:* 97

Ribosomal
P, autoantibodies to, in lupus hepatitis, *97:* 179

P2 protein, autoantigen-specific T cell proliferation induced by, in systemic lupus erythematosus, *96:* 109

RNA
mRNA, measles virus nucleocapsid, in marrow mononuclear cells in Paget's disease, *97:* 385
polymerase II, phosphorylation form of, in scleroderma, *96:* 152

Rodnan TSS
modified, observer variability in scleroderma, *97:* 241

Rome criteria
for active rheumatoid arthritis, *96:* 50

Ro/SS-A
autoantibodies to, some are antiidiotypes to anti-double stranded DNA, *98:* 100

Rotator cuff
dysfunction in rheumatoid arthritis, MRI of, *97:* 54

Runner
former, knee osteoarthritis in, *97:* 257

Running
disability development with age and, *96:* 191
musculoskeletal pain with age and, *98:* 215
osteoarthritis and, follow-up study, *96:* 190

Rupture
aorta, thoracic, in giant cell arteritis, *96:* 257
hemorrhagic, of shoulder, *96:* 205

S

Sa system
in rheumatoid arthritis, *96:* 35

Sacroiliac
joint in chronic low back pain, *96:* 5

Sacroiliitis
in spondyloarthropathy, MRI of, *96:* 267

Salivary
glands
expression of E-selectin, tumor necrosis factor-α, and mast cell infiltration in, in early systemic sclerosis, *98:* 155
Fas and *Fas* ligand expression in, in primary Sjögren's syndrome, *98:* 133
labial, in Sjögren's syndrome, common T cell receptor clonotype in, *98:* 134

Salmonella
post-*Salmonella* reactive arthritis, clinicopathology, *97:* 335
Salsalate
in rheumatoid arthritis, *97:* 118
Sarcoidosis
acid-fast L forms from blood in, growth of, *98:* 271
cardiac, masquerading as metastatic tumor, echocardiography in, *97:* 355
lymph nodes in, non-palpable supraclavicular, ultrasound-guided fine-needle aspiration cytology of, *98:* 273
recurrence in lung transplant recipient, and tumor necrosis factor-α expression by alveolar macrophages, *98:* 272
in scleroderma, *97:* 245
"Sawtooth" strategy
in rheumatoid arthritis treatment, early, outcome of, *98:* 41
Schirmer test
with nasal stimulation for reflex tearing in Sjögren's syndrome, *98:* 137
Scintigraphy
abdominal, three-phase, in lupus vasculitis of gastrointestinal tract, *97:* 177
bone
heel pain evaluation in Reiter's disease, *97:* 334
quantitative, in monostotic Paget's disease of bone, *97:* 384
in reflex sympathetic dystrophy diagnosis, *97:* 290
thallium-201
for cardiac involvement in limited systemic sclerosis, *98:* 173
perfusion defects predict subsequent cardiac dysfunction in systemic sclerosis, *98:* 175
Scleredema
as poststreptococcal complication, *96:* 185
Scleroderma, *98:* 141; *97:* 205
adhesion molecules in peripheral blood of, soluble, *96:* 160
alveolitis in, fibrosing, *96:* 172
memory T cells increase in lung interstitium in, *97:* 246
anal function in, *98:* 179
antibodies in
antihistone, and lung fibrosis, *96:* 169
antimyenteric neuronal, *96:* 149
to histone DNA complexes, more sensitive and specific for scleroderma than lupus, *96:* 153
audiovestibular involvement in, *96:* 168
autoantibodies to fibrillarin in, *98:* 159
autoantibodies to topoisomerase I and RNA polymerase II in, *96:* 152
Borrelia burgdorferi DNA is undetectable by polymerase chain reaction in skin lesions of, in North American patients, *98:* 242
breast implants and, silicone-gel, silicone granuloma in acral skin in patient with, *97:* 379
bronchoalveolar lavage fluid from, platelet-derived growth factor and transforming growth-β1 in, *97:* 214
cardiac dysfunction in, subsequent, thallium perfusion defects predict, *98:* 175
clinical aspects, *98:* 163
clinical features, *97:* 231; *96:* 164
connective tissue growth factor gene expression and skin sclerosis in, *97:* 216
cooling in, digital pressure responses to, *96:* 175
diffuse
autonomic dysfunction in, *96:* 173
pulmonary hypertension in, *98:* 168
pulmonary hypertension in, and serum anti-U3RNP antibody, *98:* 169
diltiazem in, left ventricular myocardial perfusion and function after, *98:* 176
DNA topoisomerase I inducing T cell proliferative response in, *97:* 219
elastin and collagen degradation products in urine in, cross-linked, *97:* 224
endothelial cell apoptosis in, *98:* 160
endothelial cells, class II MHC and ICAM-1 expression on, up-regulation by interferon-gamma and tumor necrosis factor-α in early disease stage, *98:* 143
eosinophil major basic protein elevated levels in, *97:* 228
exacerbation, rapid, after interleukin-2 and lymphokine activated killer cells for renal cell carcinoma, *96:* 181
exercise in, incremental, cardiorespiratory responses to, *98:* 171
fibroblasts (*see* Fibroblasts, scleroderma)

free radical-mediated injury in, *98:* 161
HLA class II genes and anticentromere antibody in, *97:* 212
iloprost in, IV, for treatment of ischemic digital ulcers and prevention of gangrene, *98:* 184
immunogenetics of, *98:* 143
immunoglobulin G antiendothelial cell autoantibodies from, inducing leukocyte adhesion to vascular endothelial cells, *97:* 205
incidence in Allegheny County, Pennsylvania, *98:* 165
interleukin-2 receptors in, soluble serum, *98:* 150
interleukin-4 levels in, elevated serum, *98:* 154
interleukin-6 secretion augmentation in collagen-stimulated peripheral blood mononuclear cells in, *96:* 162
interleukin-8 expression in, *97:* 222
interleukin-10 levels in, elevated serum, *98:* 154
interleukin-13 levels in, elevated serum, *98:* 154
intestinal ischemia in, small, *96:* 167
killer cells in, natural, and anti-scl-70 antibodies, *97:* 227
limited
  cardiac involvement in, comprehensive noninvasive assessment of, *98:* 173
  pulmonary hypertension in, *98:* 168
linear, progression to fatal systemic sclerosis in children, *96:* 164
lipoproteins isolated from, low-density, oxidation increased susceptibility of, *97:* 221
lung disease in, severe
  interstitial, therapy, *96:* 178
  restrictive, *96:* 170
lung function improvement after cyclophosphamide in, *96:* 179
lung involvement in, *98:* 166
  diagnosis, predictive value of procollagen III in, *97:* 239
model of, animal, with cutaneous fibrosis and mononuclear cell infiltration, *97:* 209
neuropathy in, autonomic and sensorimotor, *97:* 236
pathogenesis, *97:* 208; *96:* 147
pathophysiology, *98:* 143
prevalence, increased in Native American tribe in Oklahoma, *98:* 163
progressive, accelerated, in hypothenar hammer syndrome, *97:* 234
-related disorders, *98:* 141
renal failure in, and antineutrophil cytoplasmic autoantibodies, *96:* 244
renal vascular damage in, *98:* 177
salivary glands in, early expression of E-selectin, tumor necrosis factor-α, and mast cell infiltration in, *98:* 155
sarcoidosis in, *97:* 245
severe, with anti-topoisomerase I antibodies associated with HLA-DRw11 allele, *96:* 151
skin
  collagen in, type VII, transforming growth factor-β regulating, *96:* 163
  endothelin-1 localization and binding sites in, *96:* 154
  interleukin-4 expression in, *98:* 152
  thickness score in, total, observer variability in, *97:* 241
spectrum disorders, cooling in, digital vascular responses to, *98:* 183
subsets, circulating endothelin-1 levels in, *96:* 157
systemic and localized, circulating Fcγ receptor specific autoantibodies in, *97:* 213
T cells in, γδ, and anti-scl-70 antibodies, *97:* 227
therapy, *96:* 177
tumor necrosis factor-α levels in, elevated serum, and pulmonary fibrosis, *98:* 156
uranium miners exposed to quartz dust and, anti-CENP-B response of, *97:* 217
ventricular long-axis function abnormality in, *97:* 232
vesical dysfunction in, *97:* 247
von Willebrand factor, thrombomodulin, thromboxane, beta-thromboglobulin and fibrinolysis markers in, *97:* 208

Sclerosis
  cutaneous, and connective tissue growth factor gene expression in scleroderma, *97:* 216
  systemic (*see* Scleroderma)

Selectin
  E-, early expression in salivary glands in systemic sclerosis, *98:* 155

Sensorimotor
  neuropathy in systemic lupus erythematosus and scleroderma, *97:* 236

Serologic
  findings in hypocomplementemic urticarial vasculitis syndrome, *96:* 261
Sexual
  abuse in women
    with fibromyalgia, *96:* 225
    with fibromyalgia syndrome, *96:* 227
Shooters
  knee osteoarthritis in, *97:* 257
Shoulder
  arthropathy in, idiopathic destructive, *98:* 223
  rheumatoid, painful, ultrasound of, *96:* 47
  rupture of, hemorrhagic, *96:* 205
  tendon biopsy samples in organ culture producing procollagenase and tissue inhibitor of metalloproteinases, *97:* 291
Sialoadenitis
  autoimmune, immunization with carbonic anhydrase II inducing (in mice), *97:* 202
Silica
  exposure and autoimmune diseases, *97:* 370
Silicone
  blood, elevated levels, with silicone gel breast implants, *97:* 373
  gel, repeated exposure inducing delayed hypersensitivity, *97:* 371
  granuloma in acral skin in patient with silicone-gel breast implants and scleroderma, *97:* 379
  implant, *97:* 370
    breast (*see* Breast, implant, silicone)
Sjögren's syndrome, *98:* 129; *97:* 196
  anti-Ro/SS-A autoantibodies and, complete heart block in adult with, *98:* 139
  CNS disease in, anti-Ro/SSA autoantibodies in, *96:* 116
  with dorsal root ganglionitis, anti-dorsal root ganglion neuron antibody in, *97:* 199
  follow-up, long-term, *97:* 196
  interleukin-10 production in, *96:* 100
  kidney disease in, biochemical markers of, *97:* 198
  lymphoma and, malignant, *97:* 197
  primary
    autoantigen in, α-fodrin as, *98:* 131
    Fas and *Fas* ligand expression in, *98:* 133
    hepatitis C virus infection in, *98:* 135
    lymphoma development in, predictive factors for, *98:* 136
    renomegaly in, sudden onset unilateral, as initial manifestation, in teenager, *98:* 129
  T cell receptor clonotype, common, in lacrimal glands and labial salivary glands in, *98:* 134
Skeletal
  (*See also* Musculoskeletal)
  muscle in fibromyalgia, increased incidence of a resonance in phosphodiester region of ^{31}P nuclear magnetic resonance spectra in, *96:* 220
Skin
  (*See also* Cutaneous)
  acral, silicone granuloma in, in patient with silicone-gel breast implants and scleroderma, *97:* 379
  development and fibrosis, postnatal, transforming growth factor β1 and collagen gene expression during (in mice), *97:* 230
  diseases, vascular, and antiphosphatidylethanolamine antibodies, *98:* 107
  fibroblasts
    normal and systemic sclerosis, heterogeneity of collagen synthesis in, *98:* 148
    scleroderma, cultures, altered dermatan sulfate proteoglycan synthesis in, *98:* 158
  lesions
    of dermatomyositis, microvascular injury in pathogenesis of, *97:* 353
    of morphea, scleroderma, or lichen sclerosus et atrophicus, *Borrelia burgdorferi* DNA is undetectable by polymerase chain reaction in, in North American patients, *98:* 242
  scleroderma
    collagen in, type VII, transforming growth factor-β regulating, *96:* 163
    endothelin-1 localization and binding sites in, *96:* 154
    interleukin-4 expression in, *98:* 152
  thickness score, total, observer variability in scleroderma, *97:* 241
SLE (*see* Lupus, erythematosus, systemic)
Sleep
  improvement after zolpidem in fibromyalgia, *98:* 256
  after triazolam for rheumatoid arthritis, *97:* 51
Sleepiness
  daytime, after triazolam for rheumatoid arthritis, *97:* 51

Sleeping
difficulty in fibromyalgia syndrome, *98:* 253
Smoking
rheumatoid arthritis lung disease and, *98:* 26
SnRNP A and D polypeptides
lupus autoantibodies to DNA cross-react with, *96:* 108
Soccer
players, knee osteoarthritis in, *97:* 257
Sodium
fluoride, slow-release, for postmenopausal osteoporosis, *97:* 279
Soft tissue
injections, current practice survey, *97:* 297
lesions around heel in chronic inflammatory arthritis, ultrasound-guided injection of, *96:* 273
Somatic
findings and long-term outcome after whiplash injury, *97:* 298
Somatostatin
-induced modulation of inflammation in arthritis (in rabbit), *97:* 39
Spa therapy
effectiveness for chronic low back pain, *97:* 295
Specialist
rheumatology care, *97:* 19
Specialty
practice at university medical center, managed care effects on, *97:* 12
Spectroscopy
magnetic resonance, phosphorus-31, in dermatomyositis
amyopathic and myopathic, muscle dysfunction in, *96:* 279
data useful in longitudinal management, *96:* 281
Spine
bone loss
corticosteroids in rheumatoid arthritis causing, low-dose, calcium and vitamin D_3 supplementation in prevention of, *98:* 56
lumbar, postmenopausal, intermittent nasal salmon calcitonin to prevent, *97:* 276
in osteoporosis, corticosteroid-induced, etidronate reversing, *97:* 278
bone mass in postmenopausal osteoporosis, effect of alendronate over 3 years on, *98:* 226
cervical
(*See also* Neck)
injury, increased rates of fibromyalgia after, *98:* 250
osteoarthritis, pulsed electromagnetic fields for, *96:* 201
in rheumatoid arthritis, MRI of, *96:* 48
gout of, *97:* 369
pain in fibromyalgia, prevalence and treatment outcome, *97:* 282
stenosis, degenerative lumbar, history and physical exam diagnostic value in, *97:* 253
Spondylitis
ankylosing
fracture risk in, *96:* 266
indigenous to Mesoamerica, *97:* 333
juvenile-onset, early recognition of, differentiation from juvenile rheumatoid arthritis, *97:* 348
severe, methotrexate for, *97:* 331
Spondyloarthropathy, *97:* 331; *96:* 265
juvenile, synovium in, expression of tumor necrosis factor-α and -β and their receptors in, *98:* 71
long-term outcome, predictive factors for, *96:* 265
sacroiliitis of, MRI of, *96:* 267
seronegative, late onset undifferentiated, *97:* 336
Sports
weight-bearing, long-term, and risk of osteoarthritis, in women, *98:* 214
Staphylococcal
protein A column immunoadsorption therapy, leukocytoclastic vasculitis after, *97:* 318
Staphylococcus aureus
arthritis, experimental, corticosteroids plus antibiotics in, *98:* 232
nasal carriage, chronic, and higher relapse rates in Wegener's granulomatosis, *96:* 233
Stenosis
spine, lumbar degenerative, history and physical exam diagnostic value in, *97:* 253
vascular, due to atherosclerosis and vasculitis, intracranial angioplasty for, results, *97:* 326
Steroid(s)
(*See also* Corticosteroids)
-related complications in temporal arteritis, *96:* 212
requirements, perioperative, in secondary adrenal insufficiency, *98:* 52

in rheumatoid arthritis, effect of hormone replacement therapy on bone mass after, *96:* 215
-sparing effect of methotrexate in relapsing polychondritis, *98:* 210
Stiff neck
in Lyme borreliosis, early, with erythema migrans, *98:* 237
Stiffness
morning, after triazolam in rheumatoid arthritis, *97:* 51
Stomach (*see* Gastric)
Stomatitis
after methotrexate in systemic lupus erythematosus and undifferentiated connective tissue disease, *98:* 123
methotrexate-induced, allopurinol mouthwashes in, *96:* 61
Strength
training, high-intensity, effect on osteoporotic fracture risk, *96:* 208
Streptococcal
scleredema as poststreptococcal complication, *96:* 185
Stress
management in rheumatoid arthritis outcomes, *97:* 94
Stromelysin 1
levels and joint involvement in osteoarthritis, *96:* 204
Substance P
CSF level elevation in fibromyalgia syndrome, *96:* 220
Sulfasalazine
in psoriatic arthritis, *97:* 340
in rheumatoid arthritis
early, *vs.* gold, *97:* 63
juvenile, *97:* 349
with methotrexate and hydroxychloroquine, *97:* 1
vs. auranofin, efficacy and toxicity of, *98:* 43
for small intestine inflammation and blood loss, NSAID-induced, *96:* 71
Supraclavicular
lymph nodes, non-palpable, in sarcoidosis, ultrasound-guided fine-needle aspiration cytology of, *98:* 273
SWR x SJL F_1 mice
model for lupus-like disease, *96:* 115
Sympathetic
derangement, orthostatic, in fibromyalgia, *98:* 252
dystrophy, reflex, bone scintigraphy in diagnosis, *97:* 290
Synovectomy
yttrium-90 radiochemical, in chronic knee synovitis, *98:* 277
Synovial
(*See also* Synovium)
cysts, bicipital, in juvenile rheumatoid arthritis, *97:* 344
fibroblasts in rheumatoid arthritis attach and invade human cartilage when engrafted into SCID mice, *98:* 68
fluid
macrophages in rheumatoid arthritis, antiinflammatory effects of interleukin-13 on, *98:* 23
Neisseria gonorrhoeae in, polymerase chain reaction for, *96:* 309
osteoarthritic, submicroscopic crystals in, *96:* 300
membrane
hypertrophy in rheumatoid arthritis of wrist, MRI scoring of, *97:* 47
inflammation and cytokine production in early osteoarthritis, *98:* 217
rheumatoid tissue, engraftment in severe combined immunodeficiency disease (in mice), *96:* 30
T cells, Fas^{high} CD4+, apoptosis by *Borrelia*-reactive Fas $ligand^{high}$ $\gamma\delta$ T cells in Lyme arthritis, *98:* 241
tissue in Lyme arthritis, *Borrelia burgdorferi* detected by DNA amplification in, *98:* 236
Synoviocyte
collagenase gene expression, inhibition by adenosine receptor stimulation, *98:* 145
Synovitis
crystal-induced, acute, ACTH for, *96:* 297
knee, chronic, yttrium-90 radiochemical synovectomy in, *98:* 277
remitting seronegative symmetrical, with pitting edema, clinical spectrum of, *98:* 276
in rheumatoid arthritis, MRI of, *96:* 46
Synovium
(*See also* Synovial)
gene transfer to, retrovirus-mediated, in bacterial cell wall-induced arthritis (in rat), *97:* 105
rheumatoid
interleukin-13 in, *98:* 23
p53 overexpression in, *98:* 25

in rheumatoid arthritis, juvenile, expression of tumor necrosis factor-α and -β and their receptors in, *98:* 71
in spondyloarthropathy, juvenile, expression of tumor necrosis factor-α and -β and their receptors in, *98:* 71

T

T cell(s)
CD56+, impaired recovery and cytolytic function in systemic lupus erythematosus, *98:* 90
CD40 ligand hyperexpression by, in systemic lupus erythematosus, *98:* 88
CD4+ synovial, Fas^{high}, apoptosis by *Borrelia*-reactive Fas ligand^{high} γδ T cells in Lyme arthritis, *98:* 241
depletion, in rheumatoid arthritis, oligoclonal T cell populations after, *97:* 97
γδ
Borrelia-reactive Fas^{high}, in Lyme arthritis, apoptosis of Fas^{high} CD4+ synovial T cells by, *98:* 241
in scleroderma, and anti-scl-70 antibodies, *97:* 227
leukemia virus type 1, human, Tax gene, stimulation of α1 (I) procollagen gene expression in NIH-3T3 cells by, *98:* 147
of lupus erythematosus, systemic, deficient type I protein kinase A isozyme activity in, *96:* 105
memory, increase in lung interstitium in fibrosing alveolitis in scleroderma, *97:* 246
proliferation, autoantigen-specific, induced by ribosomal P2 protein in systemic lupus erythematosus, *96:* 109
proliferative response induced by DNA topoisomerase I, in scleroderma, *97:* 219
reactivity to heat shock protein 60 predicts disease remission in oligoarticular juvenile rheumatoid arthritis, *98:* 73
receptor
β-chain DNA polymorphisms in pauciarticular-onset juvenile rheumatoid arthritis, *96:* 275
clonotype, common, in lacrimal glands and labial salivary glands in Sjögren's syndrome, *98:* 134
recognizing self heat shock protein 60-kD, activation of, as protection against arthritis (in rat), *96:* 89
Takayasu's arteritis, *96:* 259
renovascular hypertension due to, *97:* 325
Tax
gene, HTLV-1, stimulation of α1 (I) procollagen gene expression in NIH-3T3 cells by, *98:* 147
Taxol
in arthritis, collagen-induced, *96:* 88
Team
managed outpatient care for early onset chronic inflammatory arthritis, *97:* 24
Tearing
reflex, decreased, and lymphocytic infiltration in lacrimal glands, *98:* 137
Teenager
Sjögren's syndrome in, primary, sudden onset unilateral renomegaly as initial manifestation of, *98:* 129
Telephone
interventions and health outcomes in rheumatoid arthritis or osteoarthritis, *98:* 10
Temperature
of arthritic knees, local heat and cold treatment for, *96:* 72
Temporal
arteritis (*see* Arteritis, giant cell)
artery biopsy in suspected giant cell arteritis, prediction of results, *96:* 16
association of cancer with polymyositis and dermatomyositis, *96:* 283
Tendinitis
calcific, in proximal thigh, *96:* 229
Tendon
shoulder, biopsy samples in organ culture producing procollagenase and tissue inhibitor of metalloproteinases, *97:* 291
Tenidap
in rheumatoid arthritis, *vs.* hydroxychloroquine and piroxicam, *97:* 127
Tenosynovitis
calcium pyrophosphate dihydrate crystal-induced, *97:* 368
tuberculous, imaging findings, *98:* 235
Testosterone
for lupus erythematosus, systemic, with Klinefelter's syndrome, *97:* 193

Thalamus
  cerebral blood flow abnormalities in, and low pain thresholds in fibromyalgia in women, *97:* 284
Thallium-201
  scintigraphy
    for cardiac involvement in limited systemic sclerosis, *98:* 173
    perfusion defects predict subsequent cardiac dysfunction in systemic sclerosis, *98:* 175
Thigh
  proximal, calcific tendinitis in, *96:* 229
Thromboembolic
  incidence in anticardiolipin-positive patients with malignancy, *97:* 151
Thrombogenic
  properties of monoclonal IgG anticardiolipin antibody in antiphospholipid syndrome (in mice), *98:* 111
β-Thromboglobulin
  in Raynaud's phenomenon and scleroderma, *97:* 208
Thrombomodulin
  marker of disease activity in systemic lupus erythematosus, *96:* 122
  in Raynaud's phenomenon and scleroderma, *97:* 208
Thrombosis
  antiphosphatidylethanolamine antibodies and, *98:* 107
  in antiphospholipid syndrome
    induction by immunoglobulin G, M and A (in mice), *97:* 141
    management, *97:* 150
  in patients with antiphospholipid antibodies, natural history and risk factors for, *98:* 113
Thromboxane
  in Raynaud's phenomenon and scleroderma, *97:* 208
Thumb
  base osteoarthritis, trapezium excision for, *96:* 203
Thymocytes
  apoptotic, antiphospholipid autoantibodies binding to, and β_2-glycoprotein-I, *98:* 108
Tibiofemoral
  joint osteoarthritis, *96:* 196
    obesity and, in women, *98:* 214
TIMP 1
  levels and joint involvement in osteoarthritis, *96:* 204
Tissue
  connective (*see* Connective tissue)
  cytokine profiles in giant cell arteritis, *98:* 188
  soft
    injections, current practice survey, *97:* 297
    lesions around heel in chronic inflammatory arthritis, ultrasound-guided injections of, *96:* 273
  synovial, *Borrelia burgdorferi* detected by DNA amplification in, in Lyme arthritis, *98:* 236
Tomography
  computed (*see* Computed tomography)
Tophaceous
  tissue samples, formalin dissolving urate crystals in, *96:* 299
Tophi
  in bi- or tripartite bones, *98:* 222
  intraarticular, in knee, CT of, *98:* 222
  in patella, *98:* 222
Topoisomerase
  I
    autoantibodies in scleroderma, *96:* 152
    DNA, causing T cell proliferative response in scleroderma, *97:* 219
Toxic
  oil syndrome, epidemic Spanish, follow-up study, *96:* 184
Toxicity
  liver, of methotrexate in rheumatoid arthritis, *96:* 58
    monitoring guidelines, *96:* 55
  of methotrexate, *98:* 123
  ocular, monitoring practices with hydroxychloroquine, *96:* 14
  of p80 fusion protein, recombinant soluble, in refractory rheumatoid arthritis, *98:* 62
  of sulfasalazine *vs.* auranofin in rheumatoid arthritis, *98:* 43
Traction
  for low back pain, non-specific, efficacy of, *97:* 292
Trainee
  study in rheumatology education and management skills in general practice, *97:* 22
Training
  high *vs.* low intensity, in well-controlled rheumatoid arthritis, *98:* 65
  physical, in fibromyalgia, in women, *96:* 228
  physicians completing in 1994, initial employment status of, *97:* 14
  resistance, progressive, effect in rheumatoid arthritis, *98:* 37

rheumatology, clinical, in an uncertain future, *96:* 12
strength, high-intensity, effect on osteoporotic fracture risk, *96:* 208
Transforming growth factor
-β regulating type VII collagen in skin in scleroderma, *96:* 163
-β1
in bronchoalveolar lavage fluid from scleroderma, *97:* 214
effect on inflammation, monosodium urate monohydrate crystal-induced acute (in rat), *98:* 220
expression during postnatal skin development and fibrosis (in mice), *97:* 230
expression in fascial fibroblasts in diffuse fasciitis with eosinophilia, *98:* 203
Transplantation
bone marrow, allogenic, from donor with systemic lupus erythematosus, *98:* 92
chondrocyte, autologous, for deep cartilage defects in knee, *96:* 197
kidney, dialysis arthropathy outcome after, *97:* 387
lung, recurrence of sarcoidosis after, and tumor necrosis factor-α expression by alveolar macrophages, *98:* 272
Trapezium
excision for thumb base osteoarthritis, *96:* 203
Trauma
spine, cervical, increased rates of fibromyalgia after, *98:* 250
Tretinoin
in POEMS syndrome, *98:* 264
Triamcinolone
hexacetonide, intraarticular, in knee osteoarthritis, *97:* 263
Triazolam
in rheumatoid arthritis, effects on sleep, daytime sleepiness and morning stiffness, *97:* 51
Trichloroethene
-induced autoimmune response (in mice), *97:* 171
Trisomy 8
Behçet's disease and myelodysplastic syndromes, *98:* 206
Trochanteric
bursitis, *98:* 248
Tryptophan
metabolism in chronic inflammatory lung disease, *97:* 210
Tuberculosis
rheumatologic manifestations of, *98:* 235
Tuberculous
arthritis and gout, *98:* 222
bursitis, imaging findings, *98:* 235
tenosynovitis, imaging findings, *98:* 235
Tumor
metastatic, cardiac sarcoidosis masquerading as, echocardiography in, *97:* 355
necrosis factor
-induced integrin activation, effect on Fcγ receptor II-mediated signal transduction, *97:* 309
receptor 75, soluble, as biological marker of disease activity in Behçet's disease, *98:* 204
receptor p80 fusion protein, recombinant soluble, in refractory rheumatoid arthritis, *98:* 62
necrosis factor-α
chimeric monoclonal antibodies to, in rheumatoid arthritis, *96:* 85
expression in salivary glands in early systemic sclerosis, *98:* 155
expression in synovia in juvenile rheumatoid arthritis and juvenile spondyloarthropathy, *98:* 71
gene expression by alveolar macrophages in lung transplant recipient with recurrence of sarcoidosis, *98:* 272
levels, after all-*trans*-retinoic acid in POEMS syndrome, *98:* 265
levels, elevated serum, in systemic sclerosis, and pulmonary fibrosis, *98:* 156
production in synovial membranes in early osteoarthritis, *98:* 217
receptors, expression in synovia in juvenile rheumatoid arthritis and juvenile spondyloarthropathy, *98:* 71
receptors, p55 and p75, serum, as markers for disease activity in juvenile chronic arthritis, *98:* 70
scleroderma fibroblasts and, *96:* 158
up-regulation of class II MHC and ICAM-1 expression on scleroderma fibroblasts and endothelial cells by, in early stage disease, *98:* 143
necrosis factor-β and its receptors, expression in synovia in juvenile rheumatoid arthritis and juvenile spondyloarthropathy, *98:* 71

Twins
lupus erythematosus in, systemic, impaired recovery and cytolytic function of CD56+ T and non-T cells in, *98:* 90
monozygotic sisters, antiphospholipid and anti-β_2 glycoprotein I antibodies in, *96:* 139

U

Ulcer
digital, ischemic, in systemic sclerosis, IV iloprost for, *98:* 184
duodenal, NSAID-induced, prevention of
famotidine for, *98:* 40
misoprostol dosage for, *97:* 116
esophageal, due to alendronate, *98:* 232
gastric
epithelial regenerative repair in, corticosteroids reducing (in rat), *97:* 130
NSAID-induced, prevention with famotidine, *98:* 40
NSAID-induced, prevention with misoprostol, *96:* 66
NSAID-induced, prevention with misoprostol, dosage, *97:* 116
intestine, indomethacin-induced, oxygen radical scavengers protecting against (in rat), *97:* 122
peptic
bleeding, risk with NSAIDs, *96:* 68
NSAID-induced, *Helicobacter pylori* infection increasing risk of, *97:* 126
Ultrasound
Doppler, color-flow, for renal vascular damage in systemic sclerosis, *98:* 177
-guided fine-needle aspiration cytology of non-palpable supraclavicular lymph nodes in sarcoidosis, *98:* 273
-guided injection of soft tissue lesions around heel in chronic inflammatory arthritis, *96:* 273
of rheumatoid shoulder, painful, *96:* 47
of synovial cysts, bicipital, in juvenile rheumatoid arthritis, *97:* 344
therapy in musculoskeletal disorders, *98:* 263
University
-based practice, more aggressive drug treatment of rheumatoid arthritis in, *97:* 70
medical center, potential effects of managed care on specialty practice at, *97:* 12
Uranium miners
exposed to quartz dust, anti-CENP-B response to, and scleroderma, *97:* 217
Urate
-lowering drugs in recurrent gouty arthritis, cost effectiveness of, *97:* 365
Uric acid
lowering effect of oxipurinol in hyperuricemia, *98:* 224
Urinary
erythrocyte/leukocyte casts appearance and onset of renal relapse in systemic lupus erythematosus, *97:* 174
Urticarial
vasculitis
autoantibodies in, *97:* 161
hypocomplementemic urticarial vasculitis syndrome, clinical and serologic findings in, *96:* 261

V

Vaccine
Lyme, protein A, safety and immunogenicity of, *96:* 293
Vaccinia
virus expressing heat shock protein 60-kD, therapeutic effect in arthritis (in rat), *96:* 90
Varicella
zoster virus causing waxing and waning vasculitis, *98:* 194
Vascular
cardiovascular fitness and health in end-stage osteoarthritis, *97:* 254
collagen disease, histopathologic spectrum of palisaded neutrophilic and granulomatous dermatitis in, *96:* 120
cutaneous diseases, and antiphosphatidylethanolamine antibodies, *98:* 107
damage, renal, in systemic sclerosis, *98:* 177
endothelial cells, leukocyte adhesion to, immunoglobulin antiendothelial cell autoantibodies from scleroderma inducing, *97:* 205
injury in systemic lupus erythematosus, pathology and pathogenesis, *97:* 168

responses, digital, to cooling, in subjects with cold sensitivity, primary Raynaud's phenomenon, or scleroderma spectrum disorders, *98:* 183
stenosis due to atherosclerosis and vasculitis, intracranial angioplasty for, results, *97:* 326
Vasculitis, *98:* 187; *97:* 305; *96:* 233
anti-endothelial cell antibodies in, pathogenic role of (in mice), *98:* 192
central nervous system, sensitivities of noninvasive tests for, *96:* 260
development in rheumatoid arthritis, factors associated with, *98:* 196
digital, secondary to rheumatoid arthritis, cervical epidural analgesia for pain of, *98:* 198
disease activity distinguished from complications of cytotoxic therapy by antineutrophil cytoplasmic antibody assay, *96:* 240
leukocytoclastic, after staphylococcal protein A column immunoadsorption therapy, *97:* 318
lupus, of gastrointestinal tract, three-phase abdominal scintigraphy in, *97:* 177
necrotizing systemic, and chronic parvovirus B19 infection, *96:* 237
polyarteritis nodosa-like, in HIV infection, *96:* 250
PR3-ANCA positive, PiZ gene of alpha-1 antitrypsin in outcome of, *97:* 312
systemic
angiotropic large cell lymphoma with mononeuritis multiplex mimicking, *97:* 320
autoantibodies to lactoferrin and histone in, *96:* 249
autoantibodies to neutrophil cytoplasmic antigen predicting relapse in, *97:* 310
myelodysplastic syndromes and, *98:* 193
Vasculitis Damage Index for, development and initial validation of, *98:* 191
urticarial
autoantibodies in, *97:* 161
hypocomplementemic urticarial vasculitis syndrome, clinical and serologic findings in, *96:* 261
vascular stenosis due to, intracranial angioplasty for, results, *97:* 326
waxing and waning, due to varicella zoster virus, *98:* 194
Vaso-occlusive disease
ocular, in antiphospholipid syndrome, *97:* 148
Vasospasm
of nipple–A manifestation of Raynaud's phenomenon, *98:* 180
Vasospastic attacks
blockade by α_2-adrenergic antagonist in idiopathic Raynaud's disease, *97:* 243
VDU
workers, musculoskeletal problems in, *98:* 246
Vein
portal, cavernous transformation as manifestation of Behçet's disease, *97:* 356
Ventricle
left, myocardial perfusion and function in systemic sclerosis after diltiazem, *98:* 176
long-axis function abnormality in scleroderma, *97:* 232
Verapamil
lupus erythematosus due to, subacute cutaneous, *98:* 118
Vertebral
fractures, existing, effect of alendronate on risk of fracture in women with, *98:* 229
Vesical
dysfunction in scleroderma, *97:* 247
Virus
DNA binding protein generating SLE-related autoimmunity to double-stranded DNA and histones, *97:* 139
Epstein-Barr
clonality in lymphomas in rheumatoid arthritis, *98:* 30
infection, in methotrexate-related B lymphoproliferative disease in rheumatoid arthritis, *97:* 88
hepatitis (*see* Hepatitis)
immunodeficiency, human (*see* HIV)
measles virus nucleocapsid mRNA in bone marrow mononuclear cells from Paget's disease patients, *97:* 385
parvovirus (*see* Parvovirus)
retrovirus-mediated gene transfer to synovium in bacterial cell wall-induced arthritis (in rat), *97:* 105

T cell leukemia virus type 1, human, Tax gene, stimulation of α1 (I) procollagen gene expression in NIH-3T3 cells by, *98:* 147
varicella zoster, causing waxing and waning vasculitis, *98:* 194
Visit
frequency, rheumatology, and changes in functional disability and pain in rheumatoid arthritis, *98:* 8
Visual
display unit workers, musculoskeletal problems in, *98:* 246
Vitamin
D levels, serum, related to progression of osteoarthritis of knee, *98:* 219
D_3 supplementation in prevention of spinal bone loss secondary to low-dose corticosteroids in rheumatoid arthritis, *98:* 56
von Willebrand factor
in Raynaud's phenomenon and scleroderma, *97:* 208

W

Walking
velocity in elderly, determinants of, *96:* 43
Weather
changes and chronic pain, *97:* 289
Wegener's granulomatosis, *97:* 305; *96:* 238
antineutrophil cytoplasmic antibody in, *97:* 314
bladder cancer and cyclophosphamide-induced cystitis in, *97:* 305
classical *vs.* non-renal, *96:* 243
cyclophosphamide in, pulse, response to, and antineutrophil cytoplasmic antibodies, *96:* 238
link with $alpha_1$ antitrypsin PiZ allele, *96:* 241
Pneumocystis carinii pneumonia in, factors associated with, *97:* 308
Staphylococcus aureus chronic nasal carriage and higher relapse rates in, *96:* 233
Weight
-bearing sports, long-term, and risk of osteoarthritis, in women, *98:* 214
lifters, knee osteoarthritis in, *97:* 257
reduction and cauda equina compression by epidural lipomatosis in obesity, *97:* 299
Werner syndrome
with osteoporosis, insulin-like growth factor in, *96:* 209
Whiplash injury
long-term outcome after, *97:* 298
White blood cell (*see* Leukocyte)
Work
disability predictors in rheumatoid arthritis, follow-up, *97:* 58
Wrist
rheumatoid arthritis in
arthrodesis in, radiolunate, radiological evolution of wrist after, *97:* 56
bone destruction in, *96:* 28
synovial membrane hypertrophy and bone erosions in, MRI scoring of, *97:* 47

Y

Yersinia
enterocolitica adhesion YadA on collagen types I and II, binding region for, *97:* 337
Yoga
-based regimen for osteoarthritis of hands, *96:* 200
Yttrium-90
radiochemical synovectomy in chronic knee synovitis, *98:* 277

Z

Zolpidem
in fibromyalgia, *98:* 255
Zoster
varicella, causing waxing and waning vasculitis, *98:* 194

Author Index

A

Aaron LA, 259
Abney E, 66
Ahonen J, 41
Aker PD, 247
Åkesson A, 158
Alarcón GS, 45, 259
Allen SH, 76
Almenoff PL, 271
Amini S, 147
Anderson JJ, 268
Anguita J, 240
Ankara, 204
Arakawa M, 148
Armadans-Gil L, 173
Arnett FC, 159, 163, 207
Asahara H, 24
Asavatanabodee P, 277
Aupperle KR, 25
Austin HA III, 127
Austin J, 10
Authier F-J, 264
Awad JA, 161

B

Babcock EA, 53
Bacon PA, 191
Baker JR, 213
Baker PR, 12
Barbas SM, 85
Barlow JD, 179
Battle RW, 168
Beardmore TD, 13
Behr J, 171
Belec L, 264
Bennett RM, 255
Berard M, 107
Berner CM, 126
Berruti V, 177
Bessette L, 249
Birch S, 15
Bjerring P, 184
Björnsson J, 188
Black DM, 229
Bluestein HG, 126
Boumba DS, 136
Bowden A, 179
Boyle DL, 145
Bradley LA, 259
Brancaccio V, 113
Breitbach SA, 53
Bremell T, 232
Brennan P, 39
Broketa G, 148
Broll H, 226
Brun JG, 69
Buckley LM, 56
Bujak DI, 237
Buoncompagni A, 70
Burckhardt CS, 255
Buskila D, 250

C

Cadena CA, 127
Campion ME, 6, 7
Candell-Riera J, 173
Capell HA, 43
Cartularo KS, 56
Caspi D, 196
Cassidy JT, 76
Cazabon JK, 110
Cervera R, 135
Chan AW, 269
Chantome R, 107
Charley MR, 150
Chary-Valckenaere I, 236
Chen C, 235
Christophidis N, 124
Cicuttini FM, 213
Cimbalnik K, 104
Clark SR, 255
Cleary ML, 30
Clerc D, 33
Cohen H, 115
Colina RE, 232
Conant EF, 166
Conte CG, 165, 175
Cooper DL, 46
Cooper SM, 168
Correa-Rotter R, 226
Coste J, 33
Cöster L, 158
Cottin V, 48
Couderc L-J, 193
Coyte PC, 11
Creamer P, 218
Creutzig A, 182
Criswell LA, 54
Crowson AN, 117
Crowson CS, 6, 7
Croxford R, 11

D

Damianovich M, 192
Danielsen R, 176
Dattwyler RJ, 239
Dave M, 115
Davis P, 277
Davitt MA, 168
de Groen PC, 231
Deighton C, 20
de Rosayro AM, 198
Desai-Mehta A, 88
de Vita S, 201
Devlin J, 34
Devogelaer JP, 226
de Vries JX, 224
Dieppe, 218
Dietrich H, 160
Dillon WI, 242
Dinant HJ, 201
Dolnikowski G, 38
Donadi EA, 96
Dornbush RL, 237
Droz D, 193
Dudl E, 109

E

Eggelmeijer F, 60
Elkayam O, 196
Elliott JE, 90
Engel EE, 150
Erdi H, 204
Erlangen, 143
Ernst B, 224
Escalante A, 13
Exley AR, 191

F

Fam AG, 221
Fata F, 209
Feinberg HL, 200
Felson DT, 219, 253
Feltkamp TEW, 97
Ferraccioli G, 201
Finazzi G, 113
Firestein GS, 25, 145
Fivenson DP, 242
Flavin DP, 270
Follansbee WP, 175
Forseter G, 237
Fossel AH, 99
Franklin BN, 68
Freund M, 182
Fries JF, 215
Fruhmann G, 171
Fujihara T, 137
Fujimoto M, 154, 156

G

Gabriel SE, 6, 7
Gallati H, 204
Gam AN, 263
Garcia-Carrasco M, 135
Gaston-Johansson F, 265
Gattorno M, 70
Geirrsson AJ, 176
George J, 192
Gertner E, 44
Giannini EH, 79
Gilburd B, 192
Gilden DH, 194
Gillot J-M, 155
Glennås A, 31
Glowniak JV, 52
Goldenberg D, 257
Goldsmith CH, 247
Goldstein R, 159
Gough A, 34
Gowin KM, 210
Green CR, 198
Greenspan SL, 230
Gridley G, 28
Groh JD, 12
Grom AA, 71
Gross AR, 247
Gruschwitz MS, 143, 160
Gudbjörnsson B, 51
Guerne P-A, 199

H

Hachulla E, 155
Halkier-Sørensen L, 184
Hama N, 102
Hamilton S, 90
Handley HH, 111
Haneji N, 131
Harris PA, 214
Harrison WB, 49
Hart DJ, 214
Hasegawa M, 154, 156
Hasunuma T, 24
Hausdorf G, 208
Hawker G, 11
Hawkey CJ, 40
Hazes JMW, 65
He J, 89
Hebbar M, 155
Heck L, 10
Heck LW Jr, 62
Hermosillo AG, 252
Herrick AL, 179
Heyes MP, 95
Hirohata S, 118
Hirsch LJ, 231
Holland S, 230
Hörkkö S, 109
Howard RF, 163
Howe G, 46
Hrycaj P, 256
Hudson N, 40
Huissoon A, 34
Hunt M, 218
Hurley J, 15
Hutchison B, 15

I

Ioannides-Demos LL, 124
Isomäki P, 23
Isshi K, 118

J

Jacobson EW, 63
Jaovisidha S, 235
Jaskowski TD, 98
Jaulhac B, 236
Jelaska A, 148
Jerez R, 208
Jiménez SA, 203
Johannsen F, 263
Johnson A, 271
Johnson RC, 239

K

Kähäri L, 203
Kaltenhäuser S, 22
Kameda H, 102
Kane GC, 166
Kanik KS, 61
Kaplan MM, 270
Karpf DB, 227
Katsikis PD, 66
Kayagaki N, 24
Kehayias JJ, 37
Keller RB, 249
Kennedy M, 253
Khan MA, 20
Kikendall JW, 232
Kikuchi K, 154, 156
Kleinschmidt-DeMasters BK, 194
Knudsrød OG, 31
Koehnke RK, 26
Kolluri S, 26
Kong L, 133
Kraag GR, 12
Kramers C, 93
Krause PJ, 238
Krayenbühl JC, 49
Kriegsmann J, 68
Kuwana M, 102
Kvien TK, 31

L

Lawlor-Smith C, 180
Lawlor-Smith L, 180
Laxer RM, 77, 105
le Cessie S, 65
Lee LA, 139
Leib ES, 56
Lenhoff S, 92
Lesser M, 271
Levy Y, 264
Lew RA, 99, 249
Linet MS, 28
Lioté F, 220
Lohela P, 273
Loizou S, 110
Loriaux DL, 52
Lu L, 88
Lubbe DF, 231
Lue FA, 255
Luft BJ, 239
Luqmani RA, 191
Luukkainen R, 23
Luyrink L, 71
Lynch D, 241

M

Magro CM, 117
Maisiak R, 10
Maitland-Ramsey L, 230
Malone CC, 104
Manthorpe R, 129
Manzi S, 116
Marcelli A, 107
Margolies G, 62
Maricq HR, 183
Marshall PS, 44
Martel S, 272
Martínez-Lavín M, 252
Martins TB, 98
Mascagni B, 177
Mason T, 74
Massonnet B, 48
Matsumoto I, 134
Matteson EL, 248
Mayskiy M, 257
McAlindon TE, 219
McCarron S, 275

McDermott E, 20
McEntegart A, 43
Meilahn EN, 116
Mellemkjær L, 28
Mendoza C, 252
Mennet P, 256
Meydani SN, 37
Miller E, 109
Mimori T, 207
Moia M, 113
Moldofsky H, 255
Moreland LW, 62
Morfeld D, 215
Mossey C, 257
Möttönen T, 41
Mously C, 255
Müller-Ladner U, 68
Muñoz E, 147
Murray KJ, 71

N

Nadelman RB, 237
Nakabayashi T, 133
Nakamura T, 131
Naparstek Y, 61
Nawrocki B, 152
Nelson AM, 74
Neumann L, 250
Nguyen K, 25
Nicholls AC, 275
Nowakowski J, 237

O

Öberg K, 51
Oddis CV, 165
Ogawa N, 133
Ohno E, 206
Ohtsuka E, 206
Okano Y, 169
Olee T, 111
Olivé A, 276
Oliver JE, 275
Ollier B, 39

P

Paimela L, 41
Papapoulos SE, 60
Park J, 210
Parke A, 122
Parker A, 217
Patel AD, 127
Pepmueller PH, 76
Persing DH, 240
Peterson LS, 74
Pétursson E, 176
Philippe B, 193
Picco P, 70
Pickford LB, 142
Pickrell MB, 139
Pierangeli SS, 111
Porter D, 43
Porter TF, 112
Prakken ABJ, 73
Pratt DS, 270
Press J, 105
Price BE, 108
Pringle M, 225
Prudhommeaux F, 220

R

Rai R, 115
Rairie JE, 116
Rall LC, 37, 38
Ramos M, 135
Ramsey-Goldman R, 88
Rathore R, 209
Rauch J, 108
Reichlin M, 100, 139
Reveille JD, 21, 159
Rijkers GT, 73
Rincón M, 240
Rivolta R, 177
Roben P, 85
Roberts WN, 53, 123
Rodríguez F, 49
Roessner K, 241
Rosen CJ, 38
Rossetti RG, 63
Rothfuss S, 223
Rubenstein J, 221
Ryan P, 124
Ryu KN, 235

S

Saag KG, 26, 54
Sacks DG, 169
Saed GM, 242
Sahlstrand P, 69
Sajjadi FG, 145
Sakiniene E, 232
Salaffi F, 201
Sallerfors B, 92
Salles AL, 142
Salloum E, 46
Salmon-Ehr V, 152
Sánchez-Guerrero J, 99
Sandoval L, 85
Satake Y, 134
Sauer H, 22
Schiff C, 209
Schiltz C, 220
Schneider R, 77
Schrepferman CG, 200
Schroder C, 98
Schumacher HR Jr, 210, 223
Schwaiblmair M, 171
Scott JC, 32
Sems KM, 54
Serpier H, 152
Sgonc R, 160
Shbeeb MI, 248
Sherman JD, 200
Sherwin R, 32
Shia MA, 108
Sholter D, 277
Sibilia J, 236
Silva LM, 96
Silver RM, 112
Simeón C-P, 173
Simms R, 268
Simms RW, 2
Singh G, 215
Skinner M, 268
Skogseid B, 51
Skopouli FN, 136
Sluiter WJ, 34
Smith M, 217, 232
Spector TD, 213, 214
Spielman A, 238
Spira A, 33
Star VL, 32
Steen VD, 150, 165, 169, 175
Stein CM, 161
Stein J, 221
Stempniak M, 82
Stohl W, 90
Strand GM, 45
Stratz T, 256
Strengell L, 273
Stuhlmüller B, 208
Sturfelt G, 92
Sullivan KE, 120
Suri D, 147

T

Taha AS, 40
Takio K, 131
Tan F, 163
Tanner SB, 161
Targoff IN, 207
Tarkowski A, 232

Tébib J, 48
Telford SR III, 238
Tetzlaff N, 188
Tikkakoski T, 273
Toivanen P, 23
Tracy IC, 45
Triantafillou S, 217
Tsubota K, 134, 137
Tucci JR, 228
Turan B, 204
Tzioufas AG, 136

U

Unemori EN, 142
Uziel Y, 77, 105

V

Vaisberg G, 250
Valter I, 183
van Booma-Frankfort C, 201
van Bruggen MCJ, 93
van de Ende CHM, 65
van de Rijn M, 30
van der Veen MJ, 201
van Eden W, 73
van Leeuween I, 112
van Leeuwen MA, 34
van Paassen HC, 60
van Rijswijk MH, 34
Varga J, 166
Variakojis D, 30
Vayssairat M, 185
Vellend H, 269
Vicent MS, 241
Vieth G, 143
Vingsbo C, 69
Vogelgesang SA, 95
Voskuyl AE, 196
Vuyyuru S, 123

W

Wagner U, 22
Walgreen B, 93
Walmsley M, 66
Walport MJ, 110
Walsh LJ, 225
Walter-Sack I, 224
Ward MM, 8
Watanabe K, 206
Webb G, 269
Weinrich MC, 183
Weinstein A, 237
Weisman MH, 126
Wellish M, 194
West B, 122
West SG, 95
Westedt ML, 196
Westergren-Thorsson G, 158
Weyand CM, 188
Williams RC Jr, 104
Wilson J, 89
Winkelstein JA, 120
Wise CM, 123
Wisnieski JJ, 120
Wolfe F, 254
Wong AL, 82
Wong CA, 225
Wong TW, 246
Worthington J, 39
Wu J, 89

X

Xu K-P, 137

Y

Yarboro CH, 61
Yaron M, 196
Yu ITS, 246

Z

Zachariae H, 184
Zack DJ, 82
Zakaoui L, 223
Zhang W, 100
Zhang Y, 219
Zurier RB, 63
Zwinderman AH, 196